Fertility and Pregnancy

Fertility and Pregnancy

An Epidemiologic Perspective

Allen J. Wilcox

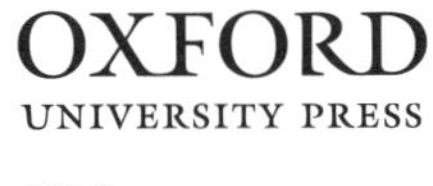

2010

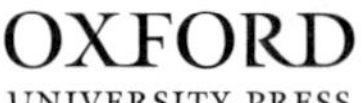

Oxford University Press, Inc., publishes works that further
Oxford University's objective of excellence
in research, scholarship, and education.

Oxford New York
Auckland Cape Town Dar es Salaam Hong Kong Karachi
Kuala Lumpur Madrid Melbourne Mexico City Nairobi
New Delhi Shanghai Taipei Toronto

With offices in
Argentina Austria Brazil Chile Czech Republic France Greece
Guatemala Hungary Italy Japan Poland Portugal Singapore
South Korea Switzerland Thailand Turkey Ukraine Vietnam

Published by Oxford University Press, Inc.
198 Madison Avenue, New York, New York 10016
www.oup.com

Oxford is a registered trademark of Oxford University Press

Library of Congress Cataloging-in-Publication Data
Wilcox, Allen J.
Fertility and pregnancy : an epidemiologic perspective / Allen J. Wilcox.
p. ; cm.
Includes bibliographical references and index.
ISBN 978-0-19-534286-4
1. Human reproduction. 2. Reproductive health. 3. Infertility—Epidemiology.
4. Pregnancy—Complications—Epidemiology. I. Title.
[DNLM: 1. Fertility. 2. Pregnancy Complications—epidemiology.
3. Reproductive Physiological Phenomena. WP 565 W667f 2010]
QP252.W55 2010
612.6—dc22 2009025396

9 8 7 6 5 4 3 2 1
Printed in the United States of America
on acid-free paper

Dedicated to

Ziggy Alden Puchowski

born 6 January 2009

who navigated the shoals
of embryonic and fetal development
while I was merely writing about them.

Preface

This book is about human reproduction. It is a story of sex (of course) and death—death on a vast scale. It is the story of unwitting survival through the fierce trials of fertilization and embryonic growth, and our drive to perpetuate this cycle by casting our particular twist of genetic fate into future generations.

What does it mean to say that this story is told from an "epidemiologic perspective"? Human biology can be approached in various ways. For example, we can focus on the things that operate consistently in every person. This is the approach of the physiologists and molecular geneticists—the laboratory scientists. However, biology is characterized not just by consistency but also by variability. To understand variability requires the study of many individuals—the approach taken by epidemiology.

The most challenging part of epidemiology (and in some ways the most fun) is to understand the reasons for human variability, including the reasons some people get a particular disease and others do not. Our detective work can go wrong, as the study of reproduction and pregnancy so richly illustrates. There are examples in these pages of misunderstandings from statistical bias, confounding, and reverse causation. Our errors can be as instructive as the things we get right. For one thing, our mistakes keep us humble. (There is not an epidemiologist alive who has not been snagged by these traps along the way.) These examples can also help us see the problems more clearly the next time we encounter them.

This book is divided into two sections. The first lays the foundations—the basic principles of reproductive physiology, demography, infectious diseases, and genetics as they apply to human reproduction. (I assume readers have been introduced to the basics of epidemiology.) The second part of the book deals with the endpoints of reproductive epidemiology—a spectrum ranging from infertility and fetal loss to birth defects and the delayed effects of fetal exposures. Some researchers make a distinction between "reproductive epidemiology" (the events of fertility and early pregnancy) and "perinatal epidemiology" (the events around delivery). These are so woven together (in my own mind, at least) that I prefer to lump them all as "reproductive epidemiology."

Now for the caveats. The story that unfolds here is my version—prejudiced by my own interests, colored by my own perspectives. When my views are in the minority, I have tried to present a fair account of the general consensus and then introduce my own dissent. I doubt I have been fully successful in keeping that distinction clear. Perhaps more worrying, my perspective (and the perspective of most researchers in this field) is overwhelmingly First World. One of the ironies of epidemiology is that our data are best where the problems are least. This is certainly true for reproductive epidemiology. Those of us privileged to work in developed countries tend to focus on the small problems close to us and neglect the huge problems elsewhere. Ninety-nine percent of maternal deaths occur in developing countries, but much of the world's literature on maternal mortality is about the other 1%. If this book were done right, most topics would have separate discussions for the developed nations and the developing nations. I have tried to acknowledge this, even if I have failed to provide it. Finally, there are countless complexities that I know I have glossed over (and still others I do not even know about). If you find yourself wanting more, the references may help direct you to some of the more subtle and difficult aspects of these topics.

A website comes with this book (www.oup.com/us/fertility). There you will find discussions of the "Puzzlers" provided at the end of this book. It's also a place to provide feedback. Please let me know about any errors, confusions, or omissions. You are also welcome to suggest additional "Unanswered questions in reproductive epidemiology" (Chapter 21). If there is another edition of this book, your input will help make it better.

But in the end, it all comes back to the beginning—conception, and the incredible events that conception sets in motion. How a speck of fertilized egg becomes a fully formed infant is, on top of everything else, a great story. Epidemiologists are lucky to be able to help tell it.

A. J. W.
Durham, North Carolina

Acknowledgments

I used to wonder how authors could possibly list so many people in their acknowledgements. Now I know.

Jeffrey House of Oxford University Press steered me wisely in conversations about what it takes to write a good textbook. When the time came, I was lucky to get William Lamsback as my editor. Bill's advice was on the mark, and his support unflagging. Regan Hofmann gave the final boost to carry the book across the finish-line.

I am grateful to administrators at the National Institute of Environmental Health Sciences (NIEHS), who allowed me to leave my research job for a year to write this book, and then allowed me to return. During that year, the University of North Carolina at Chapel Hill gave me invaluable library access. Through the university's online resources I came to appreciate how profoundly scholarly research has evolved since my dissertation in the 1970s. Instead of roaming dim and musty racks of bound medical journals, we now tap huge chunks of the world's scientific literature from the nearest computer.

Crucial translations were provided by my neighbors Pela Gereffi (Spanish) and Maurice Ritchie (German). Jan Drake at NIEHS cleared my confusion over estimates of gene mutation across generations. The cool insight by Carl Sagan on time travel was brought to my attention by my friend Ethan Loewenthal. My godson Tobin Eshelman and his colleague Katherine Naughton helped track down the inside scoop on sex sorting of sperm. Olga Basso provided the summary U.S. statistics (from public-access data files) that are the basis of Chapters 14 and 15. Julie Daniels let me try out some of this material on her reproductive epidemiology class at University of North Carolina.

Pictures are paramount. Diane Anderson of the University of Chicago provided the photographs of the legendary tablets at Women's Lying-In Hospital. Steven Schrader gave me the previously unpublished figure showing longitudinal sperm counts, and Jennie Kline dug into her original data for a new presentation of her results on miscarriage risk by mother's age. The awesome microphotographs of egg and blastocyst were provided by Stan Beyler at the University of North Carolina and Mary Francis of USC Fertility. Bob McConnaughey was graph-maker extraordinaire.

The scientific literature on infections that affect reproduction is fragmented, and so a chapter on this topic required a different approach. I was fortunate to get the help of Bill Miller (a specialist in infectious disease) and Laura Baecher-Lind (an obstetrician-gynecologist) in writing a comprehensive review of infectious disease and its effects on reproduction. The glossary at the end of the text merges and extends two glossaries Ruby Nguyen and I published in the *Journal of Epidemiology and Community Health* in 2005.

I owe a huge debt to my colleagues who provided comments on one or more chapters: Donna Baird, Cynthia Berg, Jens Peter Bonde, Abee Boyles, Michael Bracken, Pierre Buekens, William Callaghan, Ward Cates, Kaare Christensen, Sven Cnattingius, Julie Daniels, Marlene Goldman, Tine Brink Henriksen, Arthur Herbst, Sonia Hernández-Diaz, Jessica Illuzzi, Anne Marie Jukic, Jennie Kline, Michael Kramer, Shannon Laughlin, David Leon, Rolv Terje Lie, Allen Mitchell, Nigel Paneth, Jørn Olsen, Markku Sallmen, David Savitz, Laura Schieve, Gary Shaw, Rolv Skjaerven, Cheryl Stein, Jack Taylor, John Thorp, James Trussell, Michelle Williams, and Jim Zhang all gave cogent suggestions for improvements. I am still incredulous that several of my busy colleagues were willing to tackle the whole book: Cande Ananth, Anne-Marie Nybo Andersen, Olga Basso, Curt Eshelman, Matt Longnecker, and Meg McCann made major contributions to the coherence of the final product. If there are still places where I have blundered into error, it wasn't for lack of good advice.

I am humbled by the generosity of not just my colleagues and friends but of people I do not know and may never meet. A fellow in London named Jon Johnson did me the extraordinary service of resurrecting files from the 1958 British Perinatal Survey and providing the data I needed to describe the perinatal risk around the time of delivery. Matthew Payne of Emory University (whom I happened to find through a Google search) guided me to the source of an extended quote from Karl Pearson's 1907 Oxford lecture that had eluded me.

Writing a textbook is more than the assembly of information—it's an opportunity for playfulness and intuition. The best insights on harnessing those to productive use came from my daughter Lauren Puchowski and my son Joseph Wilcox, each speaking from the experience of their own intensely creative pursuits. (Lauren also provided the concept for the cover photograph.)

But more than any other single person, it is my wife Claire who (literally) made this book possible. She didn't bat an eye when I said I needed to leave my job for a year to get this done. She paid the bills, worked around endless stacks of papers at the computer, and never faltered in her loving and cheerful encouragement.

A. J. W.

Durham, North Carolina

Contents

I

FOUNDATIONS

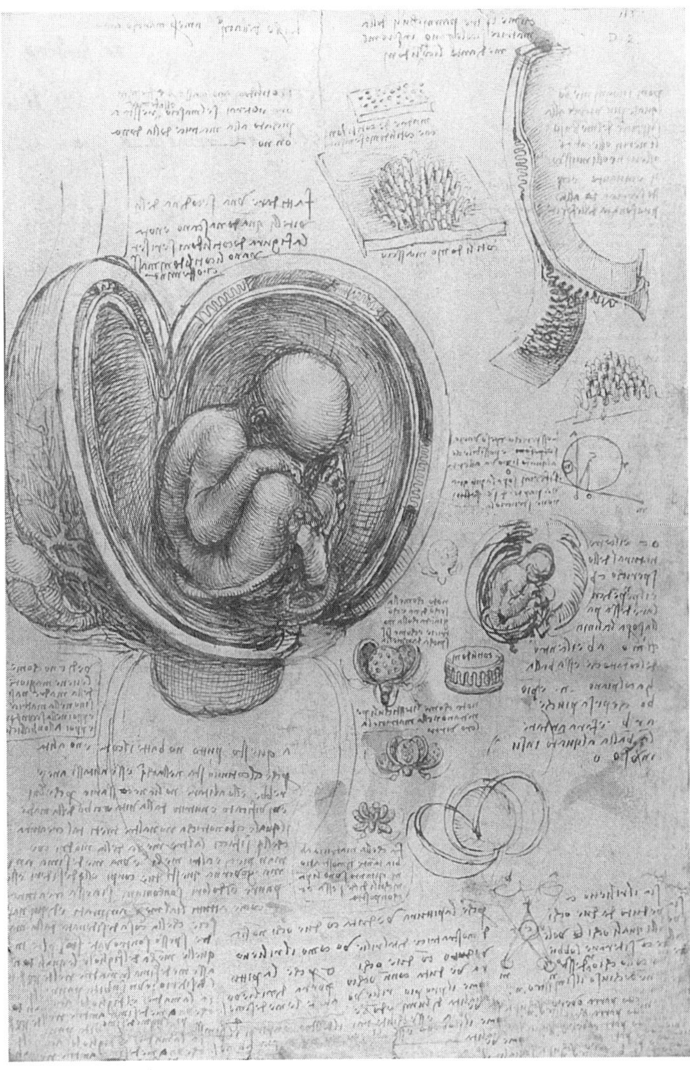

Studies of embryos by Leonardo da Vinci (Pen over red chalk 1510–1513)
(Photo by Luc Viatour)

1

The Creative Biology of Human Reproduction

The processes of procreation involve some of the oddest and most inventive mechanisms to be found in all of human biology. The ordinary rules are broken: cells change their number of chromosomes, genetically distinct cells intermix, and the usual boundaries between individuals are breached.

Of all the functions of the human body, reproduction was among the last to be understood. William Harvey grasped the essential mechanics of blood circulation in 1628, but his notions about reproduction were the stuff of fantasy. Harvey wrote that a man caused a woman to be "ignited" by fertility, "his seed so imbued with spirit and divine efficacy that it can convey fertility ... just as we see some object suddenly burst into flame from a spark struck by a flint."[1] This may sound like mysticism to modern ears, but in some respects it is no less fantastic than the biological mechanisms actually at work.

Fifty years after Harvey, Leeuwenhoek drew the first pictures of human sperm (Fig. 1-1). These living creatures clearly were not "sparks"—but what were they? Some scientists proposed that each of these tiny particles contained a baby ready to be implanted (the so-called homunculus) (Fig. 1-2). Others regarded these organisms as contaminants of the seminal fluid, like the swimming things found in pond water. This interpretation of sperm as contamination persisted into the mid-1800s.[2]

The idea that a man's sperm and a woman's egg can join to make a new person is so commonplace today that we can easily forget how radical it once seemed. It was not until Mendel's experiments on heritability (begun in the 1850s but not recognized until the early 1900s) that the equal genetic contributions of the two parents was firmly established.

Reproduction by means of sperm and ova (known collectively as gametes) makes use of unusual biological mechanisms. There is no other setting in which healthy cells go from two sets of chromosomes to one set (meiotic cell division).

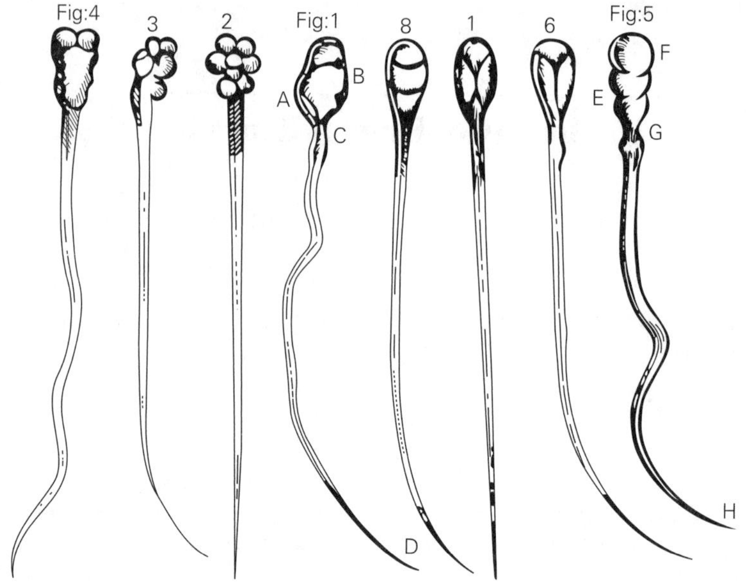

Figure 1-1. The first drawings of sperm (Antoni Leeuwenhoek's "animalcules engendered in the semen," 1679)

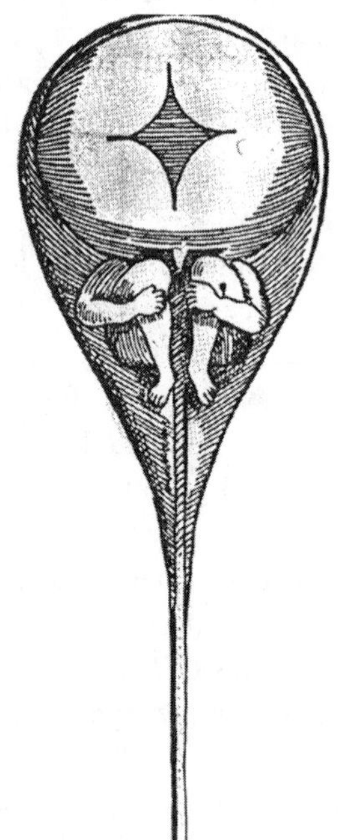

Figure 1-2. The homunculus (Nicolas Hartsoeker, 1694)

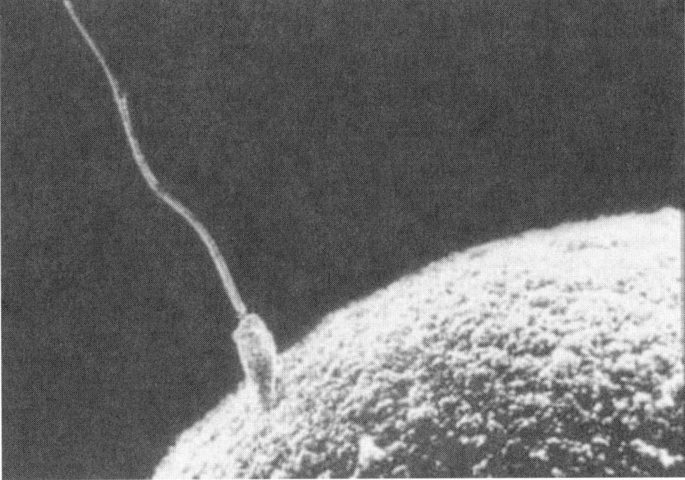

Figure 1-3. Sperm fertilizing an egg

Nowhere else in biology does a pair of genetically distinct cells combine to form a genetically new and unique cell (Fig. 1-3). Special mechanisms allow the fertilized egg—antigenically foreign to the mother—to parasitize the mother's tissue while eluding immune rejection. To explain these phenomena requires concepts of genetics and immunology and endocrinology that emerged only in the late twentieth century.

For early scientists trying to understand human reproduction, it was no help that reproductive mechanisms vary widely among species. Extrapolation from other species to humans was risky (and still is). Episodes of fertility for female domestic animals are typically signaled by vaginal bleeding, whereas women are rarely fertile while bleeding. Labor and delivery are uneventful for many species but dangerous for humans. As our observational tools have improved, even more species differences have emerged. The Y chromosome causes its carrier to be male if you are a mammal but female if you are a bird. In some species, sex is determined not by chromosomes but by ambient temperature: the gecko (a lizard) hatches as a male if the egg has been incubated at 32°C but as a female if the temperature is 25°C.[3]

The study of reproduction in other species can teach us only a limited amount about ourselves. To understand human reproduction, we must study humans. Unfortunately, the exploration of human reproduction presents its own difficulties. Research intrusions on human procreation are constrained by the privacy that surrounds this intimate domain. Ethical considerations are multiplied—although the fetus has uncertain legal status, its protection is paramount. Even with all the advances in reproductive biology that have occurred in recent decades, our grasp of human reproduction is still unfolding.

Gametogenesis

The reproductive cycle provides the classic metaphor for something that has no starting point: "the chicken or the egg." In another sense, reproduction is like a set of nested Russian dolls: the typical pregnant woman does not have symptoms of pregnancy until embryogenesis has begun, by which time her embryo may already have formed the germ cells that will produce the subsequent generation. The cells that form a woman's grandchildren may be laid down before she yet knows she is going to be a mother.

Male Gametogenesis

The germ cells (or spermatogonia) that produce sperm in the adult male are formed in the early stages of embryonic life. These male germ cells are contained in the seminiferous tubules of the testes (Fig. 1-4). At puberty, hormones released from the pituitary gland in the brain awaken the testes, which begin to produce testosterone. The germ cells undergo meiotic division (reducing their chromosomes to a single—or haploid—set per cell), and the cells proceed to develop into

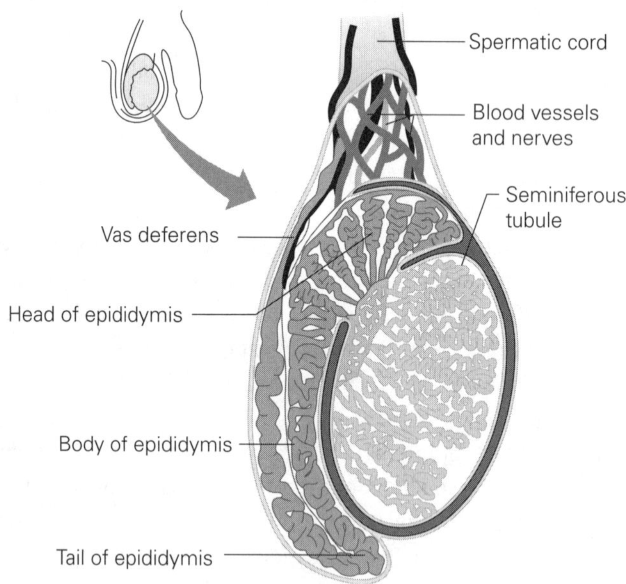

Figure 1-4. Structures of the testis

recognizable sperm. Once formed, sperm are stored in the epididymis, where they undergo their final stages of maturation. The time required for a germ cell to form a mature spermatozoan is estimated at nine weeks.[4] Sperm are vulnerable to damage during development and maturation, but once matured, sperm are robust. The fully formed sperm consists of little more than a condensed pellet of nuclear DNA (packed more densely than bone) propelled by a tail. Sperm are stored in the vas deferens until ejaculation, at which time they are mixed with seminal fluid (consisting of secretions of the prostate gland and seminal vesicles).

The production of sperm requires several conditions. One is the presence of testosterone, the male hormone produced by cells of the testis. Testosterone circulates throughout the body, but it is most highly concentrated in the compartments where sperm are produced. A second necessary condition is a temperature slightly cooler than normal body temperature. It is for this reason that the testes are suspended outside the body cavity.

A man produces roughly 100 million sperm a day, with spermatogenesis typically continuing until he dies. This production of hundreds of billions of sperm over a man's lifetime may seem profligate, but it is modest in comparison with some other creatures. Male hogs produce 16 billion sperm a day.[5]

Female Gametogenesis

As with the male germ cells, the female germ cells have their origins in embryonic life. However, the female and male germ cells take very different paths. Male germ cells are essentially dormant until puberty, at which time they begin to divide to form sperm. In contrast, the female germ cells (or oogonia) complete their major cell divisions during fetal life. The woman's lifetime supply of eggs (an estimated 7 million) will be complete by the time she reaches her sixth month as a fetus.[6]

A woman's so-called biological clock begins to tick even before she is born.[7] By the time of birth, about three-quarters of her oocytes have died, leaving a newborn girl with about 2 million eggs.[8] By the time she reaches puberty, another 80% will have died, with perhaps 400,000 still alive as the woman begins to menstruate. Ninety-five percent of those will die by the time the woman reaches age 30, leaving about 20,000.[7,9] Such drastic attrition may seem alarming, but extravagant wastefulness is the hallmark of reproduction. Roughly 400 eggs are released over a woman's reproductive lifetime and are made available for fertilization—still far more than any woman would wish to have fertilized.

The woman's physiologic role in reproduction is not simply to produce eggs but to provide a site for the fertilized egg to implant. Preparation of the site requires a finely orchestrated sequence of events, and this heightened state of readiness cannot be maintained for long. Rather, women phase in and out of this state of preparedness, in a pattern known as the menstrual cycle.

The Menstrual Cycle

The menstrual cycle is a coordinated sequence of hormone signals and tissue responses that function to bring a ripe fertilized egg into contact with a ready uterus. Consider the menstrual cycle first from the standpoint of ovarian function (Fig. 1-5). The ovary contains thousands of tiny fluid-filled cavities (or follicles), each of which holds an oocyte. Under the stimulus of the pituitary hormone FSH (follicle-stimulating hormone), a few follicles are "recruited" in each cycle and begin to grow. As these follicles grow, they produce an estrogen called estradiol. Within a few days, one of the recruited follicles becomes dominant, and the rest regress and die. The dominant follicle continues to grow, all the while producing an increasing amount of estradiol that stimulates the lining of the uterus to prepare for a possible pregnancy.

As the dominant follicle develops, it expands toward the surface of the ovary, where it becomes visible as a large blister (up to 2 cm in diameter). Ovulation occurs when the rising levels of estradiol trigger another pituitary hormone (luteinizing hormone, LH) to surge, which in turn causes the follicle to rupture and the egg to be released.

The method for transferring the ovum from the ruptured follicle (on the surface of the ovary) to the interior of the uterus seems a bit precarious (Fig. 1-6). There are two tubes (called oviducts or fallopian tubes) attached to the uterus, each with a free end that is encircled by finger-like projections called fimbria. This open end

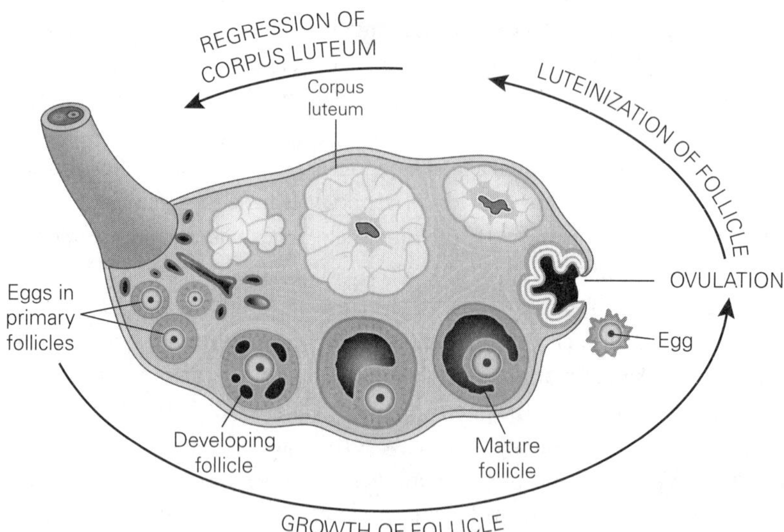

Figure 1-5. Structures of the ovary and their changes during the menstrual cycle

of the oviduct is free to wander in various directions. Around the time of ovulation, the end of the oviduct is attracted to the surface of the ovary. If all goes well, the fimbria scoop up the released ovum and usher it into the tube.

The freshly ruptured ovarian follicle quickly undergoes a drastic change. Under the influence of LH, the follicle is transformed into a small swelling of yellowish tissue called the corpus luteum. ("Corpus luteum" is Latin for "yellow body.") The corpus luteum has a highly specialized task—to produce progesterone, a hormone that alters the uterine lining. The word progesterone comes from "pro-" (in support of), "-gest-" (gestation), and "-sterone" (steroid hormone)—it is literally the hormone that supports pregnancy. Progesterone is the way that the ovary converts the endometrial lining of the uterus into a richly secretory tissue that can support the fertilized egg.

This intensive investment in the proliferation of the endometrium is not sustained for long. The production of progesterone by the corpus luteum reaches its peak 9 or 10 days after ovulation. At that point, the corpus luteum starts to go into decline, and the production of progesterone gradually falls (Fig. 1-7). If there is no hormonal signal from a fertilized egg, the corpus luteum regresses completely over the next 5 or 6 days, at which point the production of progesterone ends. The withdrawal of hormonal support leaves the richly engorged lining of the uterus to atrophy and die. This tissue sloughs from the uterus into the vagina, producing menstrual bleeding (menses). Bleeding lasts an average of 6 days, with 90% of women having menses that last from 4 to 7 days.[9] Although the number of days of bleeding varies among women, it tends to remain fairly constant for a given woman. The heaviest bleeding usually occurs on the second and third days.[10]

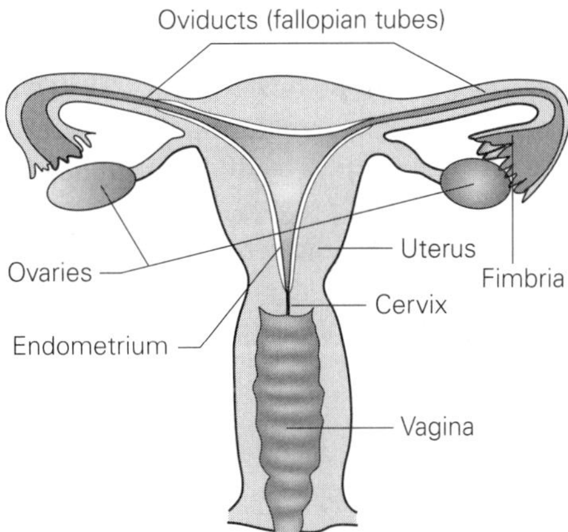

Figure 1-6. The female reproductive tract

These stages of the menstrual cycle are illustrated in Fig. 1-7. (For an excellent detailed description of these events, see Healy and Hodgen.[11]) The first day of menstrual bleeding defines day 1 of the menstrual cycle. This is also the first day of the follicular phase of the cycle, during which a new crop of follicles is developing and a dominant follicle emerges. The follicular phase ends on the day before ovulation. The day after ovulation defines the beginning of the luteal phase. The luteal phase encompasses the life cycle of the corpus luteum, with the last day of the luteal phase (and the menstrual cycle) defined as the day before the next bleeding begins.

The onset of bleeding is a convenient sign, but it is ovulation that provides the most important benchmark of the menstrual cycle. The event of ovulation ends the follicular phase and launches the luteal phase. Furthermore, it defines the days on which intercourse can produce a pregnancy (more on this in Chapter 2).

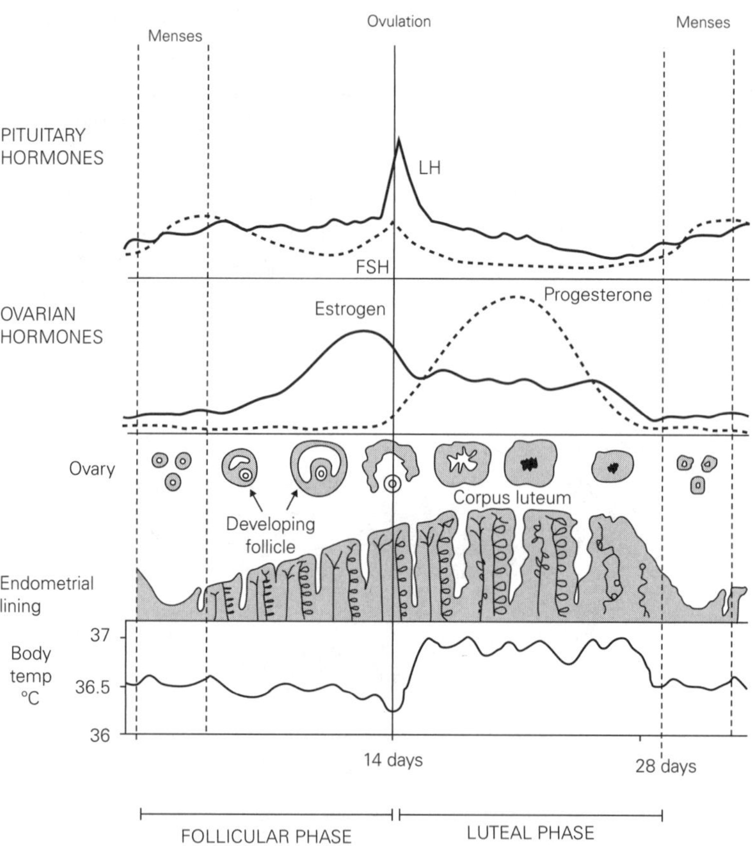

Figure 1-7. Physiologic events of menstrual cycle

The difficulty with ovulation as a benchmark is that it is largely invisible. Changes in body temperature (basal body temperature or BBT) have been used as a sign of ovulation, but individual variability makes this a poor biological marker.[12] Changes in the amount and consistency of cervical mucus is another proposed marker.[12] Although cervical mucus seems not to be a highly reliable sign of ovulation,[13] it may nonetheless be informative with regard to a woman's fertile days (Chapter 2).[14]

Variability in the Menstrual Cycle

Textbooks typically describe the "normal" or "standard" menstrual cycle as 28 days long, with ovulation on day 14. By this definition, most cycles are not normal—the menstrual cycle is highly variable. Figure 1-8 shows a typical distribution of menstrual cycle lengths for more than 18,000 menstrual cycles recorded prospectively by 700 Japanese women over 2 years. The mode is at 28 days, but only 12% of cycles are actually 28 days long. The tail of the distribution extends far to the right, producing a median of 29 days and a mean of 30 days.[13]

The menstrual cycle is especially variable among young women during the first few years of menstruation and among older women as they approach menopause.[15] This variability at the extremes of reproductive life was demonstrated in a classic study by Alan Treloar (Fig. 1-9). In 1935, Treloar and his colleagues invited several thousand college students at the University of Minnesota to keep diaries of their menstrual cycles.[16] Forty percent of these women continued to provide menstrual data until menopause, and several hundred participants enrolled their daughters at the time of their menarche. This study (perhaps the longest-running longitudinal study ever conducted) continues to the present day and comprises more than a half-million menstrual cycles.[17] Another pattern that is apparent in

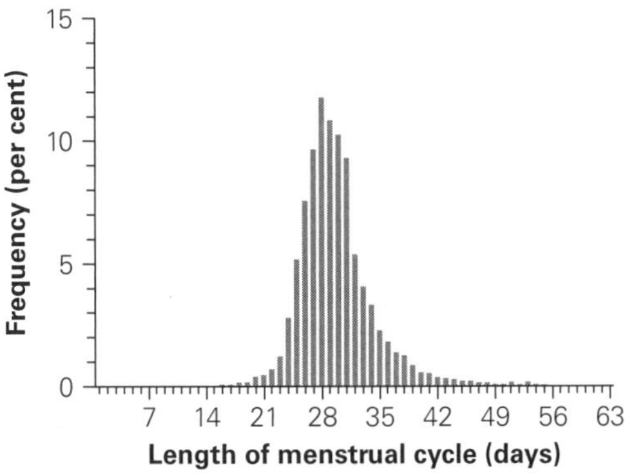

Figure 1-8. Variability in menstrual cycle length (18,084 cycles recorded by 701 women, Japan, 1958–59)[13]

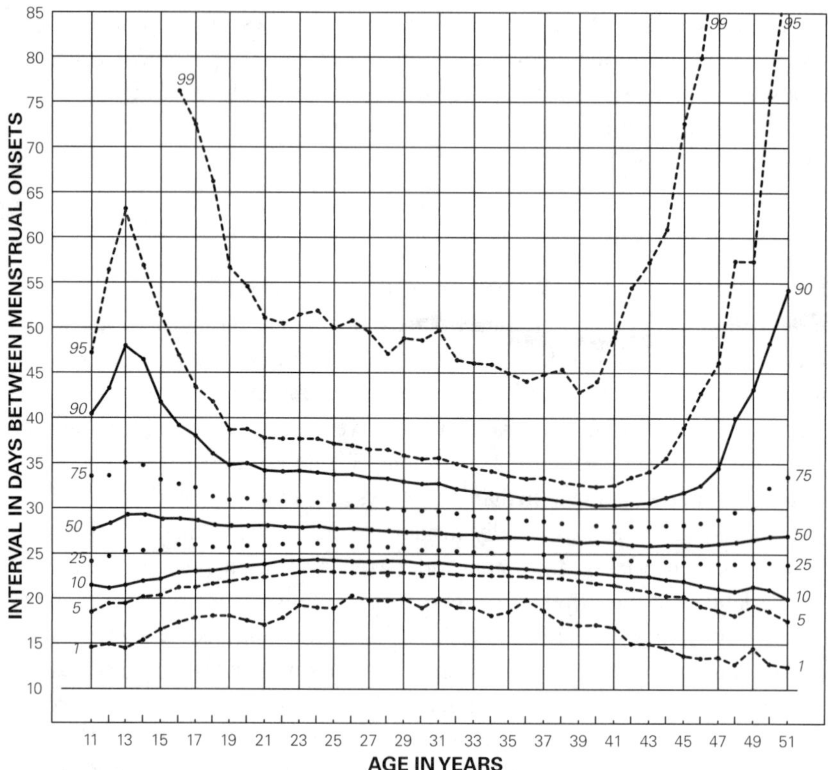

Figure 1-9. Variability in menstrual cycle length by women's age (275,947 menstrual cycles recorded by 2,702 women, United States, 1935–61).[16] Lines indicate percentiles of cycle length at each age

Figure 1-9 is the gradual shortening of menstrual cycles during the time when women have their most stable menstrual patterns (about ages 20–40). During these two decades the median cycle length falls from 29 to 27 days.[16]

Menstrual cycles vary within women as well as among women, with some women varying by only a few days from cycle to cycle and others varying by much more. Overall, within-woman variance is greater than the among-women variance.[18] Most of this variability occurs during the follicular phase (that is, the time from bleeding to ovulation). Figure 1-10 shows a distribution of follicular phases for 200 healthy women of reproductive age (most between the ages of 25 and 35).[19] (The day of ovulation in these was determined by hormone assays carried out on daily urine samples.) Length of the follicular phase ranged from 9 to

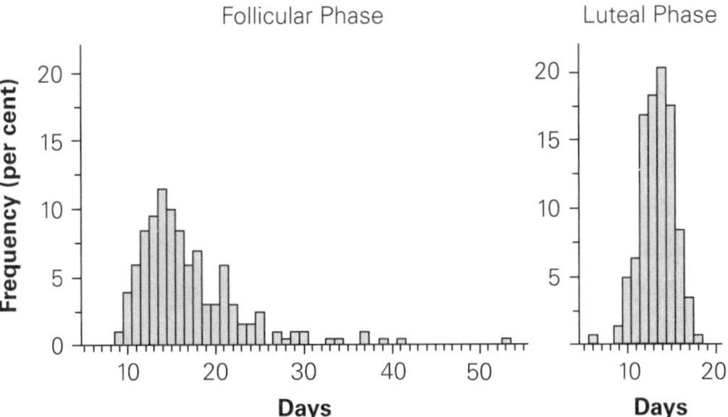

Figure 1-10. Variability in the follicular and luteal phases (217 women, North Carolina, United States, 1983–85)[19]

55 days. Only about 1% of these menstrual cycles fit the textbook picture of the "standard" menstrual cycle (28 days long, with ovulation on day 14).[20]

Compared with the follicular phase, the luteal phase is less variable (Fig. 1-10). This reflects the control of the luteal phase by the programmed death of the corpus luteum. However, this lesser variability should not be mistaken for "no variability," a condition rarely (if ever) found in biology. Although the average time from ovulation to onset of the next menses is around 14 days, the actual time is usually shorter or longer.

Menstrual cycles are not only highly variable, but they are easily disrupted. Extremes of body fat (too little or too much) can change menstrual patterns, as can changes in weight.[21] Small daily doses of synthetic hormones (such as hormonal contraceptives) are enough to shut down the process altogether. For most healthy women, menses continue for four decades or so, at which time the cycles naturally cease.

Menarche and Menopause

A young woman's first menses (known as menarche) occurs on average around age 12 or 13, although this can vary widely (Fig. 1-11).[22] A small percentage of healthy women have their first period at age 10 or younger or at age 16 or older.

There is a popular notion that girls are reaching their sexual maturity at steadily earlier ages. Some environmental pollutants have weakly hormonal properties, which has led to concerns that environmental contaminants may accelerate puberty or otherwise disrupt human development.[23] This perception is bolstered by anecdotes of breast development in 7-year-old girls or menarche in 9-year-olds—occurrences that can occur (albeit rarely) due to natural variability. There is considerable evidence to suggest that age at menarche did decline during the 1800s

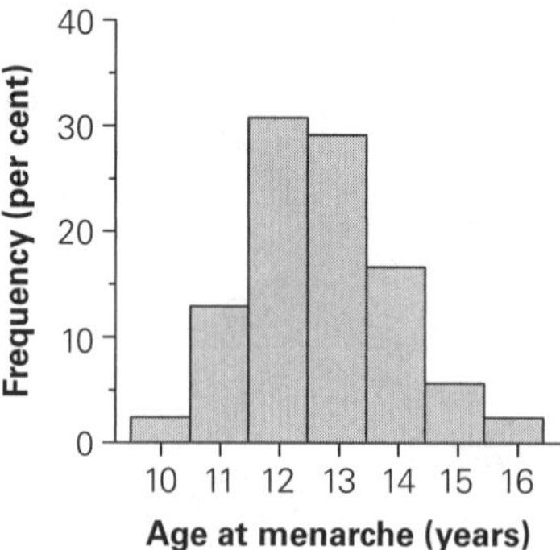

Figure 1-11. Variability in age at menarche (as recalled by 2,062 U.S. women around age 18)[22]

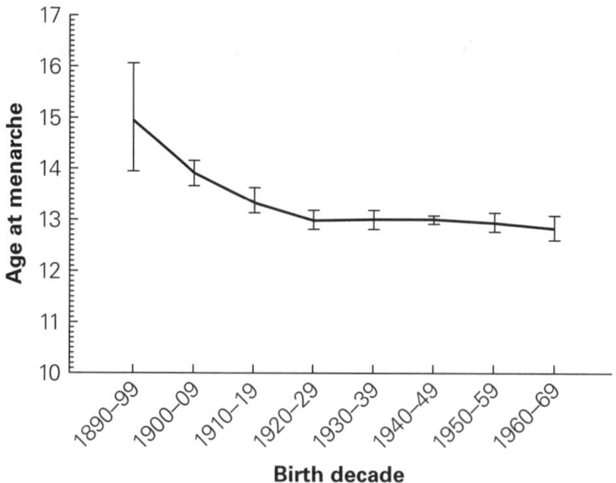

Figure 1-12. Age at menarche by birth cohort (as recalled or prospectively reported by 3,839 U.S. women) (Reprinted from Sandler et al[24])

and the first part of the 1900s (Fig. 1-12). [22,24] However, in more recent decades the trend has been negligible. In the United States, age at menarche has decreased by about 0.2 years over the past several decades, perhaps as a result of the increased prevalence of childhood obesity.[25] There is no good evidence that environmental estrogens have had a measurable impact on pubertal development.[26]

Unlike men, most women outlive their fertility. The events that precipitate the natural end of menstruation (menopause) are not well understood. One hypothesis is that menopause occurs when the ovaries' supply of eggs declines below some threshold.[27] As women approach menopause, the menstrual hormone signals

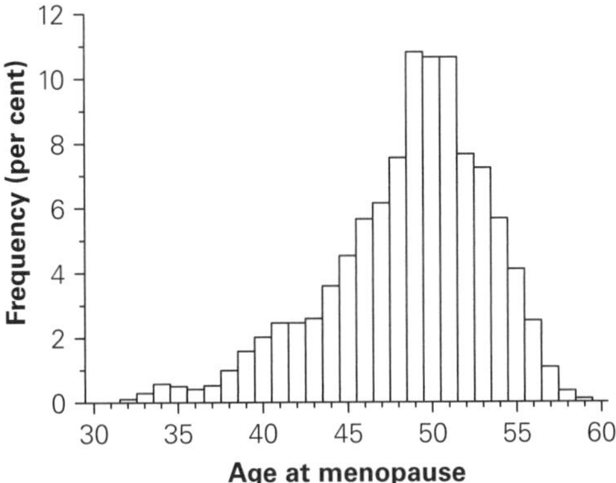

Figure 1-13. Variability in age at menopause (907 women, Finland, 1989)[15]

become weaker and less coordinated. These changes not only increase cycle variability (as in Fig. 1-9) but often produce uncomfortable symptoms. Researchers have developed various prospective definitions of the beginning of this menopausal transition, using data on menstrual variability as well as hormone measures (usually FSH, which rises as the ovarian hormones begin to falter).[24,25]

The actual event of menopause is more difficult to pinpoint than menarche, for the simple reason that first events are self-evident, whereas "last" events can be known only in retrospect. (One exception is the menopause that results from surgical removal of the ovaries, usually as part of hysterectomy.) The standard definition of menopause is 12 months or more without a menstrual cycle.[28]

Because natural menopause usually cannot be determined except in retrospect, data on age of menopause are subject to recall error. The median age at menopause is usually reported as around 51 years, with most women reporting their menopause as occurring between the ages of 45 and 55. Cigarette smoking causes earlier menopause, although the biological mechanism remains unclear.[29] Figure 1-13 presents a population-based data set from Finland.[30] In this data set, 5% of women reported their last period as occurring before age 40, which is the cutoff usually used to define premature menopause (or premature ovarian failure). Although premature menopause may result from an underlying disorder (e.g., autoimmune disease or thyroid disease), most occur without apparent cause.

When Conception Occurs

The Perilous Journey of the Fertilized Egg

In most menstrual cycles, the egg is lost in the slough of endometrial tissue at menses. There is, however, another possible outcome: pregnancy. If intercourse

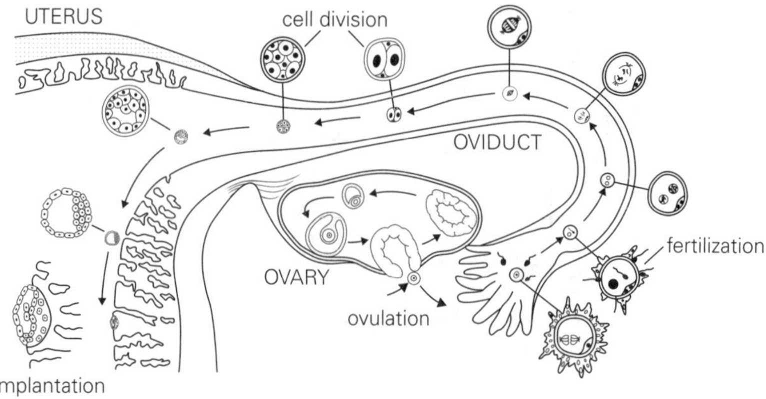

Figure 1-14. Journey of the fertilized egg[31]

has occurred during the 5 days leading up to ovulation or the day of ovulation itself, viable sperm may be present in the far end of the ovarian tubes at the time of ovulation (Fig. 1-14).

The freshly released ovum arrives in the oviduct encased in a cluster of cells brought along from the follicle. Beneath these cells lies a matrix of glycoproteins, known as the zona pellucida, that encases the ovum. The first sperm that successfully engages with the zona provokes a reaction that makes the zona impervious to other sperm.[32] At this point, the ovum finishes its second meiotic division, and expels the unneeded duplicate nucleus in a small capsule called the polar body. Meanwhile, the sperm inside the ovum loses its tail and outer covering, and its nuclear core expands as the chromosomes are unpacked. The sets of chromosomes from the sperm and egg combine, and a new and genetically unique cell is created. This newly fertilized cell immediately begins to divide.

Now the clock is ticking: the fertilized egg (or zygote) has only 10 days or so to stop the corpus luteum from going into decline. The conceptus is swept down the oviduct towards the uterus while undergoing repeated cell divisions. The challenge facing the conceptus is to be far enough along in its development that, by the time it reaches the uterus, it can invade the endometrium and secrete a hormone that will revive the corpus luteum. If the conceptus is unable to rescue the corpus luteum (and thus keep progesterone flowing), the conceptus will be lost at menses amidst the flotsam of dying endometrial tissue.

ON THE PLASTICITY OF THE EARLY CONCEPTUS. The conceptus has remarkable properties at this early stage. Even though it is genetically unique, it cannot yet be considered to be a unique individual. In the first few days of development, it is possible for the fertilized egg to separate into two parts (or more), with each genetically identical part becoming a separate person. These multiple offspring are monozygous, that is, derived from one zygote. In some species, multiple offspring are regularly produced from one fertilized egg—the armadillo routinely delivers identical quadruplets.[33]

Fraternal (or dizygotic) twins are produced when two different eggs are ovulated and fertilized in one cycle. (Higher-order multiple births can be produced by three, four, or more separate eggs, but for some reason you won't find "trizygotic" or "quadrizygotic" in a medical dictionary.)

Dizygotic twins usually develop into two individuals, but not always. On rare occasions, dizygotic twins can merge at an early stage, making a single fetus.[34] This mixture of cell lines from two genetically distinct conceptuses (known as a chimera) is compatible with healthy adulthood—even as it confounds our idea of what constitutes a "person." Once again, other species demonstrate more extreme examples. The new-world monkeys known as marmosets commonly bear chimeric dizygotic twins, with each offspring carrying cell-lines from the other twin.[35]

In yet another example of the plasticity of the early conceptus, it is possible at the 8- or 10-cell stage of development to remove a single cell for diagnostic purposes (Fig. 1-15). This maneuver cannot be performed on naturally conceived pregnancies (which are inaccessible at this stage), but it can be done for conceptions produced by in vitro fertilization (IVF). The DNA from the sampled cell can be amplified for tests of genetic disease. On this basis, parents may decide whether they wish to proceed to have the conceptus deposited into the uterus. Whether this procedure is entirely benign to the developing embryo is not yet clear.[36]

Teratomas are another strange way in which embryonic processes can go wrong. Teratomas are a type of tumor created by remnants of embryonic tissue. The cells can apparently descend from any of the three basic embryonic cell types (endoderm, mesoderm, and ectoderm). Teratomas show up anywhere in the body, although they are often near the midline—in the skull or under the spinal cord. The truly bizarre aspect of teratomas is that they can contain normal-looking tissue of just about any type, including teeth, hair, and eyeball. Most are benign.

Implantation

Returning to the journey of the fertilized egg, the conceptus moves through the oviduct toward the uterus while dividing into a cluster of inreasingly smaller cells. By the time the conceptus reaches the uterus (about 6 to 12 days after fertilization; see Fig. 1-16), it has grown into a hollow ball of cells called a blastocyst. Most of the cells of the blastocyst are trophoblasts, which are specialized cells that eventually form the placenta. At this point, the future baby is no more than a small cluster of cells inside the ball (the inner cell mass; see Fig. 1-17).

A

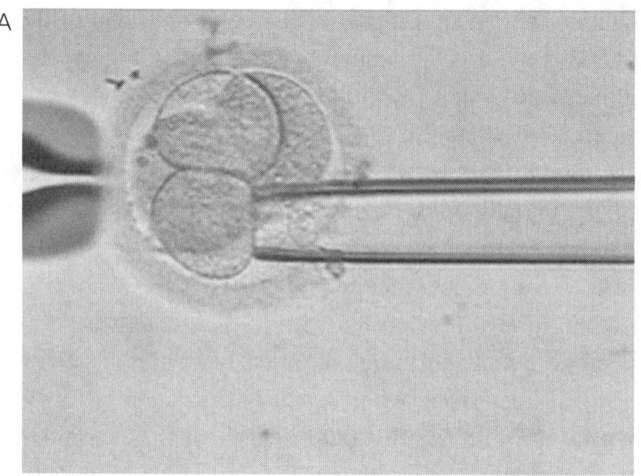

B

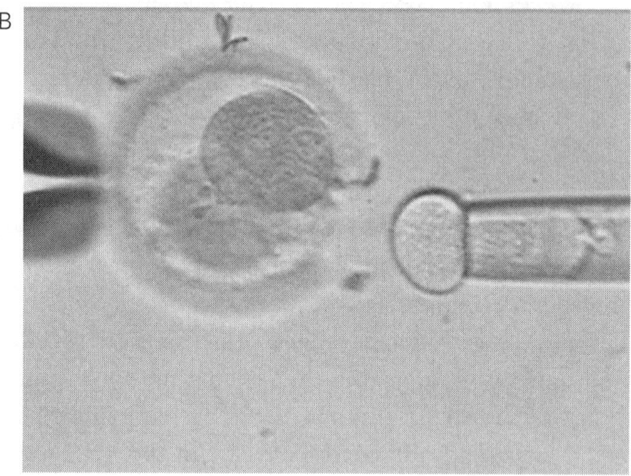

Figure 1-15. Biopsy of a human conceptus at the eight-cell stage (day 3). The holding pipette is on left, and biopsy pipette is on right, containing a cell. (Figure courtesy of Stanley Beyler, Director, Embryology and Andrology Laboratories, University of North Carolina, Chapel Hill, NC)

Once the conceptus reaches the uterus, the trophoblasts begin the process of attaching and embedding the blastocyst into the lining of the endometrium. One of the wonders of implantation is that the foreign tissue comprising the conceptus is able to successfully graft itself onto the maternal host.[38] The conceptus is antigenically distinct from the mother, and yet this invasion into maternal tissue manages not to provoke the defenses of the mother's immune system. This is all the more remarkable in light of the fact that the human trophoblast is the most invasive known; it elicits the strongest uterine response seen in any species and creates the closest possible link between the mother and the fetus.[38]

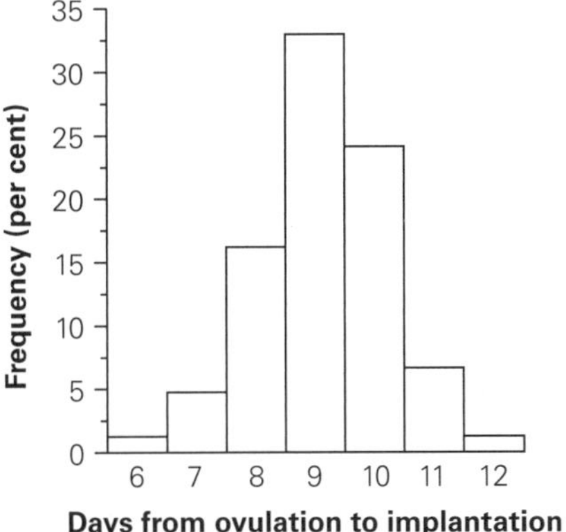

Figure 1-16. Variability in the time from conception (at ovulation) to implantation (141 naturally clinical pregnancies, North Carolina, United States, 1983–85)[37]

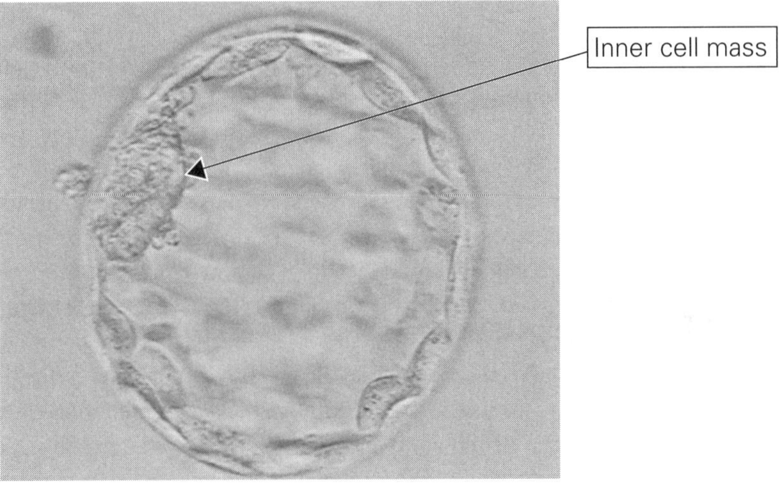

Figure 1-17. Blastocyst around the stage of implantation, with inner cell mass (Figure courtesy of Stanley Beyler, Director, Embryology and Andrology Laboratories, University of North Carolina, Chapel Hill, NC)

Human Chorionic Gonadotropin

While the trophoblast cells are invading the endometrium, they are also pumping out a hormone that is biological mimic of LH (the pituitary hormone that stimulated the corpus luteum). This mimic, known as human chorionic gonadotropin or hCG, works at the same receptor sites as LH and is produced in exponentially increasing quantities. If this surge of hCG is successful, it rescues the corpus luteum and sustains the production of progesterone for several more weeks—long enough for the developing placenta to take over hormonal control of pregnancy.

HCG is an unusual hormone in several respects. Most hormones are ephemeral, with very short half-lives—they transmit signals from one part of the body to another and then disappear. In contrast, hCG carries a signal that must be maintained for weeks without faltering. To aid in this, hCG is a highly stable molecule, with a half-life of 24 hours.

As a specific message from the conceptus, hCG is the natural candidate for pregnancy tests. Fortunately, hCG is also an easy biochemical target for assay. It is present in high concentrations in both blood and urine and can survive for days in a sample left at room temperature. Its specificity, high concentration, and robustness make hCG the universal basis for pregnancy tests. (Indeed, there are no good alternatives.) Note that because hCG is not detectable in the maternal system before the conceptus implants, there is currently no way to recognize a naturally conceived pregnancy before implantation.

Ectopic Pregnancy

The blastocyst is a desperate parasite seeking a home. It usually attaches inside the uterus, but not always. Sometimes implantation takes place in the fallopian tubes. The chances of this are increased if the tubes are damaged by previous infections.[39] A conceptus that implants in the oviduct can survive for a while, but the tube provides little room for growth. If the embryo dies without rupturing the tube, the woman may not know that conception had occurred. If the tube ruptures, the woman experiences pain and internal bleeding; rupture constitutes a surgical emergency. The rate of ectopic pregnancy is as high as 2% of all registered pregnancies in some countries.[39]

It is also possible for the fertilized egg to escape from the open end of the tube and implant outside the reproductive tract entirely. One accommodating site for implantation is the curtain of blood vessels that covers the bowels. There are rare examples of such pregnancies producing viable fetuses[40]—such pregnancies would obviously end in disaster without cesarean section because there is no natural way for the fetus to be delivered.

The Fetal-Maternal Boundary

The trophoblast cells define the boundary between fetus and mother. In the early stages of implantation, individual trophoblast cells separate from the conceptus and migrate into the endometrium, where they surround and invade the maternal spiral arteries of the uterine wall.[41] The trophoblast cells cause the arteries to relax, increasing local blood flow, which in turn bathes the newly developing blood vessels of the conceptus. Inadequate invasion of the trophoblasts at implantation can impair this transformation of the spiral arteries and thus limit the blood flow to the conceptus. This in turn can contribute to preeclampsia and other problems later in pregnancy.[41]

Trophoblast cells eventually develop into the placenta, a pie-shaped organ that mediates all exchanges between fetus and mother (Fig. 1-18). The placenta is not simply an extension of the fetus—it is a multiple-organ system with alimentary, pulmonary, renal, hepatic, and endocrine functions.[42] By six weeks after conception, the placenta has taken control of the hormonal milieu of pregnancy. The placenta produces progesterone, estrogen, placental lactogen, and other hormones. The placenta is also an active metabolic site, able to process many of the substances that cross from maternal blood.

There is a wide divergence of placental types among mammals. Some have relatively shallow invasion of the uterine tissue, and others have no invasion at all. None is more invasive than the human placenta, and there is no satisfactory animal model for studying the processes of human placentation.

Although the blood of the human mother does not actually mix with the blood of her offspring, the intimate contact between maternal blood and fetal blood vessels in the placenta allows diffusion of oxygen, nutrients, hormones, and antibodies from the mother to the developing embryo. A mother's medications or toxic

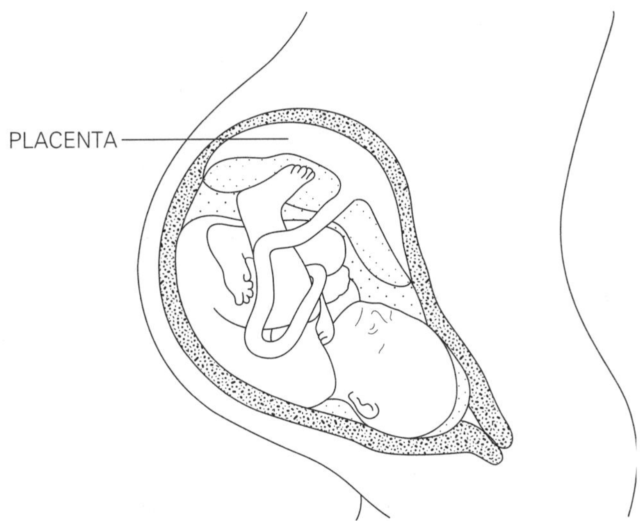

Figure 1-18. The placenta in utero

exposures can also cross this barrier, as can viruses such as cytomegalovirus and rubella—with damaging consequences for the fetus.

In the other direction, the fetus discharges its metabolic waste via the placenta. Some fetal cells also make their way into the mother's bloodstream. These fetal cells can be detected in the mother's peripheral blood (especially if the fetus is a male, allowing the cells to be more easily distinguished from the mother's own cells). Fetal cells in maternal circulation have been proposed as a source of fetal genes for prenatal genetic tests.[43] Even more promising for fetal testing is the large quantity of acellular fetal DNA found in mother's blood, presumably shed from the rapidly developing placental cells.[44]

Renegade fetal cells not only circulate in the mother's blood during pregnancy; they can settle into the mother's bone marrow as stem cells and survive for years, producing fetal blood cells in the mother long after delivery.[45] Such maternal "microchimerism" (i.e., involving a relatively small number of cells of the fetus) has been speculated to contribute to women's later risk of autoimmune diseases, although there is limited evidence to support this.[46]

On the topic of microchimerism, cells apparently cross the placenta in the other direction as well. Maternal stem cells that produce lymphocytes and blood cells are able to establish themselves in fetuses.[47] The health effects, if any, of these stowaway cells from the mother are unknown. If these maternal cell lines persist into the fetus's adult life, it could be possible for a woman to carry within her body genetically distinct cells from three generations—cells from her mother and cells from her children.

Pathologies of Placentation

Molar pregnancy (also known as hydatidiform mole) is a condition in which a placenta flourishes in the absence of a fetus. The genetics of this condition are revealing: molar pregnancies result when the maternal genetic contribution has been lost at conception, but the father's genes remain in diploid form. (A variant of molar pregnancy has one set of maternal genes and two sets of paternal genes.) These genetic observations point to the important role of paternal genes in the development of the placenta (see the discussion of gene imprinting in Chapter 5).

Molar pregnancies produce a positive pregnancy test and may at first be mistaken for an ordinary pregnancy. The classic clinical sign of molar pregnancy is painless vaginal bleeding. Although most molar pregnancies are benign and without consequence once removed, this condition can degenerate to a malignancy known as choriocarcinoma.

Other problems of the placenta include errors in its placement or attachment. Placental abruption occurs when the placenta begins to separate from the uterus before delivery. Sudden and massive bleeding into the uterus can threaten the lives of both the mother and her fetus. Another complication occurs when the placenta grows over the cervical opening (placenta previa). In this position, labor will tear the placenta from its moorings, again with the possibility of catastrophic bleeding.

After Birth

Despite its essential role during pregnancy, the placenta comes to an ignoble end. At delivery, the placenta is a half-kilogram of floppy blood-soaked tissue connected to the baby by the umbilical cord. It has no further physiologic function. Like any tissue, it is edible (for example, sautéed with onions[48]), and in other species the mother often eats the placenta after delivery. Placentas are a common ingredient in cosmetics.[49] In a few cultures, the placenta is preserved or buried with special ceremonies,[50] but more often it is simply discarded.

Science has provided another reason to save placental tissue, or at least pieces of it. The placenta is one of the most accessible of all human tissues, and can provide useful information on toxicant exposures to the fetus.[51] Substances that can be measured in placental tissue include organochloride pesticides, dioxins, and heavy metals.

The End of the Beginning

This brief overview of human reproduction does not do justice to its complexity and subtlety. Still, it provides a framework for the chapters that follow. Note especially the natural variability that characterizes nearly every aspect of reproduction—there is a bell-shaped frequency distribution of everything from age at menarche to the time of implantation. Our understanding of this variability comes from epidemiologic studies. Epidemiology is usually defined as a tool for understanding disease, but epidemiology also helps to uncover the natural workings of biology. This is nowhere more apparent than in the area of reproduction. The next chapter (on aspects of human fertility) is based almost entirely on epidemiologic observations.

References

1. Harvey W. *Disputations Touching the Generation of Animals.* Oxford: Blackwell Scientific Publications, 1981.
2. Farley J. *Gametes and Spores: Ideas about Sexual Reproduction 1750–1914.* Baltimore, MD: Johns Hopkins University Press, 1982.
3. Kolata G. Maleness pinpointed on Y chromosome. *Science* 1986;234:1076.
4. Heller CG, Clermont Y. Spermatogenesis in man: an estimate of its duration. *Science* 1963;140:184–6.
5. Amann R. A critical review of methods for evaluation of spermatogenesis from seminal characteristics. *J Androl* 1981;2(1):37–58.
6. Lintern-Moore S, Peters H, Moore GP, Faber M. Follicular development in the infant human ovary. *J Reprod Fertil* 1974;39(1):53–64.

7. Morita Y, Tilly JL. Oocyte apoptosis: like sand through an hourglass. *Dev Biol* 1999;213(1):1–17.
8. Baker TG. A quantitative and cytological study of germ cells in human ovaries. *Proc R Soc Lond B Biol Sci* 1963;158:417–33.
9. Belsey EM, Pinol AP. Menstrual bleeding patterns in untreated women. Task Force on Long-Acting Systemic Agents for Fertility Regulation. *Contraception* 1997;55(2):57–65.
10. Promislow JH, Baird DD, Wilcox AJ, Weinberg CR. Bleeding following pregnancy loss before 6 weeks' gestation. *Hum Reprod* 2007;22(3):853–7.
11. Healy D, Hodgen GD. Endocrinology of follicle growth. In: Trounson A, Wood C, eds. *In Vitro Fertilization and Embryo Transfer.* Edinburgh: Churchill Livingstone, 1984;75–93.
12. Fehring RJ. Accuracy of the peak day of cervical mucus as a biological marker of fertility. *Contraception* 2002;66(4):231–5.
13. Matsumoto S, Nogami Y, Ohkuri S. Statistical studies on menstruation: a criticism on the definition of normal menstruation. *Gunma J Med Sci* 1962;11:294–318.
14. Bigelow JL, Dunson DB, Stanford JB, Ecochard R, Gnoth C, Colombo B. Mucus observations in the fertile window: a better predictor of conception than timing of intercourse. *Hum Reprod* 2004;19(4):889–92.
15. Harlow SD, Ephross SA. Epidemiology of menstruation and its relevance to women's health. *Epidemiol Rev* 1995;17(2):265–86.
16. Treloar AE, Boynton RE, Behn BG, Brown BW. Variation of the human menstrual cycle through reproductive life. *Int J Fertil* 1967;12(1 Pt 2):77–126.
17. The TREMIN Research Program on Women's Health. Penn State Population Research Institute. Available at http://www.pop.psu.edu/tremin/tremin.html, last accessed October 27, 2009.
18. Harlow SD, Lin X, Ho MJ. Analysis of menstrual diary data across the reproductive life span: applicability of the bipartite model approach and the importance of within-woman variance. *J Clin Epidemiol* 2000;53(7):722–33.
19. Baird DD, McConnaughey DR, Weinberg CR, et al. Application of a method for estimating day of ovulation using urinary estrogen and progesterone metabolites. *Epidemiology* 1995;6(5):547–50.
20. Wilcox AJ, Dunson D, Baird DD. The timing of the "fertile window" in the menstrual cycle: day specific estimates from a prospective study. *BMJ* 2000;321(7271):1259–62.
21. Harlow SD. Menstruation and menstrual disorders: the epidemiology of menstruation and menstrual disfunction. In: Goldman MaHM, ed. *Women and Health.* San Diego: Academic Press, 2000;99–113.
22. Sandler DP, Wilcox AJ, Horney LF. Age at menarche and subsequent reproductive events. *Am J Epidemiol* 1984;119(5):765–74.
23. Colborn T, vom Saal FS, Soto AM. Developmental effects of endocrine-disrupting chemicals in wildlife and humans. *Environ Health Perspect* 1993;101(5):378–84.
24. Wyshak G, Frisch RE. Evidence for a secular trend in age of menarche. *N Engl J Med* 1982;306(17):1033–5.
25. Kaplowitz P. Pubertal development in girls: secular trends. *Curr Opin Obstet Gynecol* 2006;18(5):487–91.
26. Partsch CJ, Sippell WG. Pathogenesis and epidemiology of precocious puberty. Effects of exogenous oestrogens. *Hum Reprod* Update 2001;7(3):292–302.
27. Faddy MJ, Gosden RG, Gougeon A, Richardson SJ, Nelson JF. Accelerated disappearance of ovarian follicles in mid-life: implications for forecasting menopause. *Hum Reprod* 1992;7(10):1342–6.

28. Research on the menopause. *WHO Tech Rep Ser* 1981;670:1–120.
29. Midgette AS, Baron JA. Cigarette smoking and the risk of natural menopause. *Epidemiology* 1990;1(6):474–80.
30. Luoto R, Kaprio J, Uutela A. Age at natural menopause and sociodemographic status in Finland. *Am J Epidemiol* 1994;139(1):64–76.
31. Wilcox AJ. Early pregnancy. In: Kiely M, ed. *Reproductive and Perinatal Epidemiology*. Boca Raton: CRC Press, 1991;63–75.
32. Wassarman PM. The biology and chemistry of fertilization. *Science* 1987;235 (4788):553–60.
33. Blickstein I, Keith LG. On the possible cause of monozygotic twinning: lessons from the 9-banded armadillo and from assisted reproduction. *Twin Res Hum Genet* 2007;10(2):394–9.
34. Boklage CE. Embryogenesis of chimeras, twins and anterior midline asymmetries. *Hum Reprod* 2006;21(3):579–91.
35. Haig D. What is a marmoset? *Am J Primatol* 1999;49(4):285–96.
36. Mastenbroek S, Twisk M, van Echten-Arends J, et al. In vitro fertilization with preimplantation genetic screening. *N Engl J Med* 2007;357(1):9–17.
37. Wilcox AJ, Baird DD, Weinberg CR. Time of implantation of the conceptus and loss of pregnancy. *N Engl J Med* 1999;340(23):1796–9.
38. Moffett A, Loke C. Immunology of placentation in eutherian mammals. *Nat Rev Immunol* 2006;6(8):584–94.
39. Pisarska MD, Carson SA, Buster JE. Ectopic pregnancy. *Lancet* 1998; 351(9109): 1115–20.
40. Varma R, Mascarenhas L, James D. Successful outcome of advanced abdominal pregnancy with exclusive omental insertion. *Ultrasound Obstet Gynecol* 2003;21(2):192–4.
41. Kaufmann P, Black S, Huppertz B. Endovascular trophoblast invasion: implications for the pathogenesis of intrauterine growth retardation and preeclampsia. *Biol Reprod* 2003;69(1):1–7.
42. Beaconsfield P, Birdwood G, Beaconsfield R. The Placenta. *Sci Am* 1980;243(2):95–102.
43. Bianchi DW, Hanson J. Sharpening the tools: a summary of a National Institutes of Health workshop on new technologies for detection of fetal cells in maternal blood for early prenatal diagnosis. *J Matern Fetal Neonatal Med* 2006;19(4):199–207.
44. South ST, Chen Z, Brothman AR. Genomic medicine in prenatal diagnosis. *Clin Obstet Gynecol* 2008;51(1):62–73.
45. Lissauer D, Piper KP, Moss PA, Kilby MD. Persistence of fetal cells in the mother: friend or foe? *Br J Obstet Gynaecol* 2007;114(11):1321–5.
46. Lapaire O, Hosli I, Zanetti-Daellenbach R, et al. Impact of fetal-maternal microchimerism on women's health—a review. *J Matern Fetal Neonatal Med* 2007;20(1):1–5.
47. Jonsson AM, Uzunel M, Gotherstrom C, Papadogiannakis N, Westgren M. Maternal microchimerism in human fetal tissues. *Am J Obstet Gynecol* 2008;198(3):325 e1–6.
48. Ober WB. Notes on placentophagy. *Bull N Y Acad Med* 1979;55(6):591–9.
49. Muralidhar R, Panda, T. Useful products from human placenta. *Bioprocess Biosyst Eng* 1999;20(1):23–5.
50. Dundes L, ed. *The Manner Born: Birth Rites in Cross-Cultural Perspective*. Rowman: AltaMira, 2003.
51. Myllynen P, Pasanen M, Pelkonen O. Human placenta: a human organ for developmental toxicology research and biomonitoring. *Placenta* 2005;26(5):361–71.

2

On Getting Pregnant

For a woman to conceive, she must have intercourse close to the time of her ovulation—but how close? The number of days on which a woman can conceive depends on how long the sperm can survive in the female reproductive tract and on how long the egg is available for fertilization. As it happens, this basic reproductive information has come not from physiology or clinical studies but from epidemiology.

The year 1916 was a terrible one in Germany. More than 160,000 German soldiers had died in the disastrous Battle of the Somme, and thousands more were dying up and down the Western Front (Fig. 2-1). Not surprisingly, the country's birth rate was in decline.

Worried by the loss of young men and the falling birth rate, a young German physician named Walter Pryll carried out a research project that aimed to help replenish the population.[1] He sought to identify the days during the menstrual cycle when women were most likely to conceive. In some parts of rural Germany, weddings were scheduled for just after a woman's menses, which according to local tradition was when women were at their maximum fertility.[1] However, scientific data on this question were practically nonexistent. Pryll figured that if he could identify the most fertile days, this would help women improve their chances of conception.

As it happened, the conditions of war created an opportunity to address this question. Soldiers on the Front received occasional 1-day passes to go home. Pryll gathered data on pregnancies conceived during those brief visits. Pregnancies conceived during 1-day visits identify the fertile days of the menstrual cycle. Pryll found a total of 25 pregnancies that had resulted from 1-day visits. Under the reasonable assumption that leave days were random with regard to menstrual cycle days, the distribution of those conception days should describe the distribution of fertile days. The results are shown in Figure 2-2. Although the numbers are too

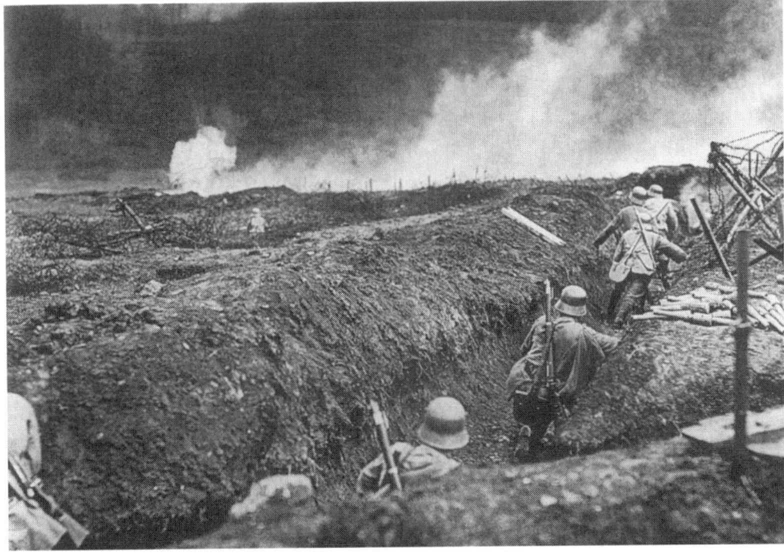

Figure 2-1. On the Western Front, World War I

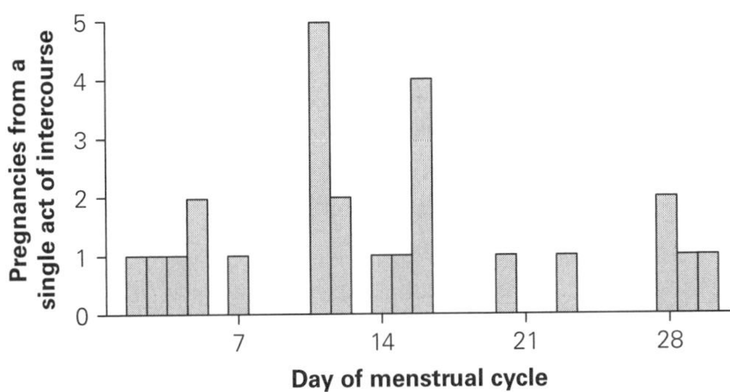

Figure 2-2. Conception days for 25 pregnancies conceived with intercourse on only 1 day of the cycle (Germany, 1917)[1]

small to provide much precision, the variability is impressive: pregnancies were conceived across a broad span of menstrual cycle days.

Pryll's unusual study underscores how hard it is under more ordinary circumstances to identify a woman's fertile days. The best evidence of whether a woman is fertile on a given day is the occurrence of conception with intercourse on that day—and on that day alone. The problem is that couples do not ordinarily have intercourse on just one particular day of a cycle. If they have intercourse on even two cycle days, then there can be no certainty as to which of the 2 days produced the pregnancy. The more cycle days with intercourse, the greater the uncertainty. Although Pryll's design was an attempt to remove this uncertainty, it is still not possible to be sure that a woman did not have intercourse on another day of the cycle—all we know is that the husband was absent on those other days.

Despite the obvious limitations of this study, decades passed before researchers were able to improve on it.

The Fertile Days of the Menstrual Cycle

A *fertile day* is defined as a day of the menstrual cycle on which unprotected intercourse is able to produce pregnancy. This does not have to be the day of ovulation, nor is it necessarily the day on which conception takes place. It is rather any day on which a spermatozoon deposited in the vagina has the possibility of fertilizing an ovum. If sperm survive for a week in the woman's reproductive tract, then the fertile days would start a week before ovulation. If the ovum were able to survive for a week after its release from a follicle, then the fertile days would last for a week after ovulation.

In 1961 the demographer R. G. Potter summarized the best available data on survival of sperm and egg to estimate the fertile window. According to Potter, "most investigators now doubt the average fertile period averages as long as 72 hours."[2] Two decades later, the World Health Organization proposed that women have 10 fertile days in every cycle, based on properties of the cervical mucus.[3] Which is correct? As it turns out, neither is.

To address this question rigorously requires daily information on ovulation, intercourse, and the resulting conceptions for a group of women. Using this approach, an epidemiologic study reported in 1995 found that the fertile days started 5 days before ovulation and ended on the day of ovulation.[4] This 6-day window has been confirmed in another population.[5] From these observations we can infer that sperm survive for up to 5 days in the woman's reproductive tract, whereas the ovum apparently dies quickly after ovulation (or becomes unavailable for fertilization, perhaps because of changes in cervical mucus that block the passage of sperm into the uterus).

It would be extremely useful for women to be able to know when their fertile days are occurring. Unfortunately, the prediction of ovulation (and thus the identification of the fertile window) is still an inexact process. Biological markers such as changes in cervical mucus have been proposed as ways to identify the six fertile days prospectively. Although most evidence suggests that such markers are not highly predictive,[6] some results appear promising.[7]

As a woman starts a new menstrual cycle, there is no way to predict with certainty when she will ovulate. It is possible, however, to make probabilistic statements about the likelihood of ovulation. Figure 1-10 in Chapter 1 shows the natural variability of ovulation in the menstrual cycle (the frequency distribution of the follicular phase length). By applying the 6-day fertile window to this distribution of ovulation, we can estimate the probability that a woman would be in her fertile days on any given day of the menstrual cycle (Fig. 2-3).[8]

Note that the probability in this figure is not a woman's chance of *conceiving* but rather her chance of being in that time window when she is *capable* of conceiving. As shown in Figure 2-3, about half of all women are in their fertile days on any given day from the eleventh to the fourteenth cycle-day. However, the chances of a fertile day are widely distributed. An estimated 2% of women are in their fertile days on day 4 of their cycle, when most women are still menstruating. Thus, the presence of menstrual bleeding is no guarantee against conception. At the other end of the cycle, around 5% of women are fertile at the beginning of their fifth week, when most women expect their next menses. Pryll's World War I study may have been limited in many respects, but the extreme range of fertile days suggested in his data is not inconsistent with data from larger and more carefully observed populations.

The Probability of Pregnancy with Intercourse on a Specific Day

Assuming that there are six fertile days in each cycle, what is the actual probability of pregnancy on these 6 days? This is a more difficult question because couples

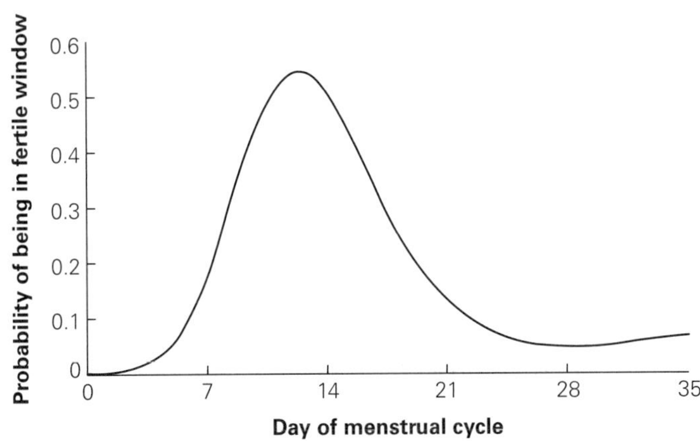

Figure 2-3. For any given day of her menstrual cycle, the probability that a woman is in the 6-day fertile window (213 women, North Carolina, 1983–85) (Reprinted from Wilcox et al[8])

vary widely in their baseline ability to conceive (see Chapter 9). However, some estimates can be made for couples on average.

The general pattern of day-specific fertility in the fertile window is shown in Figure 2-4.[9] As might be expected, the lowest probability is on the earliest day of the fertile window (presumably corresponding to the longest time that sperm can remain viable in the female reproductive tract). The highest probability is on the day before ovulation. The probability of conception fell to zero on the day after ovulation.

> **Carl Sagan and the Unintended Consequences of Time Travel**
>
> One interesting argument against the wisdom of time travel (if it were possible) is the likelihood that a step back in time would obliterate our own existence.
>
> In his book *Cosmos*,[10] Carl Sagan pointed out that even a tiny perturbation in history, centuries ago, would have a dramatic ripple effect. Consider the hundreds of millions of spermatozoa in each ejaculate. The creation of any particular person depends on fertilization by precisely one of those sperm and no others. The slightest change of environment, external or internal, would likely produce a different person from the same ejaculate. A different ejaculate would have no possibility of producing the same person. Thus, even the most trivial change, introduced far enough back in our history, would eventually cascade into a genetic rearrangement of the entire population of humanity. We and all the people we know would cease to exist. In our place would be billions of others.

These women had a 28% chance of producing a clinical pregnancy with intercourse on this peak day. This is about the same as the overall chance of getting pregnant in a given cycle.[11] Thus, intercourse on the peak fertile day doesn't appear

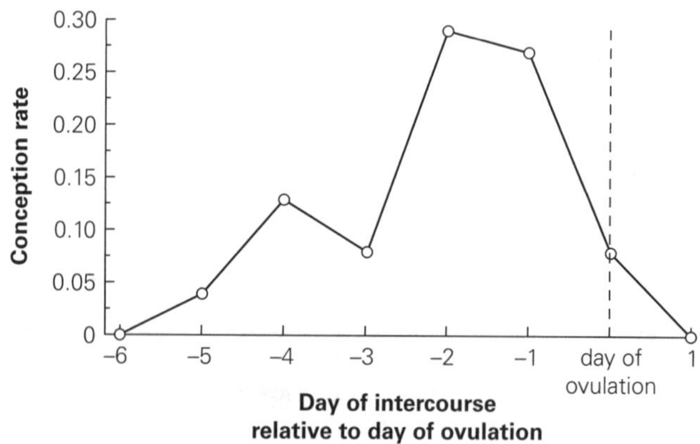

Figure 2-4. Probability of conception given intercourse on a specific day of the fertile window (144 clinical pregnancies among 221 women, North Carolina, 1983–85) (Reprinted from Wilcox et al[9])

to improve the average couple's chances of pregnancy by much. This observation may seem counterintuitive, but it probably reflects the fact that most couples of reproductive age are having intercourse often enough (two or three times a week[12]) to hit the most fertile days by chance. Also, intercourse is not entirely by chance, even among couples who pay no attention to ovulation or fertile days.

Links between Intercourse and Ovulation

There are biological mechanisms in many mammalian species to increase the chances that intercourse will take place during the female's fertile days. (The evolutionary advantages are obvious.) For some animals, the female becomes sexually attractive to males and more receptive during her fertile period. In other animals (such as cats and rabbits), causation can go in the other direction: intercourse may trigger ovulation and thus induce fertility. Neither of these mechanisms has been established in humans, although recent data suggest they both might occur.

Consider the pattern of human intercourse over the menstrual period. Even among couples who are not trying to become pregnant, intercourse reaches its peak on the most fertile days of the cycle and then declines in the luteal phase[13] (Fig. 2-5). (These data are from women who had tubal ligation or were using IUDs, and who therefore had no interest in how the timing of their intercourse might be related to their ovulation.)

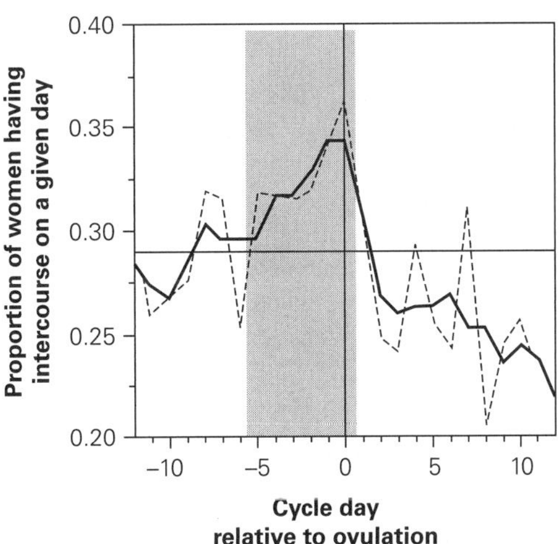

Figure 2-5. Intercourse in relation to day of ovulation (171 cycles from 68 women with tubal ligation or IUD, North Carolina, 1983–85; solid line is 3-day moving average) (Reprinted from Wilcox et al[13])

There are several possible biological mechanisms that might produce a peak of intercourse around ovulation. One possibility is that a woman has heightened sexual desire around the time of ovulation. Another is that a woman may become more sexually attractive during her fertile days. (A study of tip earnings by lap dancers supports this.[14]) Female attractiveness could be enhanced by the production of cycle-regulated pheromones.[15]

A third possibility is that intercourse accelerates the release of an egg that is already ripe for ovulation. This is difficult to determine in observational studies, although there are indirect clues. A multicenter study found that intercourse before ovulation accelerated ovulation and produced a shorter menstrual cycle.[16] Another study considered patterns of intercourse through the week. Intercourse is most likely on weekends, whereas ovulation presumably occurs randomly with regard to day of the week. If intercourse were able to trigger human ovulation, then the increased intercourse on weekends might produce increased ovulation early in the week. Preliminary data suggest this pattern.[13] These several mechanisms linking ovulation and intercourse are of course not mutually exclusive; more than one mechanism could be at work.

What is the Chance of Getting Pregnant with One Random Act of Intercourse?

In 1960, the demographer Christopher Tiezte carried out an elegant extrapolation from crude biological assumptions and concluded that women have a 2%–4% chance of conception with one random act of intercourse.[17] Forty years later, the chance of conception with one act of intercourse was calculated as 3%, based on the daily probabilities in Figure 2-4.[18]

Both estimates are flawed in that they assume intercourse is random with regard to fertile days. We now know this is not true (see Fig. 2-5). To the extent that biological mechanisms press couples toward intercourse on the fertile days, the chance of conception will be higher with a "random" act of intercourse than predicted, simply because intercourse is not completely random. Couples having daily intercourse would be unaffected by such biological influences, whereas among couples having intercourse only sporadically, those biologic mechanisms may have strong influence. Thus, the oft-heard lament from young couples who "took a chance just that once" may be true more often than is generally supposed.

How Soon Do Women Know They Are Pregnant?

SYMPTOMS OF PREGNANCY. Just as with every other aspect of reproductive biology, there is variability in the time when women start having symptoms of pregnancy. Figure 2-6 shows the cumulative proportion of women with pregnancy symptoms by time since the last menstrual period.[19] These diary data were recorded by women who were trying to get pregnant; women who are not expecting to

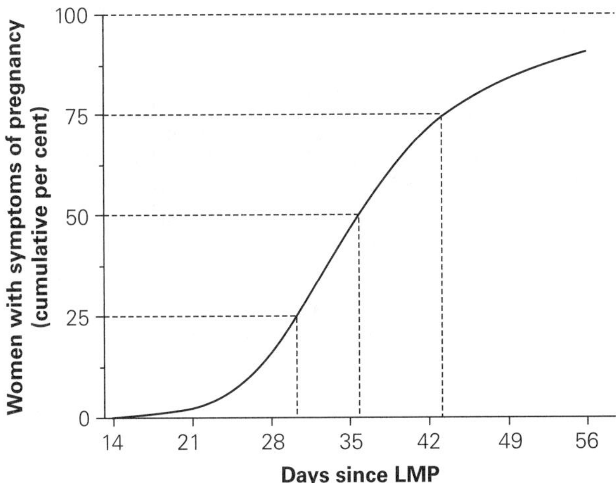

Figure 2-6. First symptoms of clinical pregnancy in relation to LMP (151 women with planned pregnancy, North Carolina, 1983–85)[19]

become pregnant might take longer to recognize their symptoms. About a quarter of women had symptoms by day 30, which is around the time when many women might also recognize that their period is late. Half of women had symptoms by 6 weeks of pregnancy, and 10% still had no apparent symptoms by 8 weeks. There is a tendency for pregnancies ending in miscarriage to produce symptoms later. Women who have no symptoms by the eighth week after the last menstrual period are twice as likely as other women to miscarry.[19]

About half of women did not yet have symptoms 3 weeks after conception.[19] By 3 weeks the neural tube has already been established, and other major organs are formed soon after.[20] Thus, women who wait for pregnancy symptoms before starting prenatal vitamins or avoiding possible toxic exposures may be acting too late to protect their baby.

PREGNANCY TESTS. Symptoms are not the only way that women discover they are pregnant. Women in many countries have access to home pregnancy test kits that can detect urinary human chorionic gonadotropin (hCG) soon after implantation. Early diagnosis of pregnancy may be useful to women, but there can be unintended consequences. For example, there is a high rate of pregnancy loss in the first week or two after implantation (discussed in Chapter 10). Women who use pregnancy tests early in their pregnancy are more likely to detect pregnancies that end in early loss, which otherwise might have been mistaken for ordinary menses.

From an epidemiologic standpoint, self-testing for pregnancy can complicate the estimation of rates of pregnancy loss. This is a problem particularly if women

A Short History of Pregnancy Tests

The idea of using urine to test for pregnancy has been around for millennia. An Egyptian papyrus from 1350 BC advises a woman to water the seeds of barley and wheat with her urine. If both types sprout, she is pregnant.[21] For women who don't want to wait for sprouts, a medical treatise from 1580 suggests that urine from a pregnant woman will turn a clean needle mottled red overnight.[21]

In 1927, researchers discovered that the urine of pregnant women could stimulate ovarian follicular development in mice.[22] This led to various pregnancy bioassays in the 1940s and 1950s in which women's raw urine was injected into mice, rabbits, or frogs, and the animals sacrificed for evidence of ovarian stimulation. These procedures are expensive and time-consuming—and not particularly reliable. The development in the 1960s of sensitive and specific assays for hCG has spared many small animals.

exposed to a possible reproductive toxin are more likely to do early testing. In that case, early testing could uncover more losses even in the absence of an effect of the toxin. To avoid such bias, an epidemiologic study would have to collect information about the use and timing of early pregnancy tests.

Although test kits are highly sensitive at detecting hCG, they are not as accurate as the package inserts state. Most instructions tell women to test for pregnancy on the "first day of their missed period." If the test result is negative, this is supposed to provide a high level of certainty that the woman is not pregnant. Such instructions do not take into account the extent to which the ovulation day (and thus the conception day) can vary among women. There are always some women who ovulate later than their usual cycle length would suggest and who therefore conceive later in their cycle than expected. Such conceptions may not have implanted even by the time a woman expects her next menses. Before implantation, there is no hCG in the mother's blood or urine and no possibility of detecting the presence of a fertilized egg. About 10% of all clinical pregnancies are undetectable on the first day of the "missed period" because of late implantation.[23] About 3% of pregnancies will still not have implanted even 1 week after the expected onset of the next period. Thus, when pregnancy test kits are used as directed (at expected onset of the next menses), there is a threat of both "false-positive" readings (in the sense of detecting pregnancies that were not going to last long enough to be clinically apparent) and false-negative readings (healthy conceptions that have not yet implanted).

The Bottom Line

Mechanisms that have developed over eons of evolution conspire to make conception happen. Most couples are able to conceive within a few months of trying and without attention to timing of intercourse or other strategies often suggested in the popular media.[24,25] For couples who have tried to conceive without success, their chances may be improved by an understanding of the fertile days. A woman who does not wish to become pregnant should be aware that in the absence of reliable information on when she ovulates, it is theoretically possible to get pregnant with intercourse on almost any day of her cycle.

References

1. Pryll W. Kohabitationstermin und kindsgeschlecht. *Muench Med Wochenschr* 1916;45:1579–82.
2. Potter RG. Length of the fertile period. *Milbank Mem Fund Q* 1961;39(1):132–62.
3. WHO. A prospective multicentre trial of the ovulation method of natural family planning. III. Characteristics of the menstrual cycle and of the fertile phase. *Fertil Steril* 1983;40(6):773–8.
4. Wilcox AJ, Weinberg CR, Baird DD. Timing of sexual intercourse in relation to ovulation. Effects on the probability of conception, survival of the pregnancy, and sex of the baby. *N Engl J Med* 1995;333(23):1517–21.
5. Dunson DB, Baird DD, Wilcox AJ, Weinberg CR. Day-specific probabilities of clinical pregnancy based on two studies with imperfect measures of ovulation. *Hum Reprod* 1999;14(7):1835–9.
6. Grimes DA, Gallo MF, Grigorieva V, Nanda K, Schulz KF. Fertility awareness-based methods for contraception: systematic review of randomized controlled trials. *Contraception* 2005;72(2):85–90.
7. Scarpa B, Dunson DB, Colombo B. Cervical mucus secretions on the day of intercourse: an accurate marker of highly fertile days. *Eur J Obstet Gynecol Reprod Biol* 2006;125(1):72–8.
8. Wilcox AJ, Dunson D, Baird DD. The timing of the "fertile window" in the menstrual cycle: day specific estimates from a prospective study. *BMJ* 2000;321(7271):1259–62.
9. Wilcox AJ, Weinberg CR, Baird DD. Post-ovulatory ageing of the human oocyte and embryo failure. *Hum Reprod* 1998;13(2):394–7.
10. Sagan C. *Cosmos*. New York: Random House, 1980.
11. Leridon H. *Human Fertility: The Basic Components*. Chicago, IL: University of Chicago Press, 1977.
12. Hornsby PP, Wilcox AJ. Validity of questionnaire information on frequency of coitus. *Am J Epidemiol* 1989;130(1):94–9.
13. Wilcox AJ, Baird DD, Dunson DB, McConnaughey DR, Kesner JS, Weinberg CR. On the frequency of intercourse around ovulation: evidence for biological influences. *Hum Reprod* 2004;19(7):1539–43.
14. Miller G, Tybur JM, Jordan BD. Ovulatory cycle effects on tip earnings by lap dancers: economic evidence for human estrus? *Evol Hum Behav* 2007;28:375–81.
15. Grammer K, Fink B, Neave N. Human pheromones and sexual attraction. *Eur J Obstet Gynecol Reprod Biol* 2005;118(2):135–42.
16. Stanislaw H, Rice FJ. Acceleration of the menstrual cycle by intercourse. *Psychophysiology* 1987;24(6):714–8.
17. Tietze C. Probability of pregnancy resulting from a single unprotected coitus. *Fertil Steril* 1960;11:485–8.

18. Wilcox AJ, Dunson DB, Weinberg CR, Trussell J, Baird DD. Likelihood of conception with a single act of intercourse: providing benchmark rates for assessment of post-coital contraceptives. *Contraception* 2001;63(4):211–5.
19. Sayle AE, Wilcox AJ, Weinberg CR, Baird DD. A prospective study of the onset of symptoms of pregnancy. *J Clin Epidemiol* 2002;55(7):676–80.
20. Moore KL, Persaud TVN. *The Developing Human: Clinically Oriented Embryology.* Philadelphia, PA: Saunders, 2003.
21. Burstein J, Braunstein GD. Urine pregnancy tests from antiquity to the present. *Early Pregnancy* 1995;1(4):288–96.
22. Ascheim S, Zondek B. Das Hormon des Hypophysenvorderlappens: Testonjekt zum Nachweis des Hormons. *Klin Wochenschr* 1927;6:248–52.
23. Wilcox AJ, Baird DD, Dunson D, McChesney R, Weinberg CR. Natural limits of pregnancy testing in relation to the expected menstrual period. *JAMA* 2001;286(14):1759–61.
24. Graham J. How to get pregnant. *Redbook* 1998;190:78.
25. Veilleux Z. He shoots, he scores! *Men's Health* 1999;94–6.

3

How Humans Control Their Fertility

A person's control of his or her fertility is an individual right as well as a matter of social and economic consequence for society at large. Personal decisions regarding fertility affect nearly all aspects of reproductive epidemiology, sometimes in obvious ways and sometimes in ways that are surprisingly subtle.

Not all population-based health research is done by epidemiologists. Much of the work summarized in this chapter is from the field of demography, a specialty of sociology that sometimes converges with epidemiology.

Fertility Control from a Global Perspective

Two hundred years ago, Thomas Malthus proposed that human populations inherently grow faster than food production.[1] In Malthus's formulation, human history is an endless cycle of population growth interrupted by starvation. The idea that population growth begets human misery was a dismal contrast to the more prevalent view at the time, that population growth was a spur to economic growth. Malthus's ideas influenced many of the important thinkers of the nineteenth century including Charles Darwin, who transformed this idea of constant struggle into the concept of natural selection.

Malthus's ideas about populations went into eclipse in the late nineteenth century, as industrialization and modernization lowered death rates (especially infant mortality) while also providing the means and wealth to sustain population growth. When the benefits of industrial development spread to the rest of the world in the twentieth century, something historically unprecedented occurred: death rates fell rapidly in areas that had high birth rates. The result was an explosion of growth (Fig. 3-1).

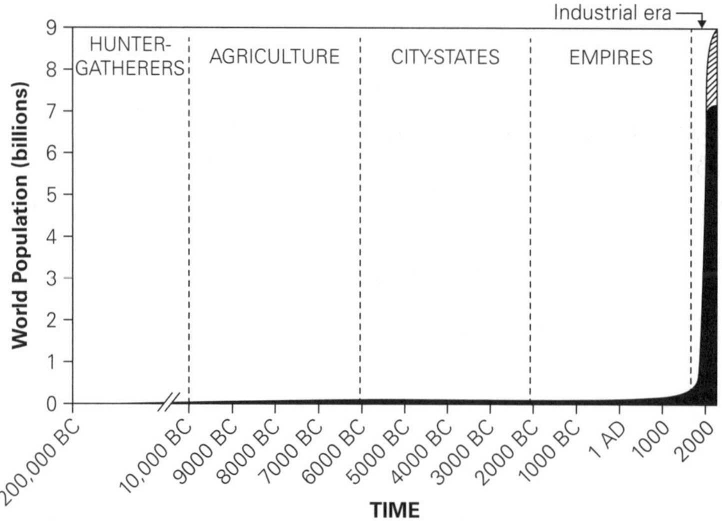

Figure 3-1. Human population growth over history. The lightly shaded area is growth projected by 2050. (Data from Kremer[2])

This population explosion led to a revival of Malthusian gloom, epitomized by the publication of *The Population Bomb* by Paul Ehrlich in 1968.[3] During the 1960s the world population was growing at a rate of 2% a year—fast enough to double in just 35 years.[2] Ehrlich proposed that this rapid population growth would soon outstrip the available food supplies, leading to widespread famine by the 1980s. International efforts were launched in the 1970s to reduce population growth by promoting family-planning methods. These efforts were focused on developing countries where birth rates were highest.

The disaster predicted by Ehrlich failed to materialize (or was it merely delayed?). The world's population did double during the 40 years after Ehrlich's book, but starvation actually decreased as a result of the industrialization of food

The Rule of 70
(or How to Compute Doubling Times in Your Head)

You can quickly estimate the time it takes a population to double in size (or your bank account to double in value) at a fixed annual rate of growth: divide 70 by the percentage annual growth as a whole number. The result is a surprisingly close approximation of the doubling time. Thus, 7% annual growth would lead to a doubling in about 10 years, whereas 10% annual growth will produce a doubling in about 7 years.

production. Meanwhile, birth rates have been falling in most parts of the world, defusing population growth as a political issue.

What Proportion of People Who Have Ever Lived Are Alive Today?

An urban myth that has circulated since the 1970s says that more people are alive today than have ever lived in the history of humankind.[4] That isn't true, or even close. The question involves guesswork, but it is possible to make a rough estimate. Assume that modern *Homo sapiens* emerged about 50,000 years ago, and that there were 5 million humans around at the dawn of agriculture 12,000 years ago. Using rough guesses about fertility and mortality, Haub has estimated that about 1 billion people lived up to the beginning of the agricultural era.[4] The population in the year 1 AD has been estimated at 300 million, so that would add another 46 billion or so in the interim. The world population passed the 1-billion mark some time after 1800, with another 44 billion in the interim. Since 1800 (when the first modern censuses were begun), there have been about 15 billion people. These total to about 106 billion humans on planet Earth.[4] With nearly 7 billion people alive today, the living comprise perhaps 7% of all past and present members of our species.

Total Fertility and Trends over Time

One measure used by demographers to summarize fertility is the *total fertility rate*. Total fertility is an artificial but useful concept—it is a projection of how many children would be born to a woman in her lifetime if she were to experience the age-specific fertility rates of a given year. (This is exactly analogous to the calculation of life expectancy based on age-specific mortality rates in a given year.) A total fertility rate of 2.1 children is regarded as *replacement level*—enough to replace the woman and her partner while allowing for the smaller number of girls than boys at birth and the small proportion of children who will not themselves reproduce. (In countries with high infant and childhood mortality, the level of fertility necessary for replacement may be higher.)

Figure 3-2 shows the distribution of total fertility rates for the world as a whole at three points in time since 1950.[5] In the early 1950s, the median total fertility (50 percent on the *Y* axis) was more than five children per woman. By the late 1970s, the median was under 4 children per woman, and in 2003 the world median reached 2.1. Although some countries continue to have high birth rates, it is nonetheless remarkable that fertility in much of the world has fallen so dramatically in such a short time—with at least half of the world now reproducing at less than replacement levels. China's one-child policy is a major contributor to this trend; total fertility rates are also approaching one child per couple in other Asian countries (Japan, Taiwan) as well as in some parts of Europe (Spain, Italy).[6] In 1994, the total fertility rate in East Germany dipped to 0.8.

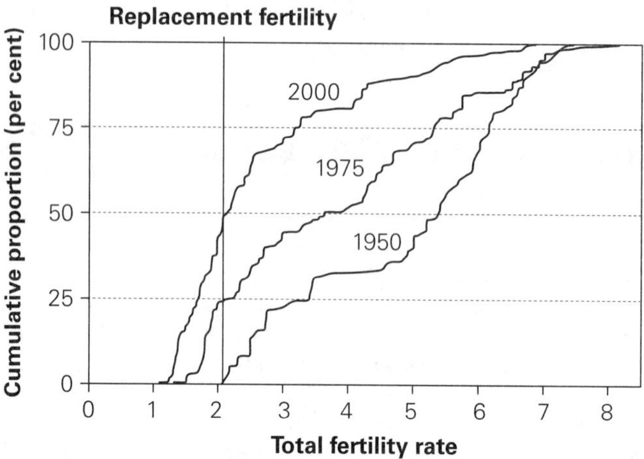

Figure 3-2. World fertility rates in 1950, 1975, and 2003 (cumulative distributions) (Adapted from Wilson and Pison[5])

Projecting Future Population Growth

Does the fact that the world is approaching replacement levels of fertility mean that the world's population has stopped growing? Not at all. There is a gap between the time when fertility reaches replacement levels and the time when growth stabilizes. This is because of the lag time that is required for a given birth cohort to reach and complete their reproductive years. This is illustrated in Figure 3-3. This graph shows the population of the Philippines stratified by sex and age. The strong pyramid pattern is characteristic of populations during times of rapid population growth and low mortality, when people are producing more than the replacement number of children.

Consider what would happen if fertility in the Philippines were immediately to fall to replacement levels. Each birth-cohort of women in the reproductive ages (shaded in the figure) would exactly replace themselves. However, the number of women of reproductive age will continue to grow for at least the next 15 years as the young women aging into this group exceed the older women aging out. It can take years for replacement levels of fertility to stop population growth.

Figure 3-4 shows the age pattern for Italy. There have been less-than-replacement levels of fertility for decades. As a consequence, even if Italy were to increase its fertility to replacement levels, the total population would continue to decline as the smaller birth cohorts move through their reproductive years.

This delayed effect of changes in fertility is why the world's population—estimated at 6.8 billion in 2009[7]—is continuing to grow even as we approach replacement levels of fertility (Fig. 3-5). The world population is projected to

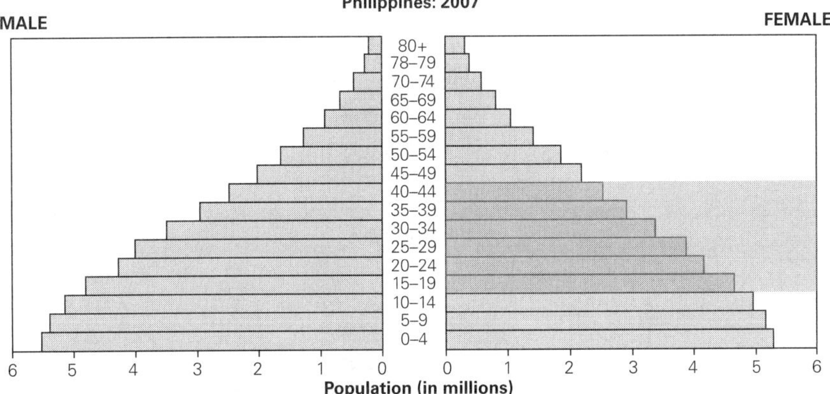

Figure 3-3. Population stratified by age and sex, Philippines 2007 (reproductive ages for women are shaded) (*Source*: U.S. Census Bureau, International Data Base)

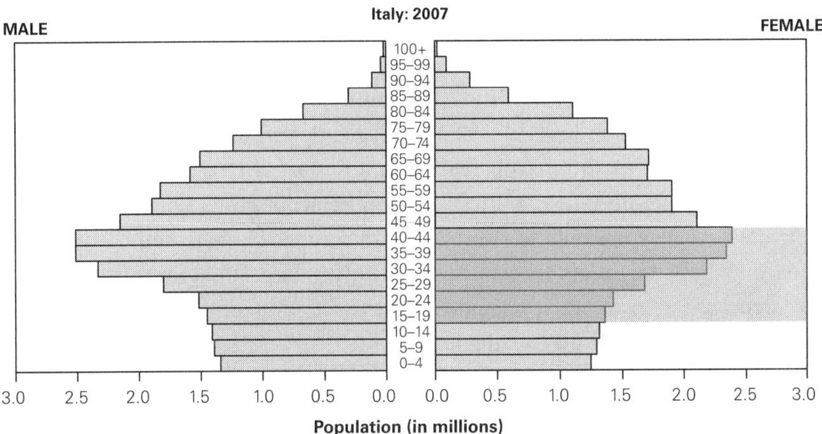

Figure 3-4. Population stratified by age and sex, Italy 2007 (reproductive ages for women are shaded) (*Source*: U.S. Census Bureau, International Data Base)

grow by more than 2 billion people by midcentury.[8] Although such predictions rest on many assumptions, they nonetheless demonstrate the tremendous momentum of population growth. Furthermore, nearly all (95%) of the world's population growth is taking place within the developing countries (Fig. 3-5).[8] Between 2005 and 2050, nine countries are expected to contribute half of the world's population growth. They are (in order of their contributions) India, Pakistan, Nigeria, Congo, Bangladesh, Uganda, the United States, Ethiopia, and China.

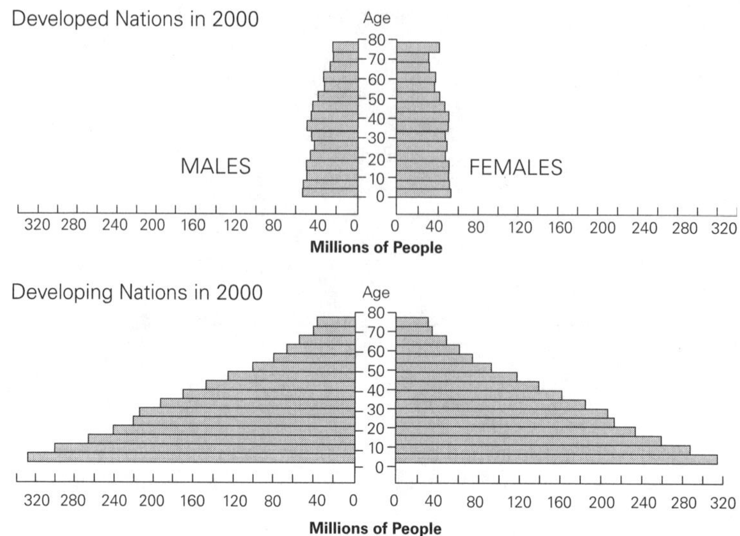

Figure 3-5. Populations stratified by age and sex for developed and developing nations, 2000 (Adapted from University of Michigan Global Change Curriculum)

While the effects of past fertility are simple to project, future changes in human fertility rates are much less certain. Fertility is determined by much more than the availability of birth control. Fertility rates started to decline in industrialized countries before effective methods of contraception had become available. Motivated couples are able to exert measurable control over their fertility even when they have few tools to help them. Still, the largest declines in birth rates have occurred after effective methods of contraception and sterilization became relatively cheap, simple and available.

Fertility Control from an Individual Perspective

We take for granted the diverse menu of birth control methods available today, but this modern convenience was hard won. Contraception inevitably raises the subject of sex, and sex can be an incendiary topic. In countries such as the United States, where Puritan values retain a foothold, the history of contraception is a history of social and political repression. Repressive policies toward birth control have in turn obstructed research and the dissemination of information. This pattern is seen even today.

Before 1900, a couple's options for preventing pregnancy were limited. Aside from abstinence, couples had the option of withdrawal before ejaculation and primitive barrier methods. The use of animal intestines as condoms dates back at least to the seventeenth century, although men used them more often to protect themselves from syphilis than from fatherhood.[9]

The first synthetic condoms were developed in the mid-1800s, after Charles Goodyear discovered vulcanization (the process that gives rubber its elasticity). The early "rubbers" were bulky contrivances with seams down the side. Although primitive by modern standards, they were still effective enough to stir up opposition. The Roman Catholic Church has had long-standing objections to any method of birth control. There were also more general concerns that birth control methods would corrupt the morals of young people. In the United States, the so-called Comstock laws enacted in the 1880s prohibited the transport of condoms—or information about contraception in any form—through the U.S. mail. Condoms were available only by prescription, "for the prevention of disease." It was not until 1972 that the U.S. Supreme Court struck down the last laws prohibiting the distribution of contraceptives to unmarried persons.

Contraceptive Methods Based on Fertility Awareness

The discovery in the 1920s that women ovulate once in midcycle led to the possibility of timed intercourse to restrict fertility.[10] In principle, women who do not wish to conceive should be able to have intercourse on any day outside their six-day fertile window without other birth control, and with no worries about becoming pregnant. The problem comes in knowing which are the fertile days. There are several approaches to identifying fertile days. The earliest methods (for example, the rhythm method) required a woman to abstain from intercourse for a long block of days during the middle of her cycle. One limitation of this approach is that the timing of ovulation is so unpredictable that extensive abstinence is needed to assure high efficacy (see Fig. 2-3 in Chapter 2).

The effectiveness of periodic abstinence as a method of birth control has been improved with basal body temperature (BBT) measurement, cervical mucus monitoring, and hormonal monitoring kits. Although none of these methods identifies the fertile days unerringly, they can substantially reduce the probability of pregnancy. With perfect use, failure rates with periodic abstinence have been reported as low as three to five pregnancies per 100 women per year.[11] (This measure is the usual method for evaluating contraceptive effectiveness—for reference, about 85 to 90 women would be expected to conceive out of 100 women using no birth control for a year.) With less perfect (and more typical) use of timed abstinence, about 25 women per 100 will conceive in a year.[11]

Barrier Methods

Rubber condoms were steadily improved in the early 1900s, and latex condoms were introduced in the 1930s. Modern condoms have the advantage of being cheap and easy to use. They also can break or slide off. With perfect use, the failure rate is estimated at 2 pregnancies per 100 women per year, and with typical use, the failure rate is around 15 pregnancies.[11]

The diaphragm is another early barrier method, and one that allowed women to more directly control their own fertility. The diaphragm is a flexible rubber shield that a woman inserts into her vagina before intercourse. Like the condom, the diaphragm blocks sperm from gaining access to the cervix. A drawback of the diaphragm is that it needs to be custom fitted and so usually requires assistance from a health professional.

The diaphragm was developed in Europe in the late 1800s but remained unavailable in the United States until Margaret Sanger illegally imported them in the 1920s. (Sanger was the founder of Planned Parenthood and is the unquestioned heroine of female reproductive rights.) The diaphragm was quickly adopted in the United States despite legal and religious obstacles, and by the 1940s, about one-third of U.S. married couples were using them. The failure rate with correct use (including spermicide) is estimated at 5 pregnancies per 100 women per year, and with typical use the failure rate is around 16 per 100.[11]

The diaphragm has fallen into general disuse since the introduction of oral contraceptives.[12] Other variations of female barrier methods are the cervical cap and the contraceptive sponge; their failure rates are in the range of 15 to 30 pregnancies per 100 women, and neither is widely used. There is a female condom—a loose-fitting sheath that is anchored externally and extends into the vagina. This device was developed in the wake of the HIV epidemic as a birth control method that could also protect women from infection. Although it does provide some degree of HIV protection, it is not a highly effective contraceptive. With perfect use, its failure rate is 5 pregnancies per 100 women per year, and, with typical use, closer to 21.[11]

Hormonal Contraceptives

Oral contraceptives are the innovation that most dramatically changed the landscape of birth control. As early as the 1940s, researchers understood the biological principles by which reproductive hormones might function as contraceptives, but no group—neither universities nor pharmaceutical companies nor governments—was willing to conduct the work necessary to develop a contraceptive pill. Margaret Sanger again came to the rescue. She introduced a wealthy woman philanthropist to physiologist Gregory Pincus in 1952. The philanthropist provided the private funding that allowed Pincus and his colleague John Rock to tackle this problem. Their collaboration produced the first oral contraceptive approved (in 1960) for human use. The pill remained illegal in some U.S. states until 1965 and was unavailable to unmarried women in some places until 1972. Today the pill is used by an estimated 100 million women worldwide.

The oral contraceptive was a unique advance in birth control: the combination of progesterone and estrogen physiologically intercepted the woman's capacity to conceive by temporarily suppressing ovulation. Oral contraceptives probably also change the endometrium and cervical mucus in ways that further discourage conception. A return to full fertility usually occurs within 3 months after discontinuing use. The failure rate is less than one per 100 users per year when used perfectly. Under more typical conditions of use (in which women occasionally forget to take a pill), the failure rate is estimated at eight per 100 users per year.

More recent formulations of oral contraceptives include a variety of synthetic progestagens and estrogens that work at much lower doses than the original formulations. Furthermore, contraceptive hormones do not necessarily need to be taken orally—routes of administration include injection, skin patch, and subcutaneous implants. The most severe side effect is stroke or heart attack related to changes in blood coagulation; these risks have been reduced with the introduction of lower-dose pills. Beneficial effects include a reduced risk of ovarian and endometrial cancer, especially among long-term users.

Intrauterine Devices

Intrauterine devices (or IUDs) are another effective method of birth control developed around the same time as the pill. These devices require medical personnel to insert the device through the cervix into the uterus. The method by which IUDs prevent conception is not fully established; the device induces a local inflammatory response that appears to decrease the survival of sperm in the uterus and perhaps also reducing the survival of the fertilized egg before implantation.[13,14] Although there were a number of forerunners, the models that made the IUD popular were the Lippes loop (introduced in 1962) and the "T" (in 1968) (Fig. 3-6). The addition of copper to the T increases its effectiveness, and almost all IUDs used today are a variant of the copper T. The IUD is the most popular reversible method of contraception in the world, with an estimated 160 million users. Failure rates are less than one per 100 women per year.

One sad story on the IUD's road to eventual success was the introduction in the United States of the Dalkon shield (Fig. 3-6). The Dalkon shield was distributed in the United States from 1971 to 1974; its use was suspended because of an associated risk of uterine infection. Several women died from complications attributed to the Dalkon shield. As a result, IUDs of any sort became unpopular in the United States and have remained so despite their acceptance elsewhere.

Breast-Feeding as a Method of Birth Control

Women's ovulation is suppressed during breast-feeding, which makes breast-feeding an effective method of birth control—up to a point. During the first 6 months or so after delivery, women who exclusively breast-feed their infants (and whose menses

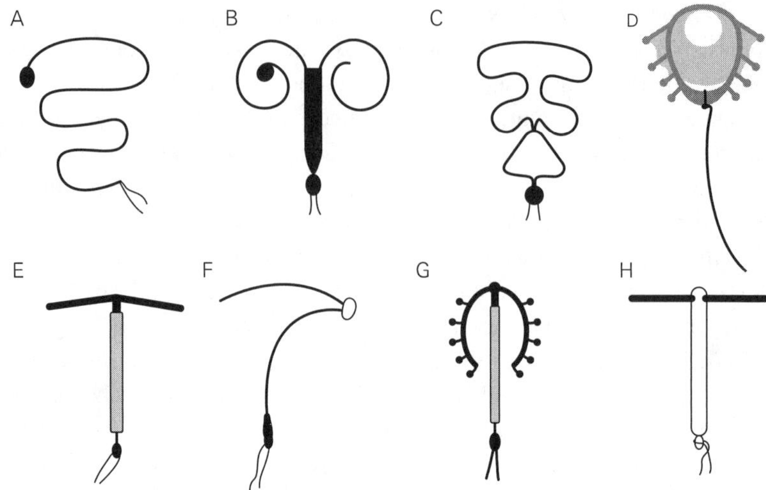

Figure 3-6. A sampler of intrauterine devices (IUDs): (A) Lippes loop, (B) Saf-T-Coil, (C) Dana-Super, (D) Dalkon shield, (E and F) copper-Ts, (G) multiload, and (H) progesterone IUD

have not resumed) have only about a 1% chance of becoming pregnant.[11] (This is known as the "lactational amenorrhea method" of birth control.) The problem is that even a brief interruption of breast-feeding can weaken the suppression of ovulation—and the first ovulation precedes menses.[11] Thus, a woman may not know her fertility has returned until she becomes pregnant again. (Conception with the first ovulation after a delivery is one reason for pregnancies with no recorded LMP.)

Sterilization

Both men and women can be permanently sterilized by relatively simple operations that cut or seal essential tubes (the oviducts in women, the vas deferens in men). Although the surgery in women is more complicated, it is also easier to reverse. Tubal ligation (in women) and vasectomy (in men) has the advantage of preserving normal hormonal function with no long-term health effects. Sterilization is more than 99% effective.

The 1960s were a watershed decade for contraception, a time when the groundwork was laid for the methods of birth control most commonly used today. Progress since then has been mostly embellishment. Truly revolutionary advances such as vaccination or male hormonal contraceptives have been proposed but without yet proving to be practical.

Table 3-1 summarizes failure rates for the most common methods of birth control. These numbers are estimates drawn from many sources and for the most part

Table 3-1 Failure rates of common types of birth control, with perfect use and with typical use

Contraception	Percentage pregnant in first year	
	Perfect use	Typical use
Sponge[a]	20	32
Spermicides	18	29
Withdrawal	4	27
Fertility awareness	5	25
Diaphragm	6	16
Male condom	2	15
Female condom	5	21
Birth control pill	0.3	8
IUD (copper T)	0.6	
Female sterilization	0.5	
Male sterilization	0.1	
None	85–90	

Source: From Trussell (2007), Table 27-1.[11]

[a]Parous women. For unknown reasons, failure rates with the sponge are lower for nulliparous women.

are only approximations. Advocates for a particular method often emphasize the method's effectiveness under optimal conditions. However, methods that require some action on the part of the couple invariably perform better with perfect usage than with typical usage.

Preferences for particular birth control methods vary widely by age and across populations. For example, IUDs are more widely used in developing nations than in the developed countries. In the United States, 2% of contracepting women use IUDs compared with 50% in China.[15] Oral contraceptives are the most popular reversible method in the United States, used by 31% of contracepting women.[12] Another 36% of U.S. contracepting women have opted for permanent sterilization (three-quarters female and one-quarter male). Fertility awareness methods and withdrawal are not widely used.

Emergency Contraception

Perhaps the most important birth control advance in recent decades has been the extension of oral hormones as a method of emergency contraception. Emergency contraception is the use of hormones by a woman after an act of unprotected intercourse. Its probable mechanism of action is to disrupt or delay ovulation.[16] The effectiveness of high doses of estrogens as emergency contraception has been known since at least the 1960s, although side effects at those high doses are unpleasant. In 1974 Yuzpe showed that two ordinary oral contraceptive pills taken after unprotected intercourse effectively reduced the risk of conception.[17] This off-label use of oral contraceptives was safe and easy, if not widely recognized.

A low-dose progestagen (levonorgestrel) has proved to be an even more effective "morning-after" pill, with few side effects.[16] In 1999, the U.S. FDA approved the use of levonorgestrel as a postcoital contraceptive. This approval predictably raised opposition. One concern has been that emergency contraception acts as an abortifacient by interfering with the survival of a fertilized egg. There is no evidence that levonorgestrel is an abortifacient.[18] Another concern (an echo of the condom argument of the late 1800s) is that a morning-after pill promotes promiscuity. Studies have found no evidence of this.[19] In 2006, emergency contraception was approved in the United States for over-the-counter use, amidst much controversy. It is presently marketed in over 50 countries.

The effectiveness of the morning-after pill is inherently difficult to estimate. A randomized clinical trial is impossible; such a trial would be unacceptable either for women who want to become pregnant or for women who do not. Estimates of efficacy have been based on average pregnancy rate for a given day of the menstrual cycle.[20] Notwithstanding the difficulties of this estimate, levonorgestrel on the day after unprotected intercourse probably prevents at least half of pregnancies that might otherwise have occurred.[21]

Pregnancy Termination

In the medical lexicon, *abortion* can refer either to the spontaneous death of a fetus before it is viable outside the uterus (miscarriage) or to the intentional termination of pregnancy (induced abortion). However, among the lay public the word abortion has become so strongly linked with induced abortion that medical usage is also changing. The word "abortion" is increasingly used only for induced abortions, while "miscarriage" is used to refer to spontaneous abortions.[22]

There is no simple or universal formula to define the occurrence of induced abortions in populations.[23] This can be defined as a percentage of all clinically recognized pregnancies, or as a ratio of abortions to live births or as abortions per 1,000 women aged 15–44 years. When abortion occurrence is compared over time or across populations, care must be taken to compare like with like. The measure used here is the ratio of abortions to live births.

The abortion ratio for the world as a whole has been estimated as 31 per 100 births.[24] As with other perinatal data, this ratio varies widely across nations. Both the lowest and the highest ratios are found in Europe (23 per 100 births in western Europe and 105 per 100 births in eastern Europe). In the United States, the ratio is 25 per 100 births.[25] Overall, abortion rates are tending to decline.[26]

Abortions are performed for reasons ranging from rape to fetal malformation to simple request by the mother. Pregnancy termination remains a highly contentious social issue in many countries, whereas in others (such as Ukraine and Japan), abortion has been a de facto method of birth control.

The laws regarding abortion also vary widely.[27] Abortion in the first trimester is provided free without questions in Italy, whereas in Chile it is illegal even as a means to save the life of the mother. Nazi Germany regarded abortion as murder, and in Nazi-occupied France a woman was guillotined for having an abortion.[28] Where abortion is restricted or illegal, it is often conducted under unsafe conditions that put women at considerable risk. In the United States, deaths related to abortion plummeted with the availability of legal abortion (Fig. 3-7).[29] WHO estimates that half of the world's abortions are unsafe, causing 68,000 deaths a year.[30] Ninety-seven percent of these unsafe abortions take place in the developing nations.[24]

MEDICAL ABORTION. There is a long history of efforts to discover herbs or other oral agents that might cause the fetus to abort.[31] In 1980 French researchers discovered mifepristone, a compound that binds competitively to the receptor for progesterone. By blocking the effects of natural progesterone in early pregnancy, mifepristone produces miscarriage with minimal risk to the mother. Taken orally within the first 7 weeks of pregnancy, a dose of mifepristone followed by a prostaglandin is more than 80% effective in terminating pregnancy.[32] Mifipristone was approved for use in France in 1988 (after much controversy), and its use has spread worldwide—along with strong opposition. There are no apparent adverse consequences of mifipristone-induced abortion on the outcome of subsequent pregnancies.[33]

SURGICAL ABORTION. In the United States, vacuum abortion is the most common surgical approach in early pregnancy, carried out with either manual syringe or

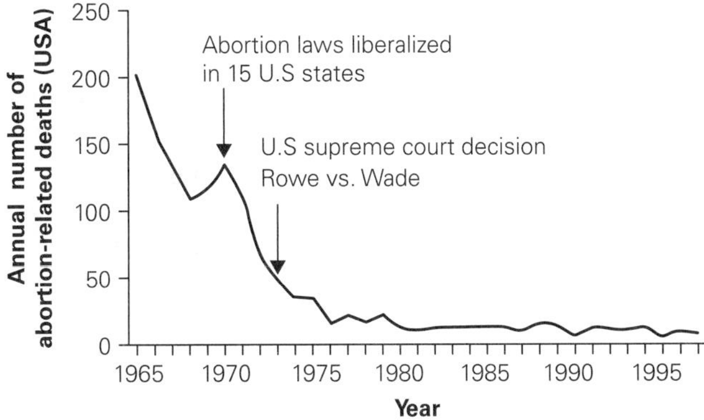

Figure 3-7. Estimated number of maternal deaths annually from induced abortion (United States, 1965–97) (*Source:* The Alan Guttmacher Institute[29])

electronic pump. Dilatation and evacuation are required after the fifteenth week of pregnancy; surgical instruments are used to widen the opening of the cervix and remove the fetus and placental tissue. The possibility of adverse effects from surgical abortion on subsequent pregnancies has been extensively explored. The consensus is that there is no increased risk of infertility, miscarriage, or ectopic pregnancies.[34] Some studies have suggested increased rates of preterm birth, although the evidence is still under debate.[35]

Prenatal Screening

Prenatal screening allows couples and their caregivers to have early information about possible problems with the fetus. Methods for prenatal screening include fetal ultrasound, maternal blood assays, amniocentesis, and chorionic villus sampling.[36] Not all fetal defects can reliably be determined prenatally; the most easily detected are major structural malformations, chromosomal abnormalities, and single-gene defects (when the gene is known). When a problem is identified, one option is to terminate the pregnancy by induced abortion.

Prenatal screening is susceptible to false-positive and false-negative results. Although the accuracy of screening generally improves as pregnancy advances, the options for termination grow correspondingly more narrow. This tradeoff between early screening and fully informative screening is the central dilemma of prenatal diagnosis, with steady efforts to improve early diagnosis.[37]

ULTRASOUND. Prenatal ultrasound is widely available in developed countries (and increasingly in developing countries). Ultrasound can detect major structural defects as well as a characteristic translucency at the back of the fetus's neck that is associated with Down syndrome. Early ultrasound can also help to establish the age of the fetus (based on fetal size), identify the presence of multiple fetuses, and detect incipient miscarriages (for example, the absence of heartbeat). Later ultrasound can show abnormalities of placental attachment.

MATERNAL SERUM MARKERS. Maternal serum can be screened for proteins derived from the fetus (alpha-fetoprotein) or from the placenta (hCG and the pregnancy-associated plasma protein-A [PAPP-A]). Specific combinations of high and low levels of these proteins are informative. For example, alpha-fetoprotein is increased in the presence of neural tube defects and reduced in the presence of Down syndrome.[38]

FETAL CELLS. A definitive diagnosis of genetic abnormalities requires fetal cells. This can be done by sampling amniotic fluid or by biopsying placental tissue (the chorionic villi). Both procedures carry a small risk of causing a healthy fetus to miscarry—probably less than 1%.[39] The detection of fetal cells or free fetal DNA in maternal blood is promising for noninvasive genetic study of the fetus, although such methods are not yet reliable enough for general use.[40]

Assisted Reproductive Technology

A discussion of fertility control would not be complete without mention of the remarkable technological advances that allow infertile couples to have children. Louise Brown, the first "test-tube" baby, was born in 1978. (She now has a son of her own, naturally conceived.) Since 1978, more than 3 million babies have been brought into the world with help from assisted reproductive technology (ART).[41]

Most ART procedures include hormonal hyperstimulation of the ovary to force the production of multiple ova. Once eggs are harvested, the most common technique is in vitro fertilization and transfer of freshly fertilized embryos into the uterus. In the United States, this procedure comprises about 75% of all cycles undergoing ART treatment.[42] Other options include the transfer of a woman's fertilized eggs from an earlier cycle (stored frozen) or the transfer of freshly fertilized eggs from another female donor. Injection of the sperm into the egg (intracellular injection of sperm, or ICSI) was developed as an attempt to overcome problems of male subfertility (Fig. 3-8). ICSI has proven so successful that it is now the preferred method for treatment of male-factor infertility.[43] The average live-birth rate per ART cycle is around 30%, with considerable variability by age of the woman, the underlying reasons for her infertility, and the types of procedures used.[44]

One unintended consequence of ART is an increase in multiple births. Although only 1% of all U.S. births are the result of ART,[42] ART pregnancies account for 16% of multiple births.[44] The effect of ART has been especially conspicuous among triplets, with ART conceptions contributing an estimated 40% of the total.[42] Indeed, the biggest risk attributable to ART seems to arise from the production of multiple fetuses. Twins and other multiple fetuses are at increased

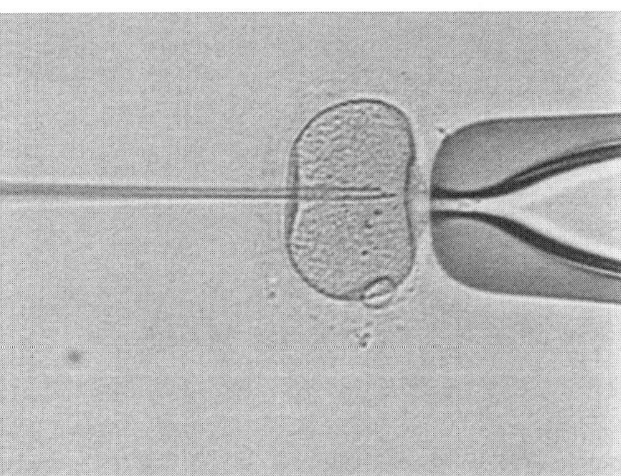

Figure 3-8. Fertilization by the injection of a spermatozoan into an egg (ICSI) (Figure courtesy of Mary M. Francis, Embryology Laboratory Director, USC Fertility, Los Angeles, CA)

risk of preterm delivery and perinatal death regardless of whether they are conceived naturally or through ART (see Chapter 13).

A further question is whether the arduous procedures of ART might indirectly damage the developing embryo and fetus. ART pregnancies are more likely to experience preeclampsia, placental abruption, and placenta previa.[45] One of the most common risks with ART is preterm delivery. Singleton babies conceived through in vitro fertilization have twice the risk of very preterm delivery compared with naturally conceived babies.[46] This could be the result of ART treatment, but it also could be caused by shared risk factors (such as occult infection) that produce both the infertility and the preterm delivery.[47] A comparison of naturally conceived babies and ART-conceived babies from the same women suggests that the excess risk of preterm lies in the women and not their treatment.[48]

A similar conundrum arises in the interpretation of low sperm counts or other signs of fertility impairment among sons conceived by ART.[49] These impairments may be the consequence of the mother's treatment, but they also could be characteristics inherited from subfertile fathers.[50] Fathers who are unable to produce offspring except through ART assistance may transmit genetic defects that make their sons infertile as well.[51]

There is some evidence to suggest a higher prevalence of birth defects among ART births.[52] This may be related to effects of treatment, but it could also be an artifact of closer scrutiny of ART deliveries, or result from an association of infertility itself with increased birth defect risk.[9]

The possibility of problems relating to gene imprinting has been raised for ART pregnancies.[53] *Imprinting* is the selective inactivation of a gene depending on whether the gene comes from the mother or the father (see Chapter 5). In vitro manipulation of the egg and sperm may interfere with these epigenetic mechanisms, although there has been no direct evidence that this is a problem.

The intracellular injection of sperm raises additional possibilities for unfavorable outcomes in ART pregnancies. This procedure allows fertilization by sperm that otherwise are impaired in their ability to penetrate the ovum. If the sperm's inability to fertilize represents a screening mechanism developed by the egg to block less-than-healthy sperm, then ICSI might be a risky procedure.[54] No such risks have yet been established.

Fertility Control from an Epidemiologic Perspective

Selective Fertility

The unprecedented level of personal control over fertility in modern times allows couples to decide whether and when they wish to become pregnant. This self-regulation of fertility becomes a filter that epidemiologists must take into account when studying reproductive outcomes. For example, in any group of pregnant women, there will be an overrepresentation of women who have no access to effective contraception, or who are uneducated in the use of birth control, or who choose to use less effective methods. The proportion of such women varies among countries. In the United States, half of all pregnancies and one-third of all births occur to women who were not actually trying to conceive.[55]

Another example of selective fertility is a couple's preference for season of delivery. Seasonal patterns in birth preference and fertility planning can lead to subtle distortions in seasonal patterns of pregnancy failure.[56] Epidemiologists sometimes examine seasonal patterns of pregnancy loss, birth defects, and other reproductive problems as a way to explore the influence of seasonally-varying factors such as infections or pollution. Such analyses need to take into account the effects of seasonal preferences in delivery.[56]

Yet another problem with selective fertility arises in evaluating the effects of aging on fertility. It is well documented that women who try to conceive at age 40 have more problems with infertility than women who attempt at age 25. However, how much of this difference reflects the selection of subfertile women at older ages? Women who have not achieved their desired family size by age 40 inevitably include some who had unprotected intercourse at younger ages or who had used imperfect methods of birth control but managed not to conceive. Women who accidentally conceived under those same conditions are, on average, more fertile, and because they are more likely to have achieved their desired family size, they are removed from the pool of women who want more children at age 40. Thus, subfertile women are overrepresented among women attempting to conceive at age 40. This selection complicates the interpretation of age effects on fertility in ways that are not easily measured or adjusted for.

The fact that couples who have not yet reached their desired family size are likely to have more pregnancies has another important consequence. Women who have had unsuccessful pregnancies in the past are more likely to have problems in future pregnancies. This overrepresentation of high-risk women among women getting pregnant can strongly distort the patterns of reproductive risk, as will be discussed in detail in Chapter 7.

Unplanned Pregnancies

The occurrence of unplanned pregnancies varies among groups, with generally low rates in northern Europe and high rates in the United States.[57] There is an extensive literature showing that women who have unplanned pregnancies have slightly poorer birth outcomes.[58] This risk presumably reflects the characteristics of the women themselves rather than the unplanned status of their pregnancy; that is, women who have less access to effective methods of birth control are more likely to be women carrying the burden of fewer economic resources, less education, and other factors associated with poor pregnancy outcomes.

Selective Abortion

Prenatal diagnosis and abortion are another important source of reproductive selection. These procedures can remove from observation fetuses that carry a defect. Neural tube defects and Down syndrome have become less prevalent at birth as a result of the availability of prenatal diagnosis and induced abortion. In interpreting changes in the birth prevalence of fetal abnormalities, it would be extremely useful to have data on fetuses that have been aborted. The issues of confidentiality surrounding induced abortion often make these data inaccessible at the population level.

References

1. Malthus RT. *On Population.* New York: Random House, 1960.
2. Kremer M. Population growth and technological change: one million B.C. to 1990. *Q J Economics* 1993;108(3):681–716.
3. Ehrlich PR. *The Population Bomb.* New York: Ballantine Books, 1968.
4. Haub C. How many people have ever lived on Earth? *Population Today* 2002;November/December:3–4.
5. Wilson C, Pison, G. More than half of the global population lives where fertility is below replacement level. *Population Societies* 2004;405 (October).
6. USCIA. *The World Factbook.* 2008.
7. World Population Clock. Available at www.census.gov/ipc/www/popclockworld.html, last accessed October 27, 2009.
8. WHO. World Population Prospects: the 2004 Revision—Highlights. United Nations 2005.
9. Youssef H. The history of the condom. *J R Soc Med* 1993;86(4):226–8.
10. Porter JF. The rhythm method of contraception. *J Reprod Fertil Suppl* 1975(22):91–105.
11. Trussell J. Contraceptive efficacy. In: Hatcher R, Trussell J, Nelson AL, Cates W, Stewart FH, Kowal D, eds. *Contraceptive Technology.* 19th Rev ed. New York: Ardent Media, 2007.
12. Mosher WD, Martinez GM, Chandra A, Abma JC, Willson SJ. Use of contraception and use of family planning services in the United States: 1982–2002. *Adv Data* 2004(350):1–36.
13. Ortiz ME, Croxatto HB, Bardin CW. Mechanisms of action of intrauterine devices. *Obstet Gynecol Surv* 1996;51(12 Suppl):S42–51.
14. Wilcox AJ, Weinberg CR, Armstrong EG, Canfield RE. Urinary human chorionic gonadotropin among intrauterine device users: detection with a highly specific and sensitive assay. *Fertil Steril* 1987;47(2):265–9.
15. d'Arcangues C. Worldwide use of intrauterine devices for contraception. *Contraception* 2007;75(6 Suppl):S2–7.
16. Brunton J, Beal MW. Current issues in emergency contraception: an overview for providers. *J Midwifery Womens Health* 2006;51(6):457–63.
17. Yuzpe AA, Thurlow HJ, Ramzy I, Leyshon JI. Post coital contraception—A pilot study. *J Reprod Med* 1974;13(2):53–8.
18. Novikova N, Weisberg E, Stanczyk FZ, Croxatto HB, Fraser IS. Effectiveness of levonorgestrel emergency contraception given before or after ovulation—a pilot study. *Contraception* 2007;75(2):112–8.

19. Polis CB, Schaffer K, Blanchard K, Glasier A, Harper CC, Grimes DA. Advance provision of emergency contraception for pregnancy prevention (full review). *Cochrane Database Syst Rev* 2007(2):CD005497.
20. Wilcox AJ, Dunson DB, Weinberg CR, Trussell J, Baird DD. Likelihood of conception with a single act of intercourse: providing benchmark rates for assessment of post-coital contraceptives. *Contraception* 2001;63(4):211–5.
21. Trussell J, Cleland, K. Levonorgestrel for emergency contraception. *Expert Rev Obstet Gynecol* 2007;2:565–76.
22. Farquharson RG, Jauniaux E, Exalto N. Updated and revised nomenclature for description of early pregnancy events. *Hum Reprod* 2005;20(11):3008–11.
23. Rossier C. Estimating induced abortion rates: a review. *Stud Fam Plann* 2004;34(2):87–102.
24. Sedgh G, Henshaw S, Singh S, Ahman E, Shah IH. Induced abortion: estimated rates and trends worldwide. *Lancet* 2007;370(9595):1338–45.
25. Elam-Evans LD, Strauss LT, Herndon J, et al. Abortion surveillance—United States, 2000. *MMWR Surveill Summ* 2003;52(12):1–32.
26. Henshaw S. Recent trends in abortion rates worldwide. *Int Fam Plann Persp* 1999;25(1):44–8.
27. Henshaw SK. Induced abortion: a world review, 1990. *Int Fam Plann Persp* 1990;16(2):59–65,76.
28. Birth Control. Encyclopedia Britannica Online, 2007; www.britannica.com/eb/article-9599, last accessed October 27, 2009.
29. *Trends in Abortion in the United States, 1973–2000.* The Alan Guttmacher Institute, 2003.
30. WHO. http://www.who.int/reproductive-health/unsafe_abortion/map.html, last accessed August 5, 2008.
31. Riddle JM. *Contraception and Abortion from the Ancient World to the Renaissance.* Cambridge, MA: Harvard University Press, 1992.
32. Sarkar NN. Mifepristone: bioavailability, pharmacokinetics and use-effectiveness. *Eur J Obstet Gynecol Reprod Biol* 2002;101(2):113–20.
33. Chen A, Yuan W, Meirik O, et al. Mefipristone-induced early abortion and outcome of subsequent wanted pregnancy. *Amer J Epidemiol* 2004;160(2):110–17.
34. Thorp JM, Hartmann KE, Shadigian E. Long-term physical and psychological health consequences of induced abortion: review of the evidence. *Obstet Gynecol Surv* 2002;58(1):67–79.
35. Thorp JM Jr, Hogue CJR, Seifer DB. Controversies in OB/GYN. Does elective abortion increase the risk of preterm delivery? *Contemporary OB/GYN* 2006;51(9):88–92.
36. de Crespigny L, Chervenak FA. *Prenatal Tests: The Facts.* Oxford, New York: Oxford University Press, 2006.
37. Ndumbe FM, Navti O, Chilaka VN, Konje JC. Prenatal diagnosis in the first trimester of pregnancy. *Obstet Gynecol Surv* 2008;63(5):317–28.
38. Wenstrom KD. First-trimester Down syndrome screening: component analytes and timing for optimal performance. *Semin Perinatol* 2005;29(4):195–202.
39. Mujezinovic F, Alfirevic Z. Procedure-related complications of amniocentesis and chorionic villous sampling: a systematic review. *Obstet Gynecol* 2007;110(3):687–94.
40. Dhallan R, Guo X, Emche S, et al. A non-invasive test for prenatal diagnosis based on fetal DNA present in maternal blood: a preliminary study. *Lancet* 2007;369(9560):474–81.

41. Editors. Assisted reproductive technologies hit all time high. *Lancet* 2006;368:2.
42. Wright VC, Chang J, Jeng G, Chen M, Macaluso M. Assisted reproductive technology surveillance—United States, 2004. *MMWR Surveill Summ* 2007;56(6):1–22.
43. Neri QV, Tanaka N, Wang A, et al. Intracytoplasmic sperm injection. Accomplishments and qualms. *Minerva Ginecol* 2004;56(3):189–96.
44. Wright VC, Schieve LA, Reynolds MA, Jeng G, Kissin D. Assisted reproductive technology surveillance—United States, 2001. *MMWR Surveill Summ* 2004;53(1):1–20.
45. Mukhopadhaya N, Arulkumaran S. Reproductive outcomes after in-vitro fertilization. *Curr Opin Obstet Gynecol* 2007;19(2):113–9.
46. Schieve LA, Cohen B, Nannini A, et al. A population-based study of maternal and perinatal outcomes associated with assisted reproductive technology in Massachusetts. *Matern Child Health J* 2007;11(6):517–25.
47. Romero R, Espinoza J, Mazor M. Can endometrial infection/inflammation explain implantation failure, spontaneous abortion, and preterm birth after in vitro fertilization? *Fertil Steril* 2004;82(4):799–804.
48. Romundstad LB, Romundstad PR, Sunde A, et al. Effects of technology or maternal factors on perinatal outcome after assisted fertilisation: a population-based cohort study. *Lancet* 2008;372(9640):737–43.
49. Jensen TK, Jorgensen N, Asklund C, Carlsen E, Holm M, Skakkebaek NE. Fertility treatment and reproductive health of male offspring: a study of 1,925 young men from the general population. *Am J Epidemiol* 2007;165(5):583–90.
50. Ramlau-Hansen CH, Thulstrup AM, Olsen J, Bonde JP. Parental subfecundity and risk of decreased semen quality in the male offspring: a follow-up study. *Am J Epidemiol* 2008;167(12):1458–64.
51. Mau Kai C, Juul A, McElreavey K, et al. Sons conceived by assisted reproduction techniques inherit deletions in the azoospermia factor (AZF) region of the Y chromosome and the DAZ gene copy number. *Hum Reprod* 2008;23(7):1669–78.
52. Reefhuis J, Honein MA, Schieve LA, Correa A, Hobbs CA, Rasmussen SA. Assisted reproductive technology and major structural birth defects in the United States. *Hum Reprod* 2009;24(2):360–6.
53. Sinclair KD. Assisted reproductive technologies and pregnancy outcomes: mechanistic insights from animal studies. *Semin Reprod Med* 2008;26(2):153–61.
54. Kurinczuk JJ. Safety issues in assisted reproduction technology. From theory to reality—just what are the data telling us about ICSI offspring health and future fertility and should we be concerned? *Hum Reprod* 2003;18(5):925–31.
55. Henshaw SK. Unintended pregnancy in the United States. *Fam Plann Perspect* 1998;30(1):24–9.
56. Basso O, Olsen J, Bisanti L, Juul S, Boldsen J. Are seasonal preferences in pregnancy planning a source of bias in studies of seasonal variation in reproductive outcomes? The European Study Group on Infertility and Subfecundity. *Epidemiology* 1995;6(5):520–4.
57. Finer LB, Henshaw SK. Disparities in rates of unintended pregnancy in the United States, 1994 and 2001. *Perspect Sex Reprod Health* 2006;38(2):90–6.
58. Mohllajee AP, Curtis KM, Morrow B, Marchbanks PA. Pregnancy intention and its relationship to birth and maternal outcomes. *Obstet Gynecol* 2007;109(3):678–86.

4

Infections and Reproduction

Laura Baecher-Lind, Allen Wilcox, and William Miller

There are physical and social barriers that help protect humans from transmission of infections. Many of these barriers are breached by the essential events of reproduction (sexual intercourse, pregnancy, and delivery). It is no wonder that the spread of infectious diseases is closely linked to the events of sex and pregnancy. We consider how infections are transmitted during human reproduction, and how infections in turn can produce infertility, infant mortality, birth defects, and other problems of reproduction.

Human reproduction provides unique opportunities for the spread of infectious agents. The mechanics of sexual intercourse, pregnancy, delivery, and breastfeeding breach physical barriers between humans that ordinarily protect against the transmission of infectious agents. Furthermore, the male and female reproductive tracts, the germ cells, and the developing fetus all have specific susceptibilities to infection. The reproductive organs can be damaged directly by sexually transmitted infections, or indirectly by organisms that have been transmitted via other routes. Delicate reproductive tissues are particularly susceptible to damage by the inflammation that can accompany even mild infection. Furthermore, the normal physiology of pregnancy induces an immunocompromised state that can add to the pregnant woman's vulnerability. The net result is that infections can interrupt reproduction at virtually any stage, ranging from the development of germ cells to the viability and ultimate survival of the newborn.

Despite the serious consequences of infection for reproduction, the interplay of infection and reproduction are not necessarily obvious. For example, malnutrition

This chapter has been adapted from a longer paper published in *Obstetrical and Gynecological Survey* ("Infections Disease and Reproductive Health," in press, 2009).

may make a person more susceptible to infection, and vice versa. Furthermore, malnutrition and infection may independently harm reproduction, producing a tangled causal pathway. When an infection is undetected, the picture can become even more complex with the infection producing reproductive problems that can be mistakenly attributed to related factors.

General Principles of Infectious Disease

Once a person is exposed to an infectious agent, the likelihood of transmission depends on several factors. One is the dose or concentration of the infectious agent per exposure. Another is virulence, usually defined as the dose necessary to infect an exposed person 50% of the time. Host susceptibility also plays a role: immunocompromised persons are at greater risk of becoming infected at a given dose and given virulence and are more likely to have severe or complicated illness if they are infected. Furthermore, immunocompromised persons are more likely to harbor high doses of a transmissible infection and thus are more likely to transmit the infection to another person.

There are four major classes of infections: bacterial, viral, fungal, and parasitic. Reproductive health can be damaged by any of these. In general, sexually transmitted viruses tend to have a lower probability of transmission per exposure (compared with bacteria or protozoa), but viruses tend to persist much longer when infection does occur.[1] The initial infection with HIV may produce transient flu-like symptoms and then be silent until the immune system fails a decade or more later. The infected person may have no symptoms in the interim, while unwittingly exposing others. Herpes simplex virus also confers lifelong infection, with extended asymptomatic periods punctuated by episodes of disease activation.

Bacterial infections are usually of shorter duration, although some organisms such as *Chlamydia trachomatis* or *Neisseria gonorrhoeae* can be asymptomatic for weeks to years. Asymptomatic bacterial infections can also become reservoirs of infectivity. Antibiotics may reduce the duration of infection, thereby reducing the infectious burden within a community. Most bacteria and protozoa can reinfect previously infected persons, whereas viral infections (once cured) tend to confer lifelong immunity.

Infectious Diseases and Reproduction: A Framework

The impact of infectious diseases on reproduction can be organized in various ways—by organism, for example, or by pathological process. This chapter is organized by the stage of reproduction at which a particular infection exerts its effects. We start with fertility, proceed through fetal life and end with birth and the neonatal period. Within each of these broad categories, we use the familiar taxonomy of bacteria, viruses, and parasites.

Table 4–1. Strength of evidence for effects of selected infectious agents on reproductive outcomes[a]

Health effects	Chlam[b]	GC[b]	GBS[b]	HIV	Syphilis	Toxo[b]	Rubella	CMV[b]	HSV[b]	Malaria	TB[b]	PD[b]	BV[b]
Male infertility	↑	↑	–	↑	–	–	–	–	–	–	↑	–	–
Female infertility	↑↑↑	↑↑↑	–	↑	–	–	–	–	–	–	↑	–	–
Miscarriage	–	–	–	–	–	–	↑	↑	↑	–	–	–	–
Birth defects	–	–	–	–	↑↑↑	↑↑↑	↑↑↑	↑↑↑	↑↑↑	–	–	–	–
Fetal infection	–	–	↑↑↑	↑↑↑	↑↑↑	↑↑↑	↑↑↑	↑↑↑	↑↑↑	↑↑↑	↑	↑	↑
Preterm delivery	↑↑	↑↑	–	–	↑↑↑	↑↑↑	↑↑↑	↑↑↑	↑↑↑	↑	↑	↑↑	↑↑
Growth restriction	–	↑	–	–	↑↑↑	↑↑↑	↑↑↑	↑↑↑	↑↑↑	↑↑	↑	–	
Intrapartum infection of the fetus	↑↑↑	↑↑↑	↑↑↑	↑↑↑	↑	–	–	↑	↑↑↑	–	–	–	–
Perinatal mortality	–	–	↑↑↑	↑	↑↑↑	↑↑↑	↑↑↑	↑↑↑	↑↑	↑↑↑	↑	–	–
Infection via breast-feeding	–	–	–	↑↑↑	–	–	–	↑↑↑	–	–	–	–	–

[a]Key: "–": evidence of no effect/no evidence of effect; "↑": some evidence of an association; "↑↑": moderate evidence of an association; "↑↑↑": strong evidence of an association.

[b]Chlam, Chlamydia; GC, Gonorrhea; GBS, Group B Streptococcus; Toxo, toxoplasmosis; CMV, cytomegalovirus; HSV, herpes simplex virus; TB, tuberculosis; PD, periodontal disease; BV, bacterial vaginosis.

Infectious diseases have been implicated in nearly every reproductive health problem (summarized in Table 4-1). However, the evidence to support some of these associations is thin or absent. Even when data are available, the extent of risk is often unclear. We focus on the more well-established associations and consider several emerging or controversial associations.

Infection of the Male Reproductive Tract

Bacteria

CHLAMYDIA. *Chlamydia trachomatis* causes urethritis in men and, if left untreated, can ascend and produce epididymitis and orchitis (inflammation of the testes).[2] It is plausible that chlamydial infection causes male infertility, but the evidence is weak.[2] Results are mixed as to whether chlamydial infection is associated with abnormal semen parameters.[3–6] In one study of infertile couples, men positive for *C. trachomatis* antibodies were less likely to achieve pregnancy, even after female tubal disease had been controlled for.[7]

GONORRHEA. The incidence of gonorrhea in the United States has been increasing in the last decade, with the highest incidence among African-American adolescents and young adults.[8] Similar to chlamydial infection, gonorrhea is thought to cause infertility secondary to orchitis, with impaired spermatogenesis as well as inflammatory changes in the vas and tubules.[9] Still, evidence for effects on male fertility is extremely limited.

TUBERCULOSIS. Tuberculosis (infection with *Mycobacterium tuberculosis*) has resurfaced as a serious public health problem, with the emergence of virulent and multi-drug-resistant strains.[10] Fourteen million people worldwide were infected with *M. tuberculosis* in 2006, 0.5 million of whom carried multi-drug-resistant strains.[10] Although pulmonary manifestations are the most common, tuberculosis can affect virtually any physiologic system including the genitourinary system. Genitourinary tuberculosis can produce male infertility through granulomas that obstruct the vas deferens and urethra.[11,12] The prevalence of this complication is unknown.

Viruses

MUMPS. Mumps is caused by a paramyxovirus and constitutes a serious threat to male fertility. Among men infected as adults, 20% to 30% will have orchitis of at least one testis, and up to 10% will have infection of both testes.[13] Once the virus reaches the testicles, a brisk inflammatory process increases testicular pressure. Half of men with orchitis are left with testicular atrophy.[13,14] In a recent review, infertility was produced in 13% of men with one affected testis and in 30–87% of men with both testes affected.[13,15] Impaired fertility is presumably secondary to postinflammatory fibrosis and germinal cell damage. Routine vaccination of children against paramyxovirus has made mumps rare in developed countries; however, as parental resistance toward pediatric vaccination grows in the United States and Europe, an increasing number of young men are vulnerable to mumps infection and consequent infertility.[15]

HIV. Damage to sperm by HIV/AIDS is one of the lesser-known consequences of this infection. HIV-infected men have substantially reduced sperm counts and increased numbers of abnormal sperm.[16] Furthermore, semen parameters of HIV-infected men become worse as the disease progresses.[17,18] To the extent that these effects on semen translate into reduced fecundability, this consequence of HIV infection may create a dilemma for HIV-discordant couples who wish to conceive. Men with advanced disease may be less fertile, requiring them to have more unprotected intercourse to impregnate their partner. In addition, the viral load per ejaculate is higher in men with advanced disease.[17]

Parasites

TRICHOMONAS. *Trichomonas vaginalis* is a common sexually transmitted protozoan that can interfere with spermatogenesis and normal sperm development. Men with trichomoniasis have been reported to have decreased sperm motility and more abnormal sperm.[19] However, long-term consequences of trichomoniasis are unknown, and overall evidence suggests that the impact on male fertility may be minimal.[20]

Infection of the Female Reproductive Tract

Bacteria

CHLAMYDIA. Up to 30% of women with a chlamydial infection progress to develop pelvic inflammatory disease, which can ascend to include the oviducts.[21–24] Chlamydial infection of the tubes causes inflammation and damage to the epithelial lining of the fallopian tubes. The cilia that line the oviducts can be destroyed, and fibrosis of the supple folds of the tubes creates blind pouches. These changes damage the propelling action of the oviducts and can completely block the tubes.[25] Even subclinical chlamydial infection can damage fertility. In a study of infertile couples, women with tubal disease were more likely to have antibodies to *C. trachomatis*.[26,27] The stronger the immune response to previous *C. trachomatis* infection, the more likely the tubal damage.[28] Although these studies suggest an association, there have not been longitudinal studies that would allow accurate estimates of the risk of infertility after *C. trachomatis* infection.[29]

Another consequence of inflammation and fibrosis of chlamydial infection is increased risk of ectopic pregnancy. Chlamydial infection accounts for about half of all tubal pregnancies worldwide.[30] In developing nations, up to 3% of ectopic pregnancies end in maternal death, 10 times more than in developed nations.[31] In light of the large number of women who do not have access to hospital care, this figure presumably underestimates the maternal mortality caused by ectopic pregnancy. With an estimated 90 million cases of chlamydial infection occurring annually,[32] the burden of chlamydia-related tubal infertility—as well as maternal mortality—may be substantial.

GONORRHEA. Although less well studied than chlamydial infection, an association between gonorrhea and tubal disease has been consistently supported in the literature.[1] As with chlamydial infection, gonoccocal infection causes inflammation and fibrosis of the oviducts. In one small study of infertile women, seropositivity for *N. gonorrhoeae* antibodies was higher for women with bilateral tubal occlusion than for women with other causes of infertility.[33] In another study, a history of gonorrhea was more common among women with tubal disease.[34]

TUBERCULOSIS. The oviducts are the most common site of genital tuberculosis in women, with granulomas producing partial or complete obstruction.[35] The endometrial cavity can also be damaged by tubercle or granuloma formation, resulting in amenorrhea and infertility.[35] Studies from Nigeria and Pakistan suggest that up to 2% of female infertility may be secondary to genitourinary TB.[36,37] Unfortunately, successful antibiotic treatment of *M. tuberculosis* does not reverse the histological changes, and most women are rendered permanently infertile.

Viruses

HIV. In endemic regions of Africa, HIV infection appears to reduce female fertility by 15%–25%, producing higher rates of involuntary childlessness and longer intervals between births.[38] HIV infection also may affect the hypothalamic-pituitary-ovarian axis and cause subfertility secondary to hormonal dysfunction. Women with HIV infection have been reported to have higher levels of follicle-stimulating hormone (a marker of ovarian failure),[39] and prolonged menstrual cycles.[39,40] However, these changes have not been observed consistently.[41,42] If HIV infection produces hormonal dysfunction, it may occur only as the disease progresses to more serious stages.[39,41]

Infection of Pregnant Women and Fetuses

Although the specific infectious agents are not clear, preterm birth has been strongly associated with infection and inflammation.[43,44] Evidence for infection is especially prevalent among the earliest preterm births.[45,46] Approximately 90% of births before 24 gestational weeks show histological evidence of chorioamnionitis in contrast to 10% of births at term.[1] (Chorioamnionitis has also been associated with cerebral palsy, independent of preterm delivery.[47])

The mechanisms responsible for preterm labor remain elusive. Infection initiates an inflammatory response that helps to trigger preterm delivery. Bacterial inoculation of the fetal membranes, placenta, or amniotic fluid increases prostaglandin production, and prostaglandins can produce uterine contractility, cervical softening and dilation, leading to preterm birth. Once initiated, labor can become self-propagating, with prostaglandins inducing a diffuse inflammatory response that stimulates a cascade of cytokines and interleukins, which in turn causes more release of prostaglandins. Despite this plausible biological pathway, it is not clear that antibiotics administered to high-risk women reduce the risk of preterm delivery.[48,49]

Bacteria

CHLAMYDIA. *Chlamydia trachomatis* has been associated with preterm birth.[1] In a large cohort study, maternal chlamydial infection increased the risk of preterm birth by 50%.[50] Chlamydial infection does not appear to be associated with growth restriction or neonatal mortality.[50,51]

GONORRHEA. Like chlamydial infection, maternal gonococcal infection has been associated with preterm birth, although studies are limited. A prospective study in a high-infection setting found that gonorrhea was associated with a sixfold increase in risk of preterm birth, and substantially lower birth weight.[52] In settings with more typical prevalence of infection, the associations are less apparent, with the strongest associations occuring for very preterm delivery.[53,54]

BACTERIAL VAGINOSIS. Bacterial vaginosis (BV) is a nonspecific overgrowth of microbes such as *Gardnerella vaginalis*, *Bacteroides*, and *Mobiluncus* and a deficit of normally prevalent *Lactobacilli*. An estimated 9%–50% of pregnant women in the United States are affected by BV, with ethnic minorities and low-socioeconomic populations more likely to be affected.[55] BV is frequently associated with preterm birth. The mechanism is thought to be through infection of fetal membranes, infection of amniotic fluids, and premature rupture of membranes. A meta-analysis found that BV was associated with a twofold increase in the odds of preterm birth[56] BV may play a role in infertility and miscarriage as well.[57]

Although these associations are well established, it is not clear that treatment of BV during pregnancy prevents preterm birth. A recent Cochrane analysis concluded that screening and treatment programs for vaginal infections (including BV) may reduce preterm birth, based on one trial that met the rigorous inclusion criteria.[58] The benefit of BV treatment is primarily among women with a history of preterm birth.[59–62] The U.S. Preventive Services Task Force concluded that routine screening and treatment of BV during pregnancy was not beneficial for average-risk pregnancies.[55]

Douching

Vaginal douching is the practice of washing the vagina with a liquid solution, usually for sanitary purposes. The rinse may consist simply of water, or water mixed with home ingredients (such as vinegar), or with preparations sold for this purpose. (Douching is sometimes also done after intercourse as a belated effort to prevent conception—with no evidence that it works.) Douching is strongly influenced by cultural norms and is more common in the United States than most other developed countries. About 20% of white women and about 50% of black women in the United States report regular douching.[63] There are no proven benefits of douching and possible risks. Health risks include increased risk of ascending reproductive-tract infections with attendant problems of infertility and poor pregnancy outcome.[63]

PERIODONTAL DISEASE. Infection of the teeth or gums is another polymicrobial infection associated with preterm delivery, although its causal role is even less certain. Periodontal disease has been associated with preterm delivery as well as with cardiovascular disease, pneumonia, and diabetes.[64–66] Nearly 40% of pregnant women in the United States have some degree of periodontitis, which is disproportionately prevalent among minority and low-socioeconomic populations.[65] Periodontitis may cause preterm delivery through low-grade bacteremia. Alternatively, the association may be confounded by other maternal characteristics associated with preterm delivery. Intervention trials have demonstrated no benefit in reducing the risk of preterm delivery.[67]

SYPHILIS. Maternal infection by *Treponema pallidum* (syphilis) is disastrous for the fetus. The organism easily crosses the placenta and infects developing fetal tissues. Approximately one million pregnancies worldwide are affected by maternal syphilis each year, with nearly half ending in miscarriage or neonatal death, and one-quarter in preterm birth. A quarter of surviving births have congenital syphilis.[68] Congenital syphilis can affect any organ system; the most commonly affected sites are bone, brain, and visceral organs.[1,69] Neonatal transmission is more likely to occur if the mother has her first infection during pregnancy or in the 4 years preceding pregnancy (during which time the spread of the spirochete through the blood is most likely).[1]

Viruses

TORCH INFECTIONS. Toxoplasmosis, rubella, cytomegalovirus (CMV), and herpes simplex virus (HSV)—collectively known as the TORCH infections—are potentially devastating infections during pregnancy, particularly when acquired during the period of organogenesis (from about the third to the sixteenth gestational week). Varicella zoster, syphilis, and parvovirus B19 are included in the TORCH acronym as "O" ("other").

With the exception of toxoplasmosis and syphilis, the TORCH infections are viral. Sequelae common to these infections include restricted fetal growth, preterm delivery, neonatal jaundice, pneumonitis, chorioretinitis and cataracts, microcephaly, mental retardation, and hearing impairment. There are emerging distinctions among these several infectious agents, and the collective "TORCH infections" are less often being regarded as a single entity.[70]

Parvovirus B19 Parvovirus B19 is perhaps the most distinctive of these agents; neonatal infection by parvovirus B19 does not cause any of the typical TORCH outcomes but rather produces miscarriage, stillbirth, and nonimmune hydrops. Among a study of Danish women, annual seroconversion rates were 1.5% during endemic periods and 13% during epidemic periods.[71] In a study of women diagnosed with parvovirus B19 during pregnancy, the risk of fetal death was estimated at 9%.[72]

Rubella Rubella was the first virus recognized as a teratogen.[73] Fetuses exposed to maternal rubella are at high risk of ocular, skeletal, and cardiac defects as well as growth restriction, microcephaly and mental retardation, hepatosplenomegaly, thrombocytopenia, and jaundice. In later life, congenital rubella syndrome can be associated with diabetes mellitus, thyroid dysfunction, panencephalitis, and psychosis.[73] As with most of the TORCH infections, neonatal morbidity is more pronounced if infection occurs early in pregnancy. Widespread childhood vaccination against rubella has substantially reduced the neonatal morbidity from rubella in developed nations, with most cases occurring among inadequately vaccinated immigrant populations. Antenatal programs routinely screen pregnant women for active antibodies against rubella; unprotected women are then vaccinated after delivery for protection in subsequent pregnancies. In less-developed regions, congenital rubella syndrome remains a substantial source of neonatal morbidity, with more than one out of four women susceptible to infection.[74]

Congenital cytomegalovirus Congenital cytomegalovirus (CMV) is one of the most common causes of neonatal and childhood disability in developed nations, affecting approximately 2 per 1000 U.S. neonates a year.[75] Clinical features include deafness, mental retardation, hepatosplenomegaly, jaundice, and pneumonitis.[75] Like rubella, CMV has more devastating effects when acquired during the first trimester of pregnancy. Women who have their first infection during pregnancy have a 30% risk of transmitting congenital disease to their fetuses, whereas women with recurrent CMV present much less risk to the fetus.[76]

Herpes simplex virus HSV is one of the most prevalent viral agents in humans, with up to 90% of the population being exposed.[77] As with most other TORCH infections, a mother's first infection confers greater risk to her fetus than recurrent infection. Approximately 0.5%–2% of pregnant women develop a primary HSV infection during pregnancy.[77,78] Transmission to the fetus can occur transplacentally as well as during delivery. Route of transmission largely determines disease presentation, with transplacental transmission resulting in "congenital herpes" and intrapartum transmission resulting in "neonatal herpes" (discussed below). Features of congenital herpes include skin vesicles, ocular damage (chorioretinitis, cataracts), and neurologic damage (seizures, intracranial calcifications).[77] Intrauterine infection may also lead to spontaneous abortion and stillbirth, although estimates of this risk vary widely.[79]

Parasites

TOXOPLASMOSIS. In contrast to the other TORCH infectious agents, toxoplasmosis is a parasitic disease caused by the protozoa *Toxoplasma gondii*. Toxoplasmosis produces its most devastating effects when primary infection occurs close to term. About one-third of women with primary infection during pregnancy deliver a neonate with toxoplasmosis. Clinical features of infected neonates include the classic triad of chorioretinitis, hydrocephaly, and intracranial calcifications.[1] Of those infants infected, 4% develop permanent neurologic sequelae or die within the first few years of life.[80]

MALARIA. Malaria remains one of the most prevalent infectious agents causing pregnancy-related and neonatal morbidity. Pregnancy itself increases a woman's susceptibility to malaria and to the more severe expressions of the disease. In sub-Saharan Africa, where malaria from *Plasmodium falciparum* is endemic, one in four women at delivery shows evidence of malarial infection.[81] These data are undoubtedly underestimates, in that they are based on diagnosis by light microscopy rather than on more sensitive measures such as polymerase chain reaction or placental histology.[81–83] Although the importance of malaria in endemic regions is apparent, its impact in nonendemic regions can also be substantial. In Northern Africa and other regions with only episodic outbreaks of malaria, 6%–14% of women seen in antenatal clinics or at delivery have malaria.[81] In regions with seasonal malaria transmission, placental malaria is seen even during the dry, less infective season, suggesting that the parasite can remain active within the placenta for many months.[84]

Maternal malaria is associated with smaller babies[83,85–88] It is not clear whether this reflects earlier delivery or fetal growth restriction; both processes may be at work.[87] Malaria-infected red blood cells and inflammatory products clog the maternal-fetal interface of the placenta, resulting in decreased sustenance to the fetus.[89] Estimates of the impact of malaria on fetal growth restriction vary;[85–87] the larger studies suggest relatively modest odds ratios of 1.4–1.7. Recent evidence indicates that nutritional status may modify this relationship. In a study in the Congo, malaria was associated with fetal growth restriction among undernourished women but not among well-nourished women.[88] Treatment of malaria during pregnancy is associated with improvement in fetal growth.[88] The maternal anemia associated with malaria may itself contribute to maternal or neonatal death. In endemic regions, an estimated 7%–26% of severe anemia is related to malaria.[81] In

Puerperal Fever

In the mid-1800s, puerperal fever (infection at delivery) killed large numbers of women who delivered in certain hospitals. Mortality was 9% in one obstetric clinic of a famous Vienna teaching hospital but—oddly—only 2% in another clinic in the same hospital. This puzzled a young immigrant physician from Hungary named Ignaz Semmelweis. He looked into differences between the clinics. The only notable difference was that physicians delivered in the clinic with high mortality rates, and midwives delivered in the clinic with low rates. During this time, a friend of Semmelweis's happened to cut himself while doing an autopsy and died of an illness similar to puerperal fever. This led Semmelweis to infer (several years before the germ theory) that doctors were transmitting something from cadavers to women that caused the fever. He instituted a practice of having doctors wash their hands in a chlorine solution when leaving the cadavers. The rate of puerperal fever in their clinic dropped to 1%. Semmelweis ought to have been a hero, but instead he was marginalized for his unorthodox views. He was admitted to a psychiatric hospital in 1865, where he died shortly thereafter at the age of 47.

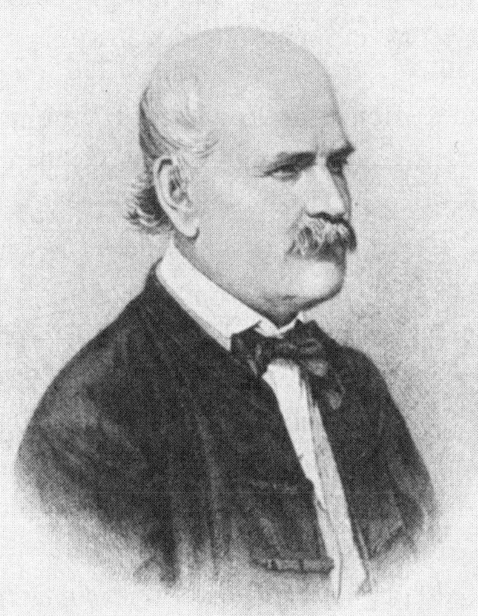

Ignaz Semmelweis, 1818–65 (copper plate engraving by Jenő Doby)

developing countries, maternal death from intrapartum or postpartum hemorrhage can occur more quickly in women who are already severely anemic.

Infection of the Neonate during Delivery

Bacteria

CHLAMYDIA. Women with active chlamydial infection at the time of vaginal delivery have a 50%–75% risk of intrapartum transmission to their neonate.[90] The most common clinical manifestation of neonatal chlamydial infection is conjunctivitis, with a risk of 18%–50% among neonates born to a Chlamydia-positive mother; the risk of neonatal pneumonitis ranges from 10%–20%.[91–93] Acquisition of Chlamydia by the infant during parturition (delivery) occurs primarily with vaginal delivery but may also occur with cesarean section, usually after prolonged rupture of membranes.[90]

GONORRHEA. *N. gonorrhoeae* is transmitted from mother to baby during delivery, with a mother-to-child transmission rate of 30%–50%.[94] Neonatal conjunctivitis is the most common gonococcal infection.[95] Application of erythromycin to the eyes of newborns has become standard prophylaxis in the United States to prevent both gonococcal and chlamydial ocular infections. Other clinical manifestations of neonatal gonorrhea include polyarticular arthritis, gonococcemia and sepsis, and genital infection.[95] In the United States, routine antenatal screening for gonorrhea and neonatal prophylaxis with erythromycin have substantially reduced the incidence of neonatal gonorrhea. In less-developed regions, neonatal gonococcal infection remains an important source of morbidity.[96]

GROUP B STREPTOCOCCUS. Before 1990, Group B Streptococcus was the leading cause of neonatal sepsis in the United States, causing early-onset neonatal infection in 2 of 1,000 babies.[97] Although the infection is usually asymptomatic in the mother, babies infected during vaginal delivery can develop pneumonia, meningitis, and sepsis, with a mortality rate of 50%.[98] In 1979, ampicillin was found to prevent vertical transmission of Group B Streptococcus.[99] Even so, it was not until 2002 when the CDC issued guidelines for screening and prophylactic antibiotic treatment that the incidence of early-onset neonatal Streptococcus infection was dramatically reduced.[98] Currently, early-onset neonatal group B Streptococcus infection occurs in approximately 0.6 of 1,000 live births in the United States.[100] Many of these cases occur in babies of women who were negative on screening.[101,102] Although routine use of prophylactic antibiotics has been successful for protecting babies against early-onset streptococcal infection, later-onset infection is still a problem, one made more difficult by the emergence of resistance to antibiotics used to treat infection.[103]

Viruses

HEPATITIS B. Perinatal transmission of the Hepatitis B virus (HBV) to the fetus is the single most important mode of HBV infection worldwide.[104] Acute maternal infection with HBV occurs in 1–2 per 1000 pregnancies, and chronic HBV infection is found in 5–15 per 1000 pregnancies.[105] Pregnancy does not exacerbate maternal HBV infection, but the virus is readily transmitted during delivery.[104,105] Current prevention strategies include adult vaccination, and administration of hepatitis B immunoglobulin and HBV vaccination to exposed infants.[105] Breastfeeding by infected mothers poses no additional threat to infants who have received adequate immunoglobulin treatment and immunization.[106]

HUMAN PAPILLOMAVIRUS. Human papillomavirus (HPV) is highly prevalent among sexually active adults—up to 40% of pregnant women may harbor HPV DNA.[107,108] The size and extent of a woman's genital warts appear to increase during pregnancy, as does the prevalence of serum HPV DNA.[107,109] Such increases may be secondary to compromise of maternal immunocompetence, or to the higher levels of estrogen and progesterone associated with pregnancy. Transmission to offspring likely results from neonatal aspiration of contaminated genital tract secretions during delivery.[110] Infected neonates may develop genital warts or laryngeal papillomas, the latter of which can cause respiratory distress.[109] Although vaginal delivery increases the risk of neonatal transmission, most newborns of infected mothers harbor HPV even when they have been delivered by cesarean section.[110]

CYTOMEGALOVIRUS. CMV can be transmitted during parturition (as well as transplacentally, as described above). Women who carry a genital cytomegalovirus infection at labor have a 30%–50% risk of transmitting the virus to their neonate.[1] The majority of infants infected at delivery remain asymptomatic. However, CMV may pose a substantial risk to infants born prematurely or who are otherwise sick, among whom infection acquired at delivery has been associated with neuromuscular disability and sepsis-like illness.[111]

HERPES SIMPLEX. Nearly 75% of pregnant women with a history of HSV can expect a reactivation of their infection during pregnancy.[112] During vaginal delivery, direct contact of the neonate to maternal herpes simplex virus can result in transmission and devastating neonatal consequences. Risk factors increasing likelihood of transmission include prolonged rupture of membranes (prolonging neonatal exposure), recent maternal acquisition of herpes infection, or disruption of the neonatal skin or mucous membranes during delivery.[113] Estimates of neonatal herpes range from 0.5 to 3 per 10,000 live births.[113] In about half of affected newborns, the infection is limited to the eyes, skin, or mouth. However, a quarter suffer infection of the central nervous system, and another quarter have broadly disseminated infection.[112,113] Mortality is 4% with central nervous system disease and 30% with disseminated disease. Of those surviving, 20% demonstrate some degree of neurologic compromise.[105] Prevention strategies include prophylactic antiviral therapy during the third trimester of pregnancy and primary cesarean delivery if lesions persist at the time of labor. Preventive efforts are limited by the fact that most neonatal herpes simplex viral infections occur in infants born of mothers without a recognized history of herpes infection.[113]

HIV. Neonates born to HIV-positive women have a 15%–25% chance of acquiring the infection during delivery in the absence of antiretroviral prophylaxis.[114] Viral transmission during delivery probably occurs through maternal-fetal microtransfusions during uterine contractions or through exposure of the baby's skin and mucous membranes during delivery.[115] Factors associated with transmission include high maternal viral load at the time of delivery, low maternal CD4 count, and extended duration of ruptured membranes before delivery.[116] In developed countries, combination antiretroviral treatment and aggressive postpartum neonatal treatment (including caesarean delivery) have reduced the rate of neonatal HIV transmission to less than 2%.[116] In developing nations, antiretroviral prophylaxis is often costly or unavailable, and neonatal HIV transmission remains common.[115]

Infection of the Neonate during Breast-Feeding

Viruses

CYTOMEGALOVIRUS. CMV is commonly carried in the breast milk of infected mothers.[117,118] Cytomegaloviral infection of the infant via breast-feeding is often limited to serologic conversion without serious infection,[119,120] although infected infants may manifest transient sepsis-like symptoms. In a prospective study of preterm infants, 15% of breast-fed infants with CMV-infected mothers became infected during breast-feeding.[118] Transmission was not associated with viral load in breast milk or frequency of breast-feeding.

HIV. HIV is present in the breast milk of infected mothers, and the infection can be transmitted to their infants. The risk of HIV transmission is about 15% for infants breast-fed through their first year.[121] Unexpectedly, the risk of HIV transmission through breast milk is lowest with exclusive breast-feeding.[122] Supplemental feeding of breast-fed infants appears to promote the transmission of HIV infection from breast milk, perhaps by increasing the susceptibility of the infant. In many developing nations, breast-feeding remains an important option because formula or clean water may not be available. Breast-feeding provides immunologic benefits against other diseases such as diarrhea or respiratory illness. WHO guidelines recommend exclusive breast-feeding through the first six months of life for infants of HIV-infected women, unless replacement feeding is acceptable, feasible, affordable and sustainable.[114] The impact of antiretroviral drugs on maternal-to-child-transmission during breast-feeding is currently under investigation.

Infectious Diseases and Causal Inference

Infections can damage reproduction in diverse ways. The complexity of these mechanisms can create confusion for epidemiologists interested in the causation of reproductive impairments. For example, chlamydial infection causes infertility through tubal scarring. By the time the infertility is manifest (often years later), the infection has usually been cleared. Meanwhile, other factors associated with chlamydial infection, such as other STIs, social habits of affected women, or environmental conditions, may mistakenly be blamed for the women's decreased fertility.

The potential for latent infections can also be confusing. Tuberculosis is a subacute to chronic infection with a small number of disseminated cases within the first year of infection. Most cases of disease occur years after the infection, often in periods of waning immunity. Pregnancy may itself contribute to activation of latent tuberculosis, which could be misinterpreted as primary infection during pregnancy.

These complexities raise challenges for epidemiologists who study reproduction. For a given infectious agent and outcome, is it prior infection, latent infection, or active infection that is most important? Is it the severity of the infection or the strength of the immune response that damages reproduction? Might noninfectious factors increase the risk of reactivation of a latent infection or increase the risk of a new infection? Are there risk factors that confound the relation of an infection with a particular outcome? Or do infections confound the study of noninfectious exposures and their relationship to fertility or pregnancy?

Taken as a whole, infections inflict their most serious damage on fertility, embryogenesis, and fetal development. Infections have less certain effects on the risk of miscarriage and impaired fetal growth. Preterm delivery, especially very preterm delivery, is emerging as an endpoint to which infections may make a major contribution. Taken as a whole, infectious diseases are at least as important to reproductive and perinatal health as the social, environmental, and genetic factors that are usually the focus of reproductive epidemiologists.

References

1. Holmes K, Sparling P, Stamm W, et al. *Sexually Transmitted Diseases*. New York: McGraw Hill, 2008.
2. Eley A, Pacey AA, Galdiero M, Galdiero F. Can *Chlamydia trachomatis* directly damage your sperm? *Lancet Infect Dis* 2005;5(1):53–7.

3. Cunningham KA, Beagley KW. Male genital tract chlamydial infection: implications for pathology and infertility. *Biol Reprod* 2008; 79(2): 180–9.
4. Veznik Z, Pospisil L, Svecova D, Zajicova A, Unzeitig V. Chlamydiae in the ejaculate: their influence on the quality and morphology of sperm. *Acta Obstet Gynecol Scand* 2004;83(7):656–60.
5. Hosseinzadeh S, Eley A, Pacey AA. Semen quality of men with asymptomatic chlamydial infection. *J Androl* 2004;25(1):104–9.
6. Vigil P, Morales P, Tapia A, Riquelme R, Salgado AM. *Chlamydia trachomatis* infection in male partners of infertile couples: incidence and sperm function. *Andrologia* 2002;34(3):155–61.
7. Idahl A, Boman J, Kumlin U, Olofsson JI. Demonstration of *Chlamydia trachomatis* IgG antibodies in the male partner of the infertile couple is correlated with a reduced likelihood of achieving pregnancy. *Hum Reprod* 2004;19(5):1121–6.
8. CDC. Sexually Transmitted Disease Surveillance 2006 Supplement, Gonococcal Isolate Surveillance Project (GISP) *Annual Report 2006*. 2008.
9. Ness RB, Markovic N, Carlson CL, Coughlin MT. Do men become infertile after having sexually transmitted urethritis? An epidemiologic examination. *Fertil Steril* 1997;68(2):205–13.
10. WHO. Global Tuberculosis Control—surveillance, planning, financing. *WHO Rep* 2008.
11. Lenk S, Schroeder J. Genitourinary tuberculosis. *Curr Opin Urol* 2001;11(1):93–8.
12. Paick J, Kim SH, Kim SW. Ejaculatory duct obstruction in infertile men. *BJU Int* 2000;85(6):720–4.
13. Masarani M, Wazait H, Dinneen M. Mumps orchitis. *J R Soc Med* 2006; 99(11):573–5.
14. Bartak V. Sperm count, morphology and motility after unilateral mumps orchitis. *J Reprod Fertil* 1973;32(3):491–4.
15. Casella R, Leibundgut B, Lehmann K, Gasser TC. Mumps orchitis: report of a mini-epidemic. *J Urol* 1997;158(6):2158–61.
16. Coll O, Lopez M, Vidal R, et al. Fertility assessment in non-infertile HIV-infected women and their partners. *Reprod Biomed Online* 2007;14(4):488–94.
17. Politch JA, Mayer KH, Abbott AF, Anderson DJ. The effects of disease progression and zidovudine therapy on semen quality in human immunodeficiency virus type 1 seropositive men. *Fertil Steril* 1994;61(5):922–8.
18. van Leeuwen E, van Weert JM, van der Veen F, Repping S. The effects of the human immunodeficiency virus on semen parameters and intrauterine insemination outcome. *Hum Reprod* 2005;20(7):2033–4; author reply 2034–5.
19. Gopalkrishnan K, Hinduja IN, Kumar TC. Semen characteristics of asymptomatic males affected by *Trichomonas vaginalis*. *J In Vitro Fert Embryo Transf* 1990;7(3):165–7.
20. Ochsendorf FR. Sexually transmitted infections: impact on male fertility. *Andrologia* 2008;40(2):72–5.
21. Paavonen J, Eggert-Kruse W. *Chlamydia trachomatis*: impact on human reproduction. *Hum Reprod Update* 1999;5(5):433–47.
22. Hafner LM, McNeilly C. Vaccines for *Chlamydia* infections of the female genital tract. *Future Microbiol* 2008;3(1):67–77.
23. Risser WL, Risser JM. The incidence of pelvic inflammatory disease in untreated women infected with *Chlamydia trachomatis*: a structured review. *Int J STD AIDS* 2007;18(11):727–31.

24. Simms I, Horner P. Has the incidence of pelvic inflammatory disease following chlamydial infection been overestimated? *Int J STD AIDS* 2008;19(4):285–6.
25. Lyons RA, Saridogan E, Djahanbakhch O. The reproductive significance of human fallopian tube cilia. *Hum Reprod Update* 2006;12(4):363–72.
26. Svenstrup HF, Fedder J, Kristoffersen SE, Trolle B, Birkelund S, Christiansen G. *Mycoplasma genitalium, Chlamydia trachomatis,* and tubal factor infertility—a prospective study. *Fertil Steril* 2008;90(3):513–20.
27. Machado AC, Guimaraes EM, Sakurai E, Fioravante FC, Amaral WN, Alves MF. High titers of *Chlamydia trachomatis* antibodies in Brazilian women with tubal occlusion or previous ectopic pregnancy. *Infect Dis Obstet Gynecol* 2007;2007:24816.
28. Akande VA, Hunt LP, Cahill DJ, Caul EO, Ford WC, Jenkins JM. Tubal damage in infertile women: prediction using chlamydia serology. *Hum Reprod* 2003;18(9):1841–7.
29. Wallace LA, Scoular A, Hart G, Reid M, Wilson P, Goldberg DJ. What is the excess risk of infertility in women after genital chlamydia infection? A systematic review of the evidence. *Sex Transm Infect* 2008;84(3):171–5.
30. Chow JM, Yonekura ML, Richwald GA, Greenland S, Sweet RL, Schachter J. The association between *Chlamydia trachomatis* and ectopic pregnancy. A matched-pair, case-control study. *JAMA* 1990;263(23):3164–7.
31. Goyaux N, Leke R, Keita N, Thonneau P. Ectopic pregnancy in African developing countries. *Acta Obstet Gynecol Scand* 2003;82(4):305–12.
32. The WHO Reproductive Health Library, Interventions for Tubal Ectopic Pregnancy. [WHO website]. Available at http://www.who.int/rhl/gynaecology/imcom2/en/, last accessed May 25, 2008.
33. World Health Organization Task Force on the Prevention and Management of Infertility. Tubal infertility: serologic relationship to past chlamydial and gonococcal infection. *Sex Transm Dis* 1995;22(2):71–7.
34. Grodstein F, Goldman MB, Cramer DW. Relation of tubal infertility to history of sexually transmitted diseases. *Am J Epidemiol* 1993;137(5):577–84.
35. Sharma JB, Roy KK, Pushparaj M, Kumar S, Malhotra N, Mittal S. Laparoscopic findings in female genital tuberculosis. *Arch Gynecol Obstet* 2008;278(4):359–64.
36. Ojo BA, Akanbi AA, Odimayo MS, Jimoh AK. Endometrial tuberculosis in the Nigerian middle belt: an eight-year review. *Trop Doct* 2008;38(1):3–4.
37. Shaheen R, Subhan F, Tahir F. Epidemiology of genital tuberculosis in infertile population. *J Pak Med Assoc* 2006;56(7):306–9.
38. Glynn JR, Buve A, Carael M, et al. Decreased fertility among HIV-1-infected women attending antenatal clinics in three African cities. *J Acquir Immune Defic Syndr* 2000;25(4):345–52.
39. Clark RA, Mulligan K, Stamenovic E, et al. Frequency of anovulation and early menopause among women enrolled in selected adult AIDS clinical trials group studies. *J Infect Dis* 2001;184(10):1325–7.
40. Chirgwin KD, Feldman J, Muneyyirci-Delale O, Landesman S, Minkoff H. Menstrual function in human immunodeficiency virus-infected women without acquired immunodeficiency syndrome. *J Acquir Immune Defic Syndr Hum Retrovirol* 1996;12(5):489–94.
41. Harlow SD, Schuman P, Cohen M, et al. Effect of HIV infection on menstrual cycle length. *J Acquir Immune Defic Syndr* 2000;24(1):68–75.

42. Seifer DB, Golub ET, Lambert-Messerlian G, et al. Biologic markers of ovarian reserve and reproductive aging: application in a cohort study of HIV infection in women. *Fertil Steril* 2007;88(6):1645–52.
43. Blanc WA. Pathology of the placenta, membranes, and umbilical cord in bacterial, fungal, and viral infections in man. *Monogr Pathol* 1981(22):67–132.
44. Chellam VG, Rushton DI. Chorioamnionitis and funiculitis in the placentas of 200 births weighing less than 2.5 kg. *Br J Obstet Gynaecol* 1985;92(8):808–14.
45. Mueller-Heubach E, Rubinstein DN, Schwarz SS. Histologic chorioamnionitis and preterm delivery in different patient populations. *Obstet Gynecol* 1990;75(4):622–6.
46. Salafia CM, Vogel CA, Vintzileos AM, Bantham KF, Pezzullo J, Silberman L. Placental pathologic findings in preterm birth. *Am J Obstet Gynecol* 1991;165(4 Pt 1):934–8.
47. Wu YW, Colford JM Jr. Chorioamnionitis as a risk factor for cerebral palsy: a meta-analysis. *JAMA* 2000;284(11):1417–24.
48. Simcox R, Sin WT, Seed PT, Briley A, Shennan AH. Prophylactic antibiotics for the prevention of preterm birth in women at risk: a meta-analysis. *Aust N Z J Obstet Gynaecol* 2007;47(5):368–77.
49. Iams JD, Romero R, Culhane JF, Goldenberg RL. Primary, secondary, and tertiary interventions to reduce the morbidity and mortality of preterm birth. *Lancet* 2008;371(9607):164–75.
50. Blas MM, Canchihuaman, FA, Alva, IE, Hawes, SE. Pregnancy outcomes in women infected with *Chlamydia trachomatis*: a population-based cohort study in Washington State. *Sex Transm Infect* 2007;83(4):314–18.
51. Germain M, Krohn MA, Hillier SL, Eschenbach DA. Genital flora in pregnancy and its association with intrauterine growth retardation. *J Clin Microbiol* 1994;32(9):2162–8.
52. Donders GG, Desmyter J, De Wet DH, Van Assche FA. The association of gonorrhoea and syphilis with premature birth and low birthweight. *Genitourin Med* 1993;69(2):98–101.
53. Elliott B, Brunham RC, Laga M, et al. Maternal gonococcal infection as a preventable risk factor for low birth weight. *J Infect Dis* 1990;161(3):531–6.
54. Christian P, Khatry SK, LeClerq SC, et al. Prevalence and risk factors of chlamydia and gonorrhea among rural Nepali women. *Sex Transm Infect* 2005;81(3):254–8.
55. Nygren P, Fu R, Freeman M, Bougatsos C, Klebanoff M, Guise JM. Evidence on the benefits and harms of screening and treating pregnant women who are asymptomatic for bacterial vaginosis: an update review for the U.S. Preventive Services Task Force. *Ann Intern Med* 2008;148(3):220–33.
56. Leitich H, Bodner-Adler B, Brunbauer M, Kaider A, Egarter C, Husslein P. Bacterial vaginosis as a risk factor for preterm delivery: a meta-analysis. *Am J Obstet Gynecol* 2003;189(1):139–47.
57. Romero R, Espinoza J, Mazor M. Can endometrial infection/inflammation explain implantation failure, spontaneous abortion, and preterm birth after in vitro fertilization? *Fertil Steril* 2004;82(4):799–804.
58. Swadpanich U, Lumbiganon P, Prasertcharoensook W, Laopaiboon M. Antenatal lower genital tract infection screening and treatment programs for preventing preterm delivery. *Cochrane Database Syst Rev* 2008(2):CD006178.
59. Brocklehurst P, Hannah M, McDonald H. Interventions for treating bacterial vaginosis in pregnancy. *Cochrane Database Syst Rev* 2000(2):CD000262.
60. McDonald HM, O'Loughlin JA, Vigneswaran R, et al. Impact of metronidazole therapy on preterm birth in women with bacterial vaginosis flora (*Gardnerella*

vaginalis): a randomised, placebo controlled trial. *Br J Obstet Gynaecol* 1997;104(12):1391–7.

61. Hauth JC, Goldenberg RL, Andrews WW, DuBard MB, Copper RL. Reduced incidence of preterm delivery with metronidazole and erythromycin in women with bacterial vaginosis. *N Engl J Med* 1995;333(26):1732–6.
62. Morales WJ, Schorr S, Albritton J. Effect of metronidazole in patients with preterm birth in preceding pregnancy and bacterial vaginosis: a placebo-controlled, double-blind study. *Am J Obstet Gynecol* 1994;171(2):345–7; discussion 348–9.
63. Martino JL, Vermund SH. Vaginal douching: evidence for risks or benefits to women's health. *Epidemiol Rev* 2002;24(2):109–24.
64. Boggess KA. Maternal oral health in pregnancy. *Obstet Gynecol* 2008; 111(4):976–86.
65. Offenbacher S, Katz V, Fertik G, et al. Periodontal infection as a possible risk factor for preterm low birth weight. *J Periodontol* 1996;67(10 Suppl):1103–13.
66. Jeffcoat MK, Geurs NC, Reddy MS, Cliver SP, Goldenberg RL, Hauth JC. Periodontal infection and preterm birth: results of a prospective study. *J Am Dent Assoc* 2001;132(7):875–80.
67. Boggess KA. Maternal oral health in pregnancy. *Obstet Gynecol* 2008; 111(4): 976–86.
68. Doroshenko A, Sherrard J, Pollard AJ. Syphilis in pregnancy and the neonatal period. *Int J STD AIDS* 2006;17(4):221–7; quiz 228.
69. Woods CR. Syphilis in children: congenital and acquired. *Semin Pediatr Infect Dis* 2005;16(4):245–57.
70. TORCH syndrome and TORCH screening. *Lancet* 1990;335(8705):1559–61.
71. Valeur-Jensen AK, Pedersen CB, Westergaard T, et al. Risk factors for parvovirus B19 infection in pregnancy. *JAMA* 1999;281(12):1099–105.
72. Prospective study of human parvovirus (B19) infection in pregnancy. Public Health Laboratory Service Working Party on Fifth Disease. *BMJ* 1990; 300(6733):1166–70.
73. De Santis M, Cavaliere AF, Straface G, Caruso A. Rubella infection in pregnancy. *Reprod Toxicol* 2006;21(4):390–8.
74. Cutts FT, Robertson SE, Diaz-Ortega JL, Samuel R. Control of rubella and congenital rubella syndrome (CRS) in developing countries, Part 1: Burden of disease from CRS. *Bull World Health Organ* 1997;75(1):55–68.
75. Ross DS, Dollard SC, Victor M, Sumartojo E, Cannon MJ. The epidemiology and prevention of congenital cytomegalovirus infection and disease: activities of the Centers for Disease Control and Prevention Workgroup. *J Womens Health (Larchmt)* 2006;15(3):224–9.
76. Kenneson A, Cannon MJ. Review and meta-analysis of the epidemiology of congenital cytomegalovirus (CMV) infection. *Rev Med Virol* 2007;17(4):253–76.
77. Sauerbrei A, Wutzler P. Herpes simplex and varicella-zoster virus infections during pregnancy: current concepts of prevention, diagnosis and therapy. Part 1: herpes simplex virus infections. *Med Microbiol Immunol* 2007;196(2):89–94.
78. Brown ZA, Selke S, Zeh J, et al. The acquisition of herpes simplex virus during pregnancy. *N Engl J Med* 1997;337(8):509–15.
79. Rawlinson WD, Hall B, Jones CA, et al. Viruses and other infections in stillbirth: what is the evidence and what should we be doing? *Pathology* 2008;40(2):149–60.
80. Thiebaut R, Leproust S, Chene G, Gilbert R. Effectiveness of prenatal treatment for congenital toxoplasmosis: a meta-analysis of individual patients' data. *Lancet* 2007;369(9556):115–22.

81. Desai M, ter Kuile FO, Nosten F, et al. Epidemiology and burden of malaria in pregnancy. *Lancet Infect Dis* 2007;7(2):93–104.
82. Steketee RW, Nahlen BL, Parise ME, Menendez C. The burden of malaria in pregnancy in malaria-endemic areas. *Am J Trop Med Hyg* 2001;64(1–2 Suppl):28–35.
83. Guyatt HL, Snow RW. Impact of malaria during pregnancy on low birth weight in sub-Saharan Africa. *Clin Microbiol Rev* 2004;17(4):760–9.
84. Brabin BJ, Romagosa C, Abdelgalil S, et al. The sick placenta-the role of malaria. *Placenta* 2004;25(5):359–78.
85. Verhoeff FH, Brabin BJ, van Buuren S, et al. An analysis of intra-uterine growth retardation in rural Malawi. *Eur J Clin Nutr* 2001;55(8):682–9.
86. Steketee RW, Wirima JJ, Hightower AW, Slutsker L, Heymann DL, Breman JG. The effect of malaria and malaria prevention in pregnancy on offspring birthweight, prematurity, and intrauterine growth retardation in rural Malawi. *Am J Trop Med Hyg* 1996;55(1 Suppl):33–41.
87. Sullivan AD, Nyirenda T, Cullinan T, et al. Malaria infection during pregnancy: intrauterine growth retardation and preterm delivery in Malawi. *J Infect Dis* 1999;179(6):1580–3.
88. Landis SH, Lokomba V, Ananth CV, et al. Impact of maternal malaria and undernutrition on intrauterine growth restriction: a prospective ultrasound study in Democratic Republic of Congo. *Epidemiol Infect* 2009;137(2):294–304.
89. Rogerson SJ, Hviid L, Duffy PE, Leke RF, Taylor DW. Malaria in pregnancy: pathogenesis and immunity. *Lancet Infect Dis* 2007;7(2):105–17.
90. Hammerschlag MR. *Chlamydia trachomatis* and *Chlamydia pneumoniae* infections in children and adolescents. *Pediatr Rev* 2004;25(2):43–51.
91. Smith JR, Taylor-Robinson D. Infection due to *Chlamydia trachomatis* in pregnancy and the newborn. *Baillieres Clin Obstet Gynaecol* 1993;7(1):237–55.
92. Brocklehurst P, Rooney G. Interventions for treating genital *Chlamydia trachomatis* infection in pregnancy. *Cochrane Database Syst Rev* 2000(2):CD000054.
93. Schachter J, Grossman M, Sweet RL, Holt J, Jordan C, Bishop E. Prospective study of perinatal transmission of Chlamydia trachomatis. *JAMA* 1986;255(24):3374–7.
94. Laga M, Meheus A, Piot P. Epidemiology and control of gonococcal ophthalmia neonatorum. *Bull World Health Organ* 1989;67(5):471–7.
95. Brocklehurst P. Antibiotics for gonorrhoea in pregnancy. *Cochrane Database Syst Rev* 2002(2):CD000098.
96. MacDonald N, Mailman T, Desai S. Gonococcal infections in newborns and in adolescents. *Adv Exp Med Biol* 2008;609:108–30.
97. CDC. Prevention of perinatal group B streptococcal disease: revised guidelines from the CDC. *Morbid Mortal Week Rep Recommendations and Reports* 2002:1–22.
98. Larsen JW, Sever JL. Group B *Streptococcus* and pregnancy: a review. *Am J Obstet Gynecol* 2008;198(4):440–8; discussion 448–50.
99. Yow MD, Mason EO, Leeds LJ, Thompson PK, Clark DJ, Gardner SE. Ampicillin prevents intrapartum transmission of group B *Streptococcus*. *JAMA* 1979; 241(12):1245–7.
100. Schrag SJ, Zywicki S, Farley MM, et al. Group B streptococcal disease in the era of intrapartum antibiotic prophylaxis. *N Engl J Med* 2000;342(1):15–20.

101. Rouse DJ, Goldenberg RL, Cliver SP, Cutter GR, Mennemeyer ST, Fargason CA Jr. Strategies for the prevention of early-onset neonatal group B streptococcal sepsis: a decision analysis. *Obstet Gynecol* 1994;83(4):483–94.
102. Yancey MK, Schuchat A, Brown LK, Ventura VL, Markenson GR. The accuracy of late antenatal screening cultures in predicting genital group B streptococcal colonization at delivery. *Obstet Gynecol* 1996;88(5):811–5.
103. Manning SD, Foxman B, Pierson CL, Tallman P, Baker CJ, Pearlman MD. Correlates of antibiotic-resistant group B *Streptococcus* isolated from pregnant women. *Obstet Gynecol* 2003;101(1):74–9.
104. ACOG Committee on Practice Bulletins. *ACOG Practice Bulletin: Viral Hepatitis in Pregnancy.* October 2007, Number 86.
105. Watts DH. Pregnancy and virally sexually transmitted infections. In: Holmes K, Sparling PF, Stamm WE, et al, eds. *Sexually Transmitted Infections*, 4th edition. New York: McGraw Hill, 2008;1572–3.
106. Hill JB, Sheffield JS, Kim MJ, Alexander JM, Sercely B, Wendel GD. Risk of hepatitis B transmission in breast-fed infants of chronic hepatitis B carriers. *Obstet Gynecol* 2002;99:1049–52.
107. Morrison EAB, Gammon MD, Goldberg GL, Vermund SH, Burk RD. Pregnancy and cervical infection with human papillomaviruses. *Int J Gynecol Obstet* 1996;54:125–30.
108. Tenti P, Zappatore R, Migliora P, Spinillo A, Belloni C, Carnevali L. Perinatal transmission of human papillomavirus from gravidas with latent infections. *Obstet Gynecol* 1999;93:475–9.
109. Watts DH. Pregnancy and virally sexually transmitted infections. In: Holmes K, Sparling PF, Stamm WE, et al, eds. *Sexually Transmitted Infections*, 4th edition. New York: McGraw Hill, 2008; 1571.
110. Tseng C-J, Liang C-C, Soong Y-K, Pao C-C. Perinatal transmission of human papillomavirus in infants: relationship between infection rate and mode of delivery. *Obstet Gynecol* 1998;91:92–6.
111. Griffiths PD, Walter S. Cytomegalovirus. *Curr Opin Infect Dis* 2005;18(3): 241–5.
112. Hollier LM, Wendel GD. Third trimester antiviral prophylaxis for preventing maternal genital herpes simplex virus (HSV) recurrences and neonatal infection. *Cochrane Database Syst Rev* 2008(1):CD004946.
113. Gupta R, Warren T, Wald A. Genital herpes. *Lancet* 2007;370(9605):2127–37.
114. Dao H, Mofenson LM, Ekpini R, et al. International recommendations on antiretroviral drugs for treatment of HIV-infected women and prevention of mother-to-child HIV transmission in resource-limited settings: 2006 update. *Am J Obstet Gynecol* 2007;197(3 Suppl):S42–55.
115. Surjushe A, Maniar J. Prevention of mother-to-child transmission. *Indian J Dermatol Venereol Leprol* 2008;74(3):200–7.
116. Welles SL, Pitt J, Colgrove R, et al. HIV-1 genotypic zidovudine drug resistance and the risk of maternal–infant transmission in the women and infants transmission study. The Women and Infants Transmission Study Group. *AIDS* 2000; 14(3):263–71.
117. Croly-Labourdette S, Vallet S, Gagneur A, et al. [Pilot epidemiologic study of transmission of cytomegalovirus from mother to preterm infant by breast-feeding]. *Arch Pediatr* 2006;13(7):1015–21.

118. Jim WT, Shu CH, Chiu NC, et al. Transmission of cytomegalovirus from mothers to preterm infants by breast milk. *Pediatr Infect Dis J* 2004;23(9):848–51.
119. Hays S. [Cytomegalovirus, breast feeding and prematurity]. *Arch Pediatr* 2007;14 Suppl 1:S2–4.
120. Neuberger P, Hamprecht K, Vochem M, et al. Case-control study of symptoms and neonatal outcome of human milk-transmitted cytomegalovirus infection in premature infants. *J Pediatr* 2006;148(3):326–31.
121. Kourtis AP, Jamieson DJ, de Vincenzi I, et al. Prevention of human immunodeficiency virus-1 transmission to the infant through breastfeeding: new developments. *Am J Obstet Gynecol* 2007;197(3 Suppl):S113–22.
122. Coovadia HM, Rollins NC, Bland RM, et al. Mother-to-child transmission of HIV-1 infection during exclusive breastfeeding in the first 6 months of life: an intervention cohort study. *Lancet* 2007;369(9567):1107–16.

5

The Genetics of Reproduction

Reproduction and genetics are intimately related. Genes choreograph conception and the development of the embryo, and in turn, fertilization and embryonic growth provide hurdles that help to weed out new gene mutations. There is a strong tendency for most perinatal problems to recur in families, which suggests that heritable genetic variants play a role.

The remarkable advances in molecular genetics affect every aspect of the study of human biology, including epidemiology. This chapter addresses aspects of genetics and gene pathology that are important to the study of reproduction.

Aneuploidy

Aneuploidy is a condition of having more or fewer than the correct number of chromosomes per cell. Aneuploidy in humans usually occurs as an error in development of the egg.[1] The defective oocytes produce a conceptus with either one copy (monosomy) or three copies (trisomy) of the affected chromosome. Most aneuploidies are fatal during early embryonic or fetal development; some trisomies survive to delivery but very few monosomies. A more severe form of aneuploidy occurs when the conceptus has a whole extra set of chromosomes (triploidy) or even two extra sets (tetraploidy). These are uniformly fatal to the developing embryo.

The occurrence of aneuploidy in human conceptuses is surprisingly common, for reasons that are not understood. About 20% of oocytes have chromosomal anomalies,[2] and aneuploidy is present in at least 5% of all conceptions—possibly much more.[1] This prevalence is at least 10 times the occurrence in other mammalian species.[3] The full extent of aneuploidy in humans is not definitely known because so many conceptuses are lost before clinical recognition (see Chapter 10). Among recognized pregnancies, aneuploidies are rapidly weeded out by natural loss. Aneuploidies comprise about 40% of all clinical miscarriages (the single most common pathology among miscarriages), 4% of stillbirths, and 0.3% of live births.[1]

The best known human aneuploidy is Down syndrome, a trisomy of chromosome 21. Chromosome 21 is the smallest of the human chromosomes, which may be one reason why trisomy 21 is less lethal than other trisomies. People with Down syndrome have a characteristic facial appearance, often resembling each other more than their family members. The syndrome is characterized by short stature, varying levels of mental impairment, and increased risk of heart defects.

Almost all the remaining aneuploidies that survive to birth involve the sex chromosomes, with disabilities that range from moderate to none. A single X chromosome (XO) produces Turner syndrome. Carriers are phenotypically female, although with underdeveloped sex characteristics and infertility. Men with an extra X chromosome (XXY) have Klinefelter syndrome, associated with mild developmental problems and reduced fertility. Women with an extra X chromosome (XXX) or men with an extra Y chromosome (XYY) usually have normal development and can be fertile.[4] These more mild genetic conditions are often discovered only by accident.

Causes of aneuploidy are not well understood. The fact that most aneuploidies have their origins in oogenesis—which is to say, during the fetal life of the mother—makes the study of their possible causes even more daunting.[3] The only factor known to be associated with risk of aneuploidy is maternal age, for reasons not understood. The prevalence of trisomy among clinically recognized fetuses rises exponentially with age.[1] There seems to be no association of aneuploidy with paternal age (although paternal age may be associated with other kinds of chromosomal deterioration).[5]

New Gene Mutations

We often discuss gene mutations as if the genes have been ruined by an error. From a broader perspective, genetic mutation is essential. (If it were not for mutations, evolution would not be possible.) Each of us carries a reshuffled sample of our ancestors' genes plus a few new, experimental varieties. In every new generation there are a few genes that mutate as they are being replicated for transfer to offspring. The human genome has 6–7 billion base pairs. The number of mutations in regions where they might affect gene function is tiny, perhaps three per person per generation.[6]

Even if a new mutation affects gene function, it is unlikely to affect phenotype because the mutation occurs alone—it is matched in the carrier by a more common form of the gene (heterozygosity). If the new mutation does have an effect in the heterozygous state, the effect is probably not good. Just as a typographical error seldom adds meaning to a sentence, a random gene mutation is unlikely to enhance the working of a human body. However, there is a small chance that the effect will actually improve the fitness of the individual (and it is this small chance on which the whole gamble of mutation rides). Such evolutionary progress is paid for by the untold number of individuals whose mutations reduced their chances of survival and reproductive success.

Gene mutations (unlike aneuploidy) occur more often in sperm than in oocytes.[7] The geneticist Lionel Penrose cleverly inferred this long before mutations could be measured. There are rare cases of children with achondroplasia (dwarfism) born to normal parents. Because achondroplasia is an autosomal dominant trait, it is not possible for an affected child to be born to unaffected parents by ordinary inheritance. Such new occurrences must therefore result from a new mutation. Penrose noted that the risk of achondroplasia in previously unaffected families was associated with older fathers but not with older mothers.[8] He inferred from this observation that new mutations occur more often in sperm than in ova.

This interpretation is biologically plausible. Mutations occur during cell division, and sperm experience many more cell divisions than ova. The spermatogonia (the stem cells that produce sperm) undergo about 30 cell divisions by the time a boy reaches puberty. After puberty the pace picks up, with spermatogonia dividing every 16 days or so. In contrast, the oocyte goes through about 22 cell divisions during the mother's fetal life and then goes into a resting state (suspended at the stage of second meiosis) until the egg is fertilized. By the time a man reaches age 20, his sperm have been through about 150 cell divisions, seven times as many as the oocytes of a 20-year-old women. By the time a man is 40, his sperm will have had 25 times more opportunities for mutation than the ova of a 40-year-old woman.

On this basis, one might expect that a man's aging would produce increased reproductive problems in his offspring related to mutations. There is surprisingly little evidence for this. One difficulty in assessing effects of father's age is that the age of the mother is strongly correlated with the age of the father. Thus, large sample sizes are required in order to remove confounding by maternal age. Large studies have suggested no increase in the risk of birth defects[9] or preterm delivery[10] with paternal age. There are preliminary data to indicate possible increases in the risk of fetal death[11] and autism.[12] Looking at the question more broadly, single-gene mutations appear to make little contribution to the major reproductive problems—certainly not as much as aneuploidy.

The Truth about Proto-Oncogenes

A class of genes known as *proto-oncogenes* provide a fundamental link between reproduction and cancer. When these genes are altered by mutation or chromosomal rearrangement, they can cause a cell to grow aggressively, producing cancer. However, the main function of these genes is during the earliest days of life, at which time they regulate essential cell proliferation and trophoblast invasion of the endometrium.[13] They also play key roles in the development of the embryo.[14] It is ironic that these genes are identified by the disease they produce after mutating, rather than by their primary functions during implantation and development. The chaotic growth of cancer can be understood as a reversion (albeit in a disorganized way) to the cells' embryonic urge to grow rapidly.

It is too bad that reproductive biologists didn't discover these genes before the cancer biologists. If they had, the proto-concogenes might be more aptly known as trophogenes (genes that control growth), giving reproductive biology its rightful place in the understanding of cancer pathology.

Inherited Genetic Variants

From the standpoint of human health, the most important gene variations are not new mutations (which are rare) but gene variants that are passed from parents to offspring and accumulate in the population. Some of these variants are highly penetrant alleles, producing traits that follow the rules of Mendelian transmission. These "simple" traits can occur either when the allele is present as a single copy (dominant) or as two copies (recessive). An example of a trait that follows the dominant pattern is Huntington disease, a progressive and devastating neurologic disease that emerges in adulthood. Persons with this illness have a 50% chance of transmitting the allele—and thus the disease—to their offspring. (The American folk singer Woody Guthrie died of Huntington disease, but his son Arlo has escaped the illness.)

Recessive traits require two copies of the disease allele. Thus, a person affected by a recessive trait cannot pass the trait to offspring unless the partner is at least heterozygous for the allele. When both parents are heterozygous carriers, they will appear phenotypically normal but 25% of their offspring will be affected. Examples of recessive traits are cystic fibrosis and albinism.

These simple genetic diseases are dramatic, but they are also uncommon. The main focus of genetic epidemiology has shifted to the so-called complex diseases, which are more prevalent and impose a larger health burden on the population.[15] Most noninfectious diseases (including cardiovascular diseases, cancers, neurologic diseases, and birth defects) tend to recur in families, but without following a pattern of Mendelian transmission. A combination of many genetic variants is presumed to contribute to these complex diseases, interacting with environmental factors and with other genes. The discovery of specific genetic variants associated with common diseases has turned out to be more difficult than first anticipated.[16] One problem is that the possibilities of false-positive findings are rife.[17]

In the search for genes that contribute to complex illnesses, the magnitude of family recurrence risk can be an indication of the strength (and thus the detectability) of a genetic contribution. From this perspective, perinatal problems may offer better targets for genetic studies than many adult diseases. The risk of the common cancers (such as colon or breast cancer) is increased two- to threefold when a sibling has also been diagnosed.[18] In contrast, the average birth defect has a sevenfold risk among siblings, reaching as high as 50-fold for certain defects.[19] If all other factors are equal, the search for a genetic association would be more promising among diseases with high familial recurrence.

Multifactorial/Threshold Model

The multifactorial/threshold model provides a theoretical framework for the joint action of multiple genes. This model assumes there is a continuum of vulnerability to a given disease, with the disease expressed only when a certain threshold of risk has been crossed.[20] Vulnerability in this context can result from the presence of multiple gene variants as well as environmental insults. With enough risk factors present, a person will be pushed over the threshold into disease. Although this concept was developed in the context of birth defects, it could in principle apply to any illness with multiple causes.

Factors That Affect Gene Function

Studies tend to focus narrowly on the way in which a certain gene variant increases the risk of a given disease. However, the same gene variant may have different functions in different contexts and at different stages of life, acting as a liability under some conditions and offering benefits in others.[21] The possibility of multiple functions should be considered especially for gene variants that have become relatively common in the population. One way that a variant becomes common is by conferring a crucial adaptive advantage in survival and reproduction, even though it may also be associated with risk of disease. Furthermore, there are mechanisms that diversify the effects of a given allele, thus complicating its indictment as a disease gene. Some of those mechanisms are described here.

Heterozygote Advantage

Some genes have a different health effect when present in one copy than when present in two. A well-known example is hemoglobin S. A person who carries two copies of this allele is likely to have sickle-cell disease. However, persons who are heterozygous for the allele (carrying only one copy) do not have the disease and, furthermore, have an advantage over noncarriers in their ability to survive an acute bout of malaria.[22] In regions where malaria is endemic, the advantage of being a heterozygous carrier can be substantial.

Heterozygote advantage could be suspected for any disease allele that has become relatively common in populations. For example, the recessive allele that causes cystic fibrosis has probably survived by giving the heterozygotes resistance to a major infectious disease, possibly typhoid fever.[23] With typhoid no longer a widespread scourge, this hypothesis is difficult to test. The vast improvements in human living conditions over the past 10,000 years may have made many of the former heterozygote advantages less apparent.

Alternative Splicing

It was once dogma that a single gene produces a single protein. In fact, a single gene may produce tens, or hundreds, or even thousands of subtly different protein products by means of *alternative splicing*, a mechanism by which segments of messenger RNA are rearranged to convey different messages.[24] Alternative splicing helps to explain how humans can produce so many proteins (estimated to be a million or more) from only 25,000 or 30,000 genes.

Epigenetics and Gene Inactivation

Yet another way in which a given gene can expand its repertoire of effects is through the phenomenon of epigenetics. Until recently, the function of a gene was thought to be determined entirely by its DNA sequence. We now know that gene expression (a crucial aspect of gene function) can be affected by changes *upon* (*epi-*) the gene that do not alter the DNA sequence. Epigenetic effects can be produced in several ways, including the attachment of methyl groups to particular parts of the DNA molecule. Such methylation is often associated with gene inactivation and is useful in modulating gene expression. Methylation can accumulate over the course of a person's lifetime, or it can be inherited. Methylation patterns that are laid down during the development of the sperm or ovum are known as *imprinting*.

IMPRINTING. The classic Mendelian model of inheritance assumes that the effect of a gene does not depend on which parent has contributed the gene. Imprinting is an exception to this rule. Specific patterns of DNA methylation for certain genes can be imposed during the development of the sperm or the oocyte and preserved in the conceptus. These genes will therefore behave differently depending on whether they were inherited from the father or from the mother. Although relatively few genes are imprinted by the parents, these genes can have substantial effects on placental and fetal development.[25]

The development of the placenta and the fetus is a dynamic process in which some genes promote growth and others suppress growth. Many of the genes that are imprinted (that is, inactivated) by the father are genes that tend to restrict placental and fetal growth. By inactivating those genes, the father gives more influence to other genes (from either the father or the mother) that promote fetal growth. (Note that the effect of gene imprinting is an implied double-negative: imprinting by the father increases fetal growth by suppressing his genes that suppress growth.) Similarly, the maternally imprinted genes are those that tend to increase placental and fetal growth, and their inactivation leads to a smaller fetus. Smaller fetuses do not tax the maternal system as severely as larger ones, and they offer less threat to the life of the mother at delivery.

Theoretical biologist David Haig has suggested that this contest between maternal and paternal genes in fetal growth represents the father's interest in a healthy fetus regardless of the risk to the mother, whereas the mother more judiciously balances the benefits for the fetus against her own well-being and that of her other children (who may or may not have the same father).[26] The placenta in particular tends to be influenced by paternal imprinting, as befits an organ that exists for the benefit of the fetus rather than the mother.

Regardless of its evolutionary roots, the process of imprinting has some remarkable consequences. One example can be seen in conceptuses that are occasionally formed with two complete sets of chromosomes from the father rather than one set from each parent. (This could happen, for example, if an ovum is fertilized by two sperm and the maternal contribution is lost.[27]) The resulting conceptus has a double dose of paternally imprinted genes, which promotes a rapid overgrowth of the placental tissue in the absence of a viable fetus. This condition is known as hydatidiform mole, or molar pregnancy. Such pregnancies end in miscarriage or must be surgically removed.

Imprinting explains a curious pair of syndromes, both caused by deletion of the same segment of chromosome 15. One is Angelman syndrome, characterized by severe developmental disability and disorders of movement. This syndrome occurs when the deletion occurs in the chromosome inherited from the mother. If the same segment is missing from the chromosome inherited from the father, then Prader-Willi syndrome is produced (marked by overeating and developmental delays).[28] The deleted region contains important imprinted genes, which presumably explains the different expressions of disease when the genes are missing.

Disorders related to imprinted alleles could be suspected in any disease associated with inheritance of a gene from one parent but not the other. Type 1 diabetes (insulin-dependent) has been reported to be more common among the children of affected fathers than affected mothers.[29] Other diseases that may fall into this category include autism, schizophrenia, retinoblastoma, and male infertility.[30]

Are Monozygotic Twins Genetically Identical?

It is well known that monozygotic twins are not necessarily the same in all respects. For example, one can have a malformation at birth while the other is unaffected. Monozygotic twins also differ in their risk of disease throughout their lifetimes. Environmental factors presumably play a role in these differences; epigenetic differences may also contribute. It appears that a person's patterns of gene methylation change over time. Such changes may be influenced by external exposures (such as diet), and perhaps by errors in the transmission of methylation patterns across successive cell divisions.[31] The consequence is that as monozygotic twins become older, they diverge in their patterns of gene expression and thus become less "genetically" similar as time goes by.[32]

Concerns have been raised about the possibility that the methods of reproductive technology may disturb imprinting processes among the resulting offspring.[30] Even if associations are found between assisted conception and imprinting disorders among offspring, the interpretation is not straightforward—an association could be caused by the disturbance of DNA methylation by in vitro procedures or by preexisting problems in methylation (especially of sperm) that have made fertility treatment necessary.

EPIGENETIC TRANSPLACENTAL EFFECTS. There has been fascinating speculation on ways in which exposures—particularly in utero exposures of the fetus—might affect methylation and gene expression in the adult.[25,33] Although these mechanisms could in principle be important to human health, this possibility remains largely hypothetical.

X INACTIVATION IN FEMALES. There is one example of gene suppression that occurs exclusively in females. Every woman has two X chromosomes, but only one is active in any given cell. Around the time that the female conceptus implants, individual cells begin to inactivate one or the other of their X chromosomes. This leaves only a single active X chromosome (which could be from either the mother or the father) in each cell. This X inactivation, which is presumably random, produces two different cell lines in the embryo. Females thus grow up as genetic mosaics for the X chromosome. Unlike men, who carry the same X chromosome in all their cells, women have the advantage of heterozygosity of the X chromosome, even though this heterozygosity operates among cells within a given woman rather than within each cell. One consequence is that diseases caused by gene variants on the X chromosome are generally more serious in males than in females,[34] presumably because males missing an essential gene product from their particular X chromosome lack the backup of a second X chromosome.

Mitochondrial DNA

The discussion so far has been on nuclear DNA, that is, genetic material contained within the nucleus of the cells. However, not all DNA is in the cell nucleus. Mitochondria are tiny organelles in the cell cytoplasm that carry their own DNA.[35] Each mitochondrion contains a ring of DNA that is similar to the DNA in certain bacteria, suggesting that mitochondria are the descendents of ancient bacteria that acquired a symbiotic relationship with our ancestral cells. Mitochondria are our cells' power source—they produce the chemical energy that keeps cell metabolism running. Mitochondria replicate independently of cell replication and according to the energy requirements of the cell. The number of mitochondria in a cell varies from one to several thousand, depending on the cell type.

Mitochondrial DNA passes from generation to generation through the mother, via the cytoplasm of the oocyte. (Sperm have no cytoplasm.) For this reason, the mitochondrial genes provide a marker of matrilineal descent, just as the Y chromosome provides a marker of patrilineal descent (for men, at least). Mitochondrial transmission is a possible explanation (along with imprinting) for observations of maternal transmission of disease risk in families. However, diseases caused by genetically defective mitochondria do not necessarily show maternal transmission; many arise as new mutations.[36] Rare syndromes associated with mutations in mitochondrial DNA include deafness[37] and an assortment of neurodegenerative diseases.[35]

Genetic Studies of Perinatal Disease

Whole textbooks are devoted to genetic epidemiology, and the study designs available to explore the associations of genes with illness. Perinatal outcomes are particularly well suited to genetic studies for several reasons, including the generally high recurrence of specific perinatal problems in families. This recurrence risk suggests a strong contribution of genetic variation (see, for example, Tables 7-1 and 7-2 in Chapter 7).

A structural advantage of genetic studies of perinatal diseases is that the biological parents are likely to be available after birth, and they are likely to be motivated to participate in etiologic studies if their child is affected. One particular design for genetic studies (the case-parent triad approach) takes advantage of this availability of parents.

Case-Parent Triads

The case-parent triad design is an example of case-only studies, which are made possible by the rigid structure of Mendelian transmission of genes from parents to offspring. For any given gene, an offspring receives two of the four alleles carried by its two biological parents. The parents transmit these alleles randomly to their offspring. However, when offspring are selected for having a given disease,

The Legacy of Genghis Khan (1162–1227)

Genghis Khan ruled a vast empire that at its peak (in the early 1200s) stretched from modern-day Hungary and Poland to China and Korea. A writer 40 years after Genghis Khan's death estimated that the emperor had 20,000 living descendants. This might be dismissed as a fawning tribute to a powerful conqueror except for a curious recent discovery. About 8% of Y chromosomes sampled from a large region of central Asia trace back to a single individual who lived roughly a thousand years ago. Such genetic clusters can sometimes happen by chance in homogeneous populations that arise from a small group, but this specific chromosome has been reported in 16 populations including the Han Chinese, the largest ethnic group in the world. The cluster seems to have originated in Mongolia and is distributed across the regions of the former Mongol Empire.[38] George Washington was merely the father of one country. Genghis Khan seems to have been the father of many.

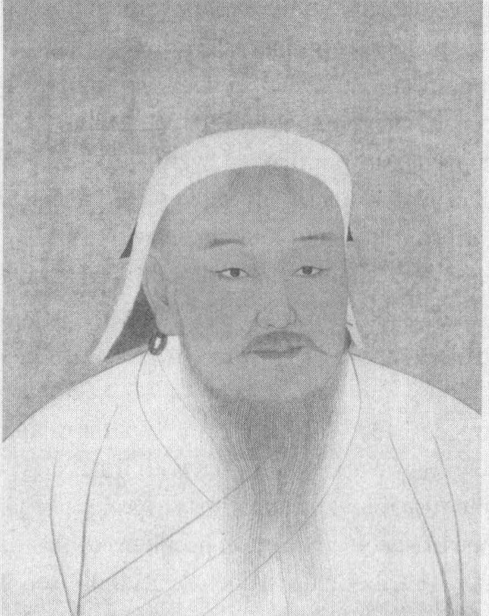

Genghis Khan

they will carry an excess of alleles that cause the disease (Fig. 5-1). In an unselected population, half of offspring with the parents shown in the figure would be expected to carry *Aa* and the other half *AA*. To the degree that allele *a* confers risk of the disease, the affected offspring with this set of parents will more often carry *Aa* than *AA*. (This excess of the causative allele is analogous to the excess of smokers found among a group of persons with lung cancer.) Thus, to the extent that a given allele is found in cases more than would be predicted by the distribution of the allele in parents, the allele is associated with the disease.

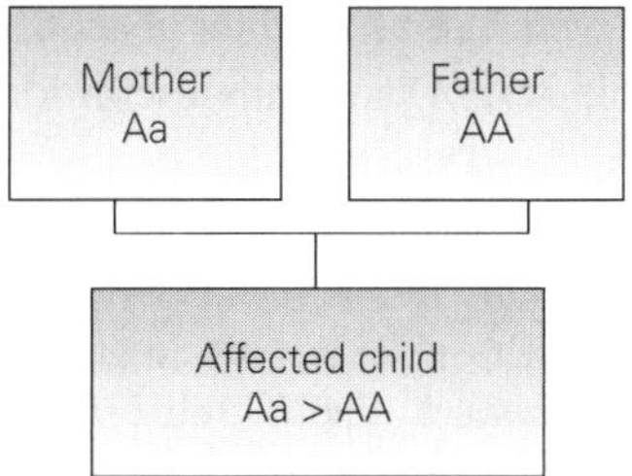

Figure 5-1. The expected allele distribution when allele *a* increases the risk of the disease, and families are selected as having an affected child.

The relative risk associated with the allele can be directly estimated within the triad design. This is done by comparing the observed frequency of alleles in cases with the expected frequency (based on the alleles of their parents). This provides a true relative risk, with no rare-disease assumption necessary.[39] Another analytic approach to the analysis of these case-parent-triad data is the transmission disequilibrium test (TDT).[40] One limitation of the TDT (for epidemiologists, at least) is that the test provides a *p*-value but no relative risk estimate.

The case-triad approach can be extended to genes that work through the phenotype of the pregnant woman to affect disease risk in her fetus.[41] For example, a maternal gene might cause a mother to metabolize an environmental exposure into a toxic form that crosses the placenta. In this case, the maternal genome would be associated with disease in the fetus regardless of whether the fetus inherited the allele.

The case-parent triad approach can be combined with the case-control design (recruiting controls and their parents). Such combined designs overcome disadvantages of either design separately: the case-control aspect of the study allows confirmation of Mendelian transmission (an essential assumption of the case-parent analysis), whereas the case-parent aspect of the design is resistant to distortion by population stratification (a weakness of case-control studies).[42] Although the

Are You and I Related? Probably

Make that "definitely!" Any two human beings can find a common ancestor if they go back far enough. (After all, if you're willing to go back *far* enough, you and your rose bush have a common ancestor.) What people often do not realize is how recently our common ancestors lived. Even if you are a Masai born on the Serengeti, you and I (an American with European roots) almost certainly have a common ancestor who lived within the last 3,500 years, and maybe as recently as 2,000 years ago.[43] Even more remarkable, if we go back 7,000 years, we all have the *same* ancestors. That is, going back just 350 generations or so, you and I and Nelson Mandela and Mao Zedong all come from the same set of forefathers and foremothers.

Have a good day, cousin!

case-parent design can in principle be used for genetic studies of any disease, the family structure makes this design especially useful for perinatal studies.

References

1. Hassold T, Abruzzo M, Adkins K, et al. Human aneuploidy: incidence, origin, and etiology. *Environ Mol Mutagen* 1996;28(3):167–75.
2. Martin RH. Meiotic errors in human oogenesis and spermatogenesis. *Reprod Biomed Online* 2008;16(4):523–31.
3. Hassold T, Hall H, Hunt P. The origin of human aneuploidy: where we have been, where we are going. *Hum Mol Genet* 2007;16 Spec No. 2:R203–8.
4. Egozcue S, Blanco J, Vendrell JM, et al. Human male infertility: chromosome anomalies, meiotic disorders, abnormal spermatozoa and recurrent abortion. *Hum Reprod* Update 2000;6(1):93–105.
5. Sloter E, Nath J, Eskenazi B, Wyrobek AJ. Effects of male age on the frequencies of germinal and heritable chromosomal abnormalities in humans and rodents. *Fertil Steril* 2004;81(4):925–43.
6. Drake JW, Charlesworth B, Charlesworth D, Crow JF. Rates of spontaneous mutation. *Genetics* 1998;148(4):1667–86.
7. Crow JF. The origins, patterns and implications of human spontaneous mutation. *Nat Rev Genet* 2000;1(1):40–7.
8. Penrose L. Parental age and mutation. *Lancet* 1955;269:312–13.
9. Kazaura M, Lie RT, Skjaerven R. Paternal age and the risk of birth defects in Norway. *Ann Epidemiol* 2004;14(8):566–70.
10. Basso O, Wilcox AJ. Paternal age and delivery before 32 weeks. *Epidemiology* 2006;17(4):475–8.
11. Nybo Andersen AM, Hansen KD, Andersen PK, Davey Smith G. Advanced paternal age and risk of fetal death: a cohort study. *Am J Epidemiol* 2004;160(12):1214–22.
12. Reichenberg A, Gross R, Weiser M, et al. Advancing paternal age and autism. *Arch Gen Psychiatry* 2006;63(9):1026–32.
13. Ferretti C, Bruni L, Dangles-Marie V, Pecking AP, Bellet D. Molecular circuits shared by placental and cancer cells, and their implications in the proliferative, invasive and migratory capacities of trophoblasts. *Hum Reprod Update* 2007;13(2):121–41.
14. Adamson ED. Oncogenes in development. *Development* 1987;99(4):449–71.
15. Peyser PA, Burns TL. Approaches to quantify the genetic component of and identify genes for complex traits. In: Khoury MJ, Little J, Burke W, eds. *Human Genome Epidemiology.* Oxford: Oxford University Press, 2004;38–57.
16. Dong LM, Potter JD, White E, Ulrich CM, Cardon LR, Peters U. Genetic susceptibility to cancer: the role of polymorphisms in candidate genes. *JAMA* 2008;299(20):2423–36.
17. Wacholder S, Chanock S, Garcia-Closas M, El Ghormli L, Rothman N. Assessing the probability that a positive report is false: an approach for molecular epidemiology studies. *J Natl Cancer Inst* 2004;96(6):434–42.
18. Hemminki K, Li X, Sundquist K, Sundquist J. Familial risks for common diseases: etiologic clues and guidance to gene identification. *Mutat Res* 2008;658(3):247–58.
19. Lie RT, Wilcox AJ, Skjaerven R. A population-based study of the risk of recurrence of birth defects. *N Engl J Med* 1994;331(1):1–4.
20. Fraser FC. The William Allan Memorial Award Address: evolution of a palatable multifactorial threshold model. *Am J Hum Genet* 1980;32(6):796–813.

21. Wilcox AJ. Benefits of "harmful" genes. *Epidemiology* 1996;7(4):450–1.
22. Aidoo M, Terlouw DJ, Kolczak MS, et al. Protective effects of the sickle cell gene against malaria morbidity and mortality. *Lancet* 2002;359(9314):1311–2.
23. Dean M, Carrington M, O'Brien SJ. Balanced polymorphism selected by genetic versus infectious human disease. *Annu Rev Genomics Hum Genet* 2002;3:263–92.
24. Park JW, Graveley BR. Complex alternative splicing. *Adv Exp Med Biol* 2007;623:50–63.
25. Cutfield WS, Hofman PL, Mitchell M, Morison IM. Could epigenetics play a role in the developmental origins of health and disease? *Pediatr Res* 2007;61(5 Pt 2):68R-75R.
26. Haig D. Genetic conflicts in human pregnancy. *Q Rev Biol* 1993;68(4):495–532.
27. Jones WB. Gestational trophoblastic disease: what have we learned in the past decade? *Am J Obstet Gynecol* 1990;162(5):1286–95.
28. Horsthemke B, Wagstaff J. Mechanisms of imprinting of the Prader-Willi/Angelman region. *Am J Med Genet* A 2008;146A(16):2041–52.
29. Harjutsalo V, Reunanen A, Tuomilehto J. Differential transmission of type 1 diabetes from diabetic fathers and mothers to their offspring. *Diabetes* 2006;55(5):1517–24.
30. Paoloni-Giacobino A. Epigenetics in reproductive medicine. *Pediatr Res* 2007;61(5 Pt 2):51R-57R.
31. Bjornsson HT, Fallin MD, Feinberg AP. An integrated epigenetic and genetic approach to common human disease. *Trends Genet* 2004;20(8):350–8.
32. Wong AH, Gottesman, II, Petronis A. Phenotypic differences in genetically identical organisms: the epigenetic perspective. *Hum Mol Genet* 2005;14 Spec No 1:R11–8.
33. Pembrey M. Human inheritance, differences and diseases: putting genes in their place. Part II. *Paediatr Perinat Epidemiol* 2008;22(6):507–13.
34. Migeon BR. The role of X inactivation and cellular mosaicism in women's health and sex-specific diseases. *JAMA* 2006;295(12):1428–33.
35. Orth M, Schapira AH. Mitochondria and degenerative disorders. *Am J Med Genet* 2001;106(1):27–36.
36. Thorburn DR. Mitochondrial disorders: prevalence, myths and advances. *J Inherit Metab Dis* 2004;27(3):349–62.
37. Kokotas H, Petersen MB, Willems PJ. Mitochondrial deafness. *Clin Genet* 2007;71(5):379–91.
38. Jobling MA, Tyler-Smith C. The human Y chromosome: an evolutionary marker comes of age. *Nat Rev Genet* 2003;4(8):598–612.
39. Weinberg CR, Wilcox AJ, Lie RT. A log-linear approach to case-parent-triad data: assessing effects of disease genes that act either directly or through maternal effects and that may be subject to parental imprinting. *Am J Hum Genet* 1998;62(4):969–78.
40. Ewens WJ, Li M, Spielman RS. A review of family-based tests for linkage disequilibrium between a quantitative trait and a genetic marker. *PLoS Genet* 2008;4(9):e1000180.
41. Wilcox AJ, Weinberg CR, Lie RT. Distinguishing the effects of maternal and offspring genes through studies of "case-parent triads." *Am J Epidemiol* 1998;148(9):893–901.
42. Vermeulen SH, Shi M, Weinberg CR, Umbach DM. A hybrid design: case-parent triads supplemented by control-mother dyads. *Genet Epidemiol* 2008.
43. Rohde DL, Olson S, Chang JT. Modelling the recent common ancestry of all living humans. *Nature* 2004;431(7008):562–6.

6

Evolutionary Biology and Eugenics

The concepts of evolutionary biology are essential to a full understanding of reproduction. Indeed, successful reproduction and survival of the offspring is the very definition of evolutionary fitness. But as history has proved, fitness and natural selection are also concepts that are subject to stunning abuse.

Evolutionary theory is a profoundly elegant principle that binds together all of biology. Evolutionary processes are particularly relevant to the topics of this book. Fertility and early pregnancy are filters through which every new genetic variation must pass. Selection seems especially stringent during the first half of pregnancy when at least one-third of human conceptions are lost.

All else being equal, genetic variants that improve the chances of successful reproduction will become more prevalent, whereas those that decrease reproduction will fade away. That being the case, it is curious that reproductive problems typically have an increased probability of recurrence in families, which suggests the presence of stable, heritable gene variants that contribute to the risk. How have these genes survived the selection against them? One possibility is that genes contributing to a risk (say, preeclampsia) also have other effects that provide the carrier with evolutionary advantages.[1] Such counterbalancing effects are seen in other areas of human health, as in the sickle cell allele discussed in the previous chapter.[2]

Conversely, what is good for the fetus may not necessarily be good for that individual late in life. If a genetic variant were to improve survival of the embryo, perhaps through more rapid growth, it might not matter (from an evolutionary perspective) if that same gene variant were to increase the person's risk of cancer or heart disease many decades later.

Similarly, specific gene variants may help in one setting and hinder in another. They may be bad for one generation and good for the next. Genetic variability is like a life insurance policy for the whole species. As with life insurance, gene variability exacts a small steady cost year-by-year while providing the possibility of major payoffs in a crisis. The crisis would be an abrupt change in our environment, for example the introduction of a new and virulent infectious agent. Even though many might die, the few who happen to have genetic resistance to the infection would allow the species as a whole to continue. Thus, the usefulness of any given allele depends on its circumstances. Genetic "perfection" has no meaning outside an impossibly narrow context.[3] Although this may seem self-evident, it has not always been regarded so.

The Birth of Eugenics

It was 150 years ago that Charles Darwin published his book *On the Origin of Species by Means of Natural Selection.*[4] The title captures the thesis: Darwin proposed the radical idea that species are not permanent but rather are part of a dynamic process driven by heredity and natural selection. Species change. Even our own species is changing.

Darwin's ideas had a huge effect on the intellectuals of his day. One important convert was his half-cousin, Francis Galton. In the wake of Darwin's discoveries, Galton became fascinated with the implications of evolutionary theory for humans (which Darwin had only hinted at). Galton conducted large-scale studies to measure human variation in such characteristics as height and span. In the process, he developed such essential statistical concepts as correlation and regression to the mean.

With Galton's encouragement, the theory of evolution gave new emphasis to heredity as an influence over all human characteristics. Environment, upbringing, education, and social opportunity took a back seat to the principle that "like begets like"—successful parents produce genetically successful children. In 1883, Galton coined the word "eugenics" and proposed that the practice of late marriage and few children among Britain's upper classes was a genetic disadvantage for the population as a whole. Galton suggested that society's best and the brightest, by limiting their own fertility, were failing to pass their superior capacities to their fair share of the next generation.[5]

Galton's most brilliant protégé was Karl Pearson, the founder of mathematical statistics. Pearson shared Galton's fascination with measurement and the analysis of data. Using Galton's voluminous data on the heights of men and their sons, Pearson developed the concept of linear regression, and he introduced a measure of correlation (Pearson's r) that we still use. Pearson was an idealist who advocated women's rights and whose socialist principles led him to decline a knighthood. He was also a eugenicist (Fig. 6-1).

In 1907, Karl Pearson gave a lecture at Oxford University in which he presented his views on genetics. He began his lecture by stating that researchers should not

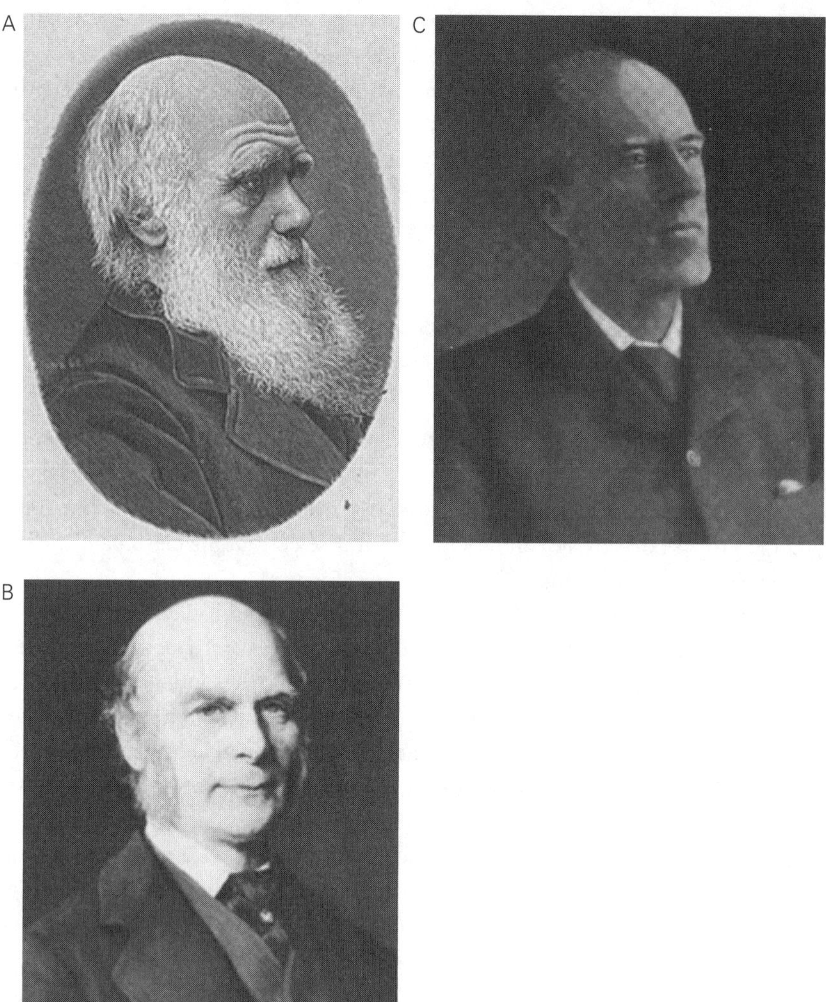

Figure 6-1. From evolution to eugenics (A) Charles Darwin (1809–82), (B) Francis Galton (1822–1911), (C) Karl Pearson (1857–1936)

study haphazard collections of individuals but rather whole populations, using "actuarial methods applied to biological data."[6] In this he articulated a central tenet of modern epidemiology. (Pearson also influenced the field of epidemiology in other ways. Pearson taught Bradford Hill, who developed the familiar guidelines for inferring causation in observational studies. Hill in turn persuaded Richard Doll to enter the field of epidemiology,[7] and in the last half of the twentieth century Doll became its most eminent practitioner.)

In his Oxford lecture, Pearson went on to present what he called the "two great principles" of human genetics. The first was the inheritance of measurable physical characteristics. This principle was a direct legacy of Francis Galton and his collections of physical measurements. The second principle was the correlation in heredity of unlike imperfections. Pearson drew on a diverse (and flawed) body of research that suggested certain problems seemed to cluster in individuals. Babies with birth defects not only had a higher risk of having other birth defects but were more likely to be mentally retarded and to become criminals or prostitutes. In Pearson's view, the fact that ostensibly heritable diseases were concentrated in a minority of the population was grounds for social action:

> [In considering] the habitual criminal, the tuberculous, the insane, the mentally defective, the diseased from birth or from excess, there can be little doubt of their unfitness. Here every remedy... which reduces their chances of parentage, is worthy of consideration.... The duty of the man of science is to... waken the conscience of his countrymen.[6]

Pearson didn't specify what "remedies" he had in mind to reduce the chances of parentage, but he didn't have to. In the same year (1907), the U.S. State of Indiana made it legal to sterilize mental patients, criminals, and paupers without their permission.[8] Twenty-eight other U.S. states soon followed.

In 1913, Theodore Roosevelt wrote:

> Some day, we will realize that the prime duty, the inescapable duty, of the good citizen of the right type, is to leave his or her blood behind him in the world; and that we have no business to permit the perpetuation of citizens of the wrong type.[9]

By the 1920s, hundreds of colleges and universities in the United States were offering eugenics courses that exhorted young citizens of the "right type" to reproduce. Meanwhile, the U.S. Supreme Court ruled that involuntary sterilization of the "wrong type" was constitutional. At least 40,000 U.S. citizens were forcibly sterilized.[10]

In 1907, the same year that Pearson gave his Oxford lecture, a young artist was seeking admission to the Academy of Arts in Vienna. He applied twice and failed both times. He was reduced to living in a homeless shelter. In 1925, he published a book called *My Struggle,* which became a best-seller. From its title, this could be the inspirational story of an artist who pursued his vocation against all odds. It was not. In fact, the following excerpt from his book suggests that the artist was paying more attention to distinguished professors such as Karl Pearson:

> The demand that defective people be prevented from propagating equally defective offspring is a demand of the clearest reason and, if systematically carried out, represents the most humane act of mankind. It will spare millions of unfortunate people sufferings they don't deserve, and consequently will lead to a rising improvement of health as a whole."[11]

The artist was Adolf Hitler, and the book *Mein Kampf.* In 1933, the year that Hitler became Germany's Chancellor, Germany established "genetic health courts" that imposed sterilization on German citizens who were judged to be unfit. The "unfit" included thousands of people with birth defects. The Germans carried out 400,000 forced sterilizations.[10]

In 1938, a German researcher conducted an epidemiologic study of the recurrence risk of facial clefts as part of his medical thesis. His data showed that 47% of all babies with cleft lip or cleft palate were born into families with an affected member—yet one more piece of evidence used to justify the eugenics creed.[12] The researcher was Joseph Mengele, later known as the "angel of death" for his experiments on children at Auschwitz.

The Death of Eugenics?

The proximity of eugenics to medical research is discomfiting. After the end of the Second World War, there was a backlash against the collection of certain kinds of population-based data. In most European countries (but not the United States), it became illegal to collect data on race or ethnicity as part of any official record, including vital statistics. Researchers distanced themselves from the principles of eugenics and anything associated with it.

The final irony is that eugenics had not been based on good science. For example, Pearson's second "great principle" of genetics (the "correlation in heredity of unlike imperfections") is not a valid generalization. This can be seen in the familial recurrence risks of various types of birth defects, which are largely independent of one another (Table 7-2). Of course, there are factors associated with low socioeconomic status (illness, crime, poverty) that do cluster in families—but for much more complex reasons than simple inheritance.

Eugenics took hold of the scientific and popular imagination not merely because of its supposed logic but because of its deep appeal to powerful prejudices about class and race. This is not an isolated historical incident. Science, and the interpretations of science, are never isolated from the values of the society in which science is conducted.

Today, the modern revolution in molecular genetics has inspired a resurgence of genetic determinism. Although no one claims eugenic intentions, there have been suggestions (carefully phrased) that genetic engineering might improve human capacities. Genetics in combination with the application of artificial reproductive technology has been proposed not just as a way to avoid rare and devastating genetic diseases but as a way to acquire offspring with particular attractive characteristics—so-called "designer" children.[13]

Once again, the evidence for these claims is scanty. The more we learn about gene functions, the less "deterministic" genes turn out to be. The actions of our genes are entwined with each other and with our environment in ways far more subtle and intricate than we would have thought possible even a decade ago. It no longer seems within our grasp to predict with certainty how complex phenotypes (such as intelligence or athletic ability) arise from genotype. To fully understand this would require an integration of biology, mathematics, engineering, and computation at a level that we can barely imagine.[14] Genetic manipulation of complex sets of genes certainly remains possible, but its full consequences are virtually impossible to predict—much less control.

Family Planning and the Neo-eugenists

Eugenic views motivated no less a hero than Margaret Sanger, champion of modern-day birth control methods and founder of Planned Parenthood. In her words, "More children from the fit, less from the unfit—that is the chief issue of birth control."[8] Although eugenics was roundly rejected after World War II, an enthusiasm emerged in the 1970s for controlling population growth at any cost. Spurred by apocalyptic visions of overpopulation and sustained by confidence in their own wisdom, policy makers launched international programs that in some cases (and incredibly) included sterilization without consent.[15]

International family-planning programs are a vital component of maternal and child health programs. Even so, the ease with which certain family planning programs violated human rights in the pursuit (once again) of apparently laudable purposes serves to remind us, in the words of William Faulkner, that "the past is never dead. It's not even past."[16]

References

1. Wilcox AJ. Benefits of "harmful" genes. *Epidemiology* 1996;7(4):450–1.
2. Dean M, Carrington M, O'Brien SJ. Balanced polymorphism selected by genetic versus infectious human disease. *Annu Rev Genomics Hum Genet* 2002;3:263–92.
3. Wilcox AJ. *Quest for the Perfect Human has Severe Flaws.* Los Angeles, CA: LA Times. 2000.
4. Darwin C. *On the Origin of Species by Means of Natural Selection.* Mineola, NY: Dover Publications, 2006.
5. Galton F. Eugenics: its definition, scope, and aims. *Am J Sociol* 1904;10(1):1–25.
6. Pearson K. *The Scope and Importance to the State of the Science of National Eugenics.* Eugenics Laboratory Lecture Series. London: University College, 1909.
7. Darby S. A conversation with Sir Richard Doll. *Epidemiology* 2003;14(3):375–9.
8. Sandel MJ. *The Case against Perfection: Ethics in the Age of Genetic Engineering.* Cambridge, MA: Harvard University Press, 2007.
9. Black E. *War Against the Weak: Eugenics and America's Campaign to Create a Master Race.* Emeryville, CA: Thunder's Mouth Press, 2003.
10. Bachrach S. In the name of public health—Nazi racial hygiene. *N Engl J Med* 2004;351(5):417–20.
11. Hitler A. *Mein Kampf.* Boston, MA: Houghton Mifflin, 1998.
12. Wyszynski DF. Fifty years after the Nuremberg Nazi Doctors' Trial: reviewing how the laws of the Third Reich applied to individuals with oral clefts. *Plast Reconstr Surg* 1998;101(2):519–27.

13. Green RM. *Babies by Design: The Ethics of Genetic Choice.* New Haven, CT: Yale University Press, 2007.
14. Silverman PH. Rethinking genetic determinism. *The Scientist* 2004:32–3.
15. Connelly M. *Fatal Misconception: The Struggle to Control World Population.* Cambridge, MA: Belknap Press, 2008.
16. Faulkner W. *Requiem for a Nun.* New York: Random House, 1951.

7

Heterogeneity of Risk

Most reproductive risks vary widely in populations, with some couples at low risk and others at high risk. One of the most important dynamics in reproductive epidemiology is the way that previous pregnancy outcomes can affect selective control of fertility to distribute high- or low-risk couples in misleading ways.

The underlying risk of any given disease varies in the population. This is the basis of epidemiology: if there were no high-risk people to contrast with low-risk, we would have no opportunity to identify the factors associated with the higher risk. Reproductive epidemiology provides an added window on this heterogeneity in that we can frequently observe recurrence risk. Couples typically have more than one pregnancy in their lifetimes and thus are exposed to reproductive risks multiple times. The larger the relative risk of recurrence, the stronger the underlying heterogeneity of risk in the population.

Heterogeneity and Recurrence Risk

Figure 7-1 represents a hypothetical population of people distributed along a spectrum of risk for a disease. A few people are at very low risk, and a few are at very high risk, with the bulk of the population clustered in the middle. The vertical arrow shows the median risk.

The exact risk for a particular person is rarely known. However, we can learn something about a person's risk by whether or not he or she gets the disease. As time passes, the disease risk will express itself (Fig. 7-2). Some portion of the population will contract the disease. High-risk people are more likely to get the disease—although not all people who get the disease are at high risk. A few affected people are low-risk individuals who just had bad luck. Even though

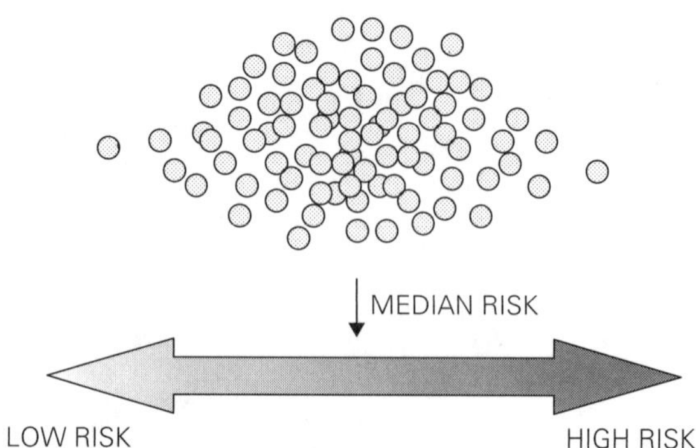

Figure 7-1. Heterogeneity of risk among a population with heterogeneous risk

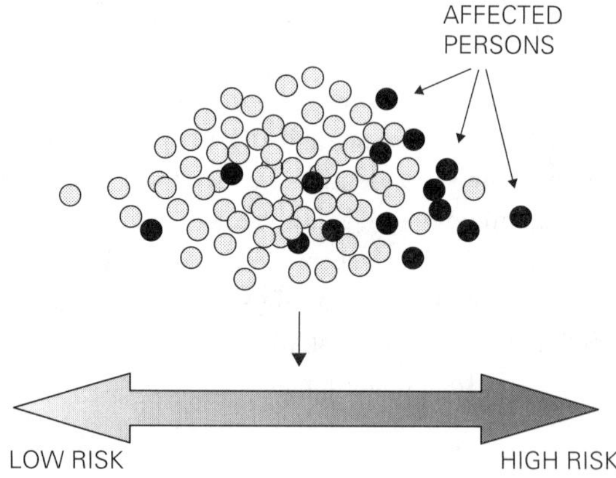

Figure 7-2. Occurrence of disease in a population

occurrence of disease is not a perfect predictor of individual risk, the median risk for the affected group is higher than that for the base population (Fig. 7-3).

Now imagine that the group of affected people is cured and that we observe them for an additional period of time. Even if we assume the second occurrence of the disease is not affected by the first occurrence, occurrence will be higher in the previously affected group than in the original population. No one has changed his or her position on the risk scale—everyone has exactly the same risk in the second period as they did in the first. They are at "high risk" for second occurrence

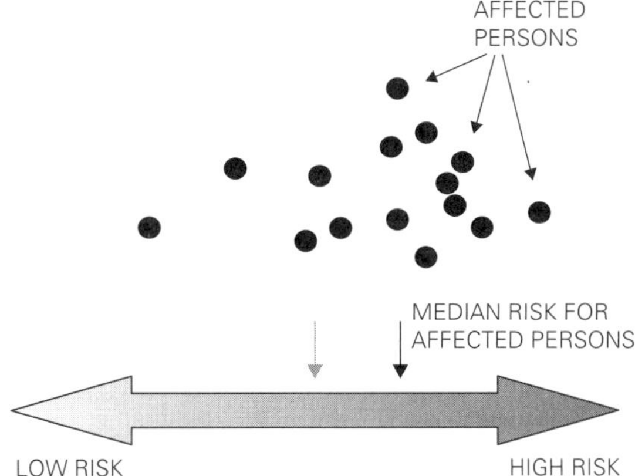

Figure 7-3. Median risk among affected persons

simply because the first occurrence identified them as being (on average) higher-risk people.

The difference between the median risk for the base population (Fig. 7-1) and the median risk for the selected group (Fig. 7-3) is a measure of recurrence risk—the subject of this chapter. Recurrence risk is often expressed as a ratio (recurrence risk divided by occurrence risk). For reproductive outcomes, recurrence risk ratios are commonly in the range of 2 to 10 and can range up to 50 or more for specific types of birth defects.

The size of the recurrence risk ratio depends on the extent of the population heterogeneity. If the risk were completely homogeneous (with every person having the same risk), then recurrence risk would be exactly the same as occurrence risk. (There also would be no work for epidemiologists because there would be no opportunity to contrast low- and high-risk people.) The greater the heterogeneity in risk, the more likely it is that we can discover factors associated with that risk.

Assumption of Risk Independence

We have made a crucial assumption about risk, namely, that having the disease once does not change the chances of getting the disease again. There are areas of epidemiology where this assumption does not hold. For example, many infectious diseases confer immunity, so that the occurrence of the disease directly reduces the chances of the affected person having it again. There are some diseases that increase the chance of their recurrence by making the affected person more susceptible; for example, infection can damage a heart valve, making the valve more vulnerable to further infection. As a general rule, reproductive problems do not directly increase or decrease subsequent risk.

Examples

Reproductive epidemiology provides abundant examples of recurrence risks higher than occurrence risks.[1] Table 7-1 presents recurrence risk ratios for various causes of perinatal mortality. The researchers used data from Norway to consider a woman's risks and recurrence risks for specific kinds of perinatal death of her offspring.[2] The first column shows the major causes of death among first births. The next columns show the relative risks of those causes of death in second births, conditional on the outcome of the mothers' first birth. (The reference group is mothers whose first baby survived.) Among women whose first pregnancy ended in early stillbirth, there was a 22-fold higher risk of early stillbirth in second pregnancies. These women also had increased relative risks of other causes of fetal or infant death, although none as high. This pattern is seen for each cause of death: recurrence risk for the specific cause is usually higher than that for other causes. Infant morbidity, including developmental disabilities, also has high recurrence risk in families.[3]

What artifacts could contribute to these associations? The categories of perinatal causes of death are not always mutually exclusive (for example, a stillborn infant may also have birth defects). Some doctors or some hospitals may prefer certain diagnoses over others, which could increase the apparent recurrence risk. Also, the presence of a particular diagnosis in a woman's previous pregnancy may

Table 7-1. Relative risk of recurrence of mortality by specific causes in second birth, given the cause of death in the first birth[a]

	Relative risks for specific causes of death in second birth					
Outcome of first birth	Early stillbirth	Late stillbirth	"Birth related"	Birth defects	SIDS	All other
Survivor (ref.)	1.0	1.0	1.0	1.0	1.0	1.0
Early stillbirth	22	4.7	16	2.1	2.0	5.5
Late stillbirth	2.6	4.6	3.0	1.9	—	2.6
"Birth related"	4.5	1.9	13	1.8	—	3.2
Birth defects	2.5	1.7	—	7.2	—	—
SIDS	—	—	—	—	5.8	—
All other	3.9	2.0	5.9	—	—	—

[a]Medical Birth Registry of Norway, 1967–88 (from Oyen et al[2]). No rates are shown for cells with fewer than five cases; shaded cells on the diagonal are relative risk for recurrence of the same outcome; remaining cells are relative risk of a different outcome.

Table 7-2 Relative risk of recurrence of specific birth defects in the second birth, given the occurrence of a birth defect in the first birth[a]

	Relative risk of recurrence in second birth	
Outcome of first birth	Similar defect	Dissimilar defect
No defect in first birth	1.0 (ref.)	1.0 (ref.)
Clubfoot	7	1.4
Genital defect	5	1.5
Limb defect	11	2.4
Cardiac defect	6	1.1
Cleft lip with or without cleft palate	31	1.2

[a]Medical Birth Registry of Norway, 1967–89 (from Lie et al.[4]).

increase the chance that her doctor will use the same diagnosis with a subsequent perinatal loss. Such biases may contribute to the observed patterns, although they are unlikely to explain the large recurrence risks entirely.

There is a strong pattern of recurrence risk for birth defects as well. Table 7-2 shows the recurrence relative risks for types of birth defects in second births given the presence of the defect in the mother's first baby. Here the risks are even more specific: the relative risks for recurrence of the same type of defect range from 5 to 31, whereas the relative risks for dissimilar defects in affected families are all less than 3. Similar patterns of increased risk of recurrence are found for most reproductive outcomes.

Underlying Causes of Recurrence Risk

What can recurrence risk tell us about the underlying causes of reproductive problems? The causes of recurrence risk are no different from the causes of risk in general, except that the causes of recurrence risk must persist over time. The most persistent of all risk factors is of course a person's genome. Recurrence risk has been studied most intensively in the context of families (pedigree studies), in which risk is traced among first-degree, second-degree, and more distant relatives as a way to describe the presumed genetic features of a disease. (In pedigree studies, genes are assumed be the complete explanation for recurrence in families.)

It can be a mistake to attribute all recurrence risk to genes; shared environment can also play a role. Especially in sibling studies (in which "recurrence" is measured among children of the same parents) (Tables 7-1 and 7-2), there could be dietary patterns, environmental conditions, or personal behaviors of the mother that expose a series of pregnancies to a consistent risk. Evidence for environmental factors can be seen in a study of couples whose first baby had a birth defect. The recurrence risk of the birth defect in the next child is lower if the parents move to a different municipality after the first birth.[4] Whatever the mechanism for this observation, it is probably not genetic. Perinatal recurrence risk can be regarded as woman-specific, or as couple-specific (in which case recurrence risk would be restricted to a woman's pregnancies by the same father). Recurrence risk that changes when one or the other parent changes partner suggests a genetic etiology—although the possibility of important environment changes with a change in partner cannot be excluded.

The Interpretation of Recurrence Risk

In reproductive studies, recurrence risk is seldom if ever a case of one unfavorable outcome causing another. This confusion is evident in clinical literature. Studies have been conducted "to determine the harmful effect of abnormal pregnancy outcome on the immediately following pregnancy."[5] A paper titled "Influence of past reproductive performance on risk of spontaneous abortion,"[6] found that women with one miscarriage were at high risk for having another. The authors concluded that "the outcome of a woman's first pregnancy has profound consequences for all subsequent pregnancies." Perhaps the authors didn't mean this literally, but the suggestion that one miscarriage causes another is misleading. Simple simulations with plausible assumptions about heterogeneity can replicate the observed associations with no need for inventive causal mechanisms.[7] A miscarriage reveals a woman's high intrinsic risk; it does not create it.

That said, recurrence risk can be a rich source of insight about causation. A classic example comes from the study of birth defects. There is a spectrum of facial clefts going from cleft lip only, to cleft lip and palate, to cleft palate only. Are these a continuum of outcomes from the same etiologic mechanism, or do they represent distinct groups? Based only on structural pathology, the answer is not obvious. A Danish surgeon named Fogh-Andersen unlocked the answer by keeping careful records of families over decades.[8] These records showed that cleft palate by itself had high recurrence in families, but these families were unlikely to have a baby with cleft lip. Conversely, families affected by cleft lip were likely to have other family members with cleft lip (sometimes with cleft palate and sometimes without), but rarely with cleft palate alone. Fogh-Anderson inferred two distinct categories of facial clefts, a finding that has since been confirmed through studies of embryonic facial development.

Furthermore, this understanding of subcategories of facial clefts is essential for studying the causes of clefts. The two types of facial clefts tend to have different risk factors.[9,10] If the two kinds of clefts are grouped, this dilutes the possibility of identifying a risk factor that affects only one type. Thus, recurrence risk can help separate etiologically distinct diseases that may otherwise appear similar.

Conversely, recurrence risk can show links between seemingly unrelated outcomes, suggesting the presence of shared biological causes. This has been shown for stillbirth risk, which is much higher among women whose previous baby was preterm and small for gestational age, suggesting that the causes of stillbirth are related to the causes of fetal growth restriction and preterm delivery.[11]

Recurrence risk data can be useful in other ways. For example, geneticists who are interested in studying birth defects may have a better chance (all else being equal) of identifying genetic causes of cleft palate (which has a sibling recurrence relative risk of 56)[12] than, say, cardiac defects (with a recurrence relative risk of 6).[4]

Recurrence Risk across Generations

Another type of familial "recurrence risk" is the risk that parents transmit their own conditions to their offspring. Risk across generations raises complications of interpretation not found in sibships. (For example, the recurrence of lethal birth defects can be studied in sibships but not across generations.) Even so, data across generations extends the possibilities for understanding causal pathways.

Birth Weight

Several authors have noted the heritability of fetal growth restriction or macrosomia.[13,14] Seen in another light, these observations are simply another example of Galton's studies on the inheritance of continuous characteristics. As

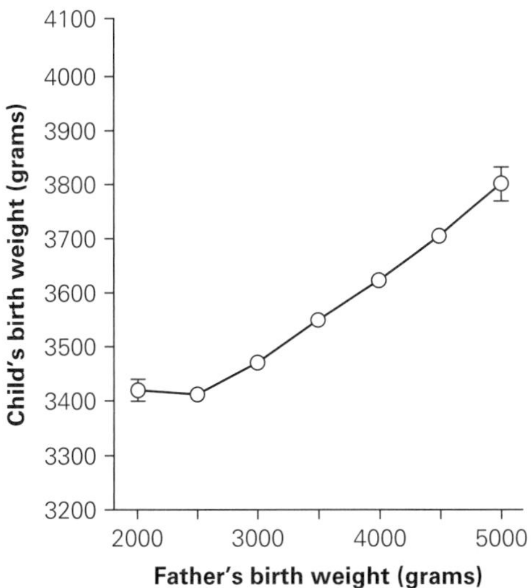

Figure 7-4. Relation of father's birth weight to child's birth weight (Norway, 1967–2003) (bars indicate 95% confidence intervals, which are too narrow to be visible at most points) (Reprinted from Lie et al[15])

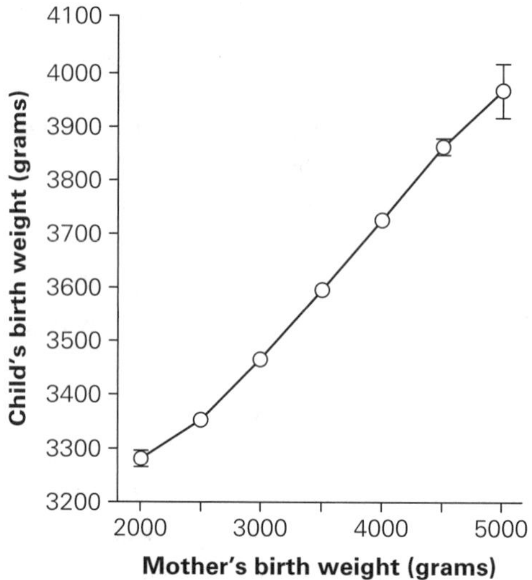

Figure 7-5. Relation of mother's birth weight to child's birth weight (Norway, 1967–2003) (bars indicate 95% confidence intervals) (Reprinted from Lie et al[15])

shown in Fig. 7-4, there is a nearly linear relationship between father's birth weight and weight of his offspring (an increase of about 125 g in offspring birth weight per kilogram of father's birth weight).[15] The simplest explanation is that certain genes that influenced the fetal growth of the father are passed to his offspring.

The same analysis for mothers and their offspring shows an even stronger pattern (Fig. 7-5). For every kilogram difference in maternal birth weight, there is a more than 250-g difference in the weight of her offspring.[15] Part of this inheritance is presumably the same as with the father: certain genes that influence fetal weight are passed from the parent to the offspring. Where does the additional contribution of the mother come from?

Imprinted genes may explain part of this difference (see Chapter 5). Additional heritable factors may also play a role. A mother's own size directly contributes to the size of her fetus in that larger women apparently allow more space for the fetus to grow. (A study of donated ova found that the baby's birth weight was associated with the carrier mother's height and weight more than with the egg donor's height and weight.[16]) To the extent that a woman's birth weight is correlated with her adult size,[17] a mother's adult phenotype may be an additional genetic pathway in the association of her birth weight with her offspring's birth weight. Another possibility (although less likely) could be environmental factors that are shared between mothers and daughters.

Preterm Delivery

The recurrence of preterm delivery offers an interesting contrast to the pattern seen with birth weight. Here, the association is entirely through the mother

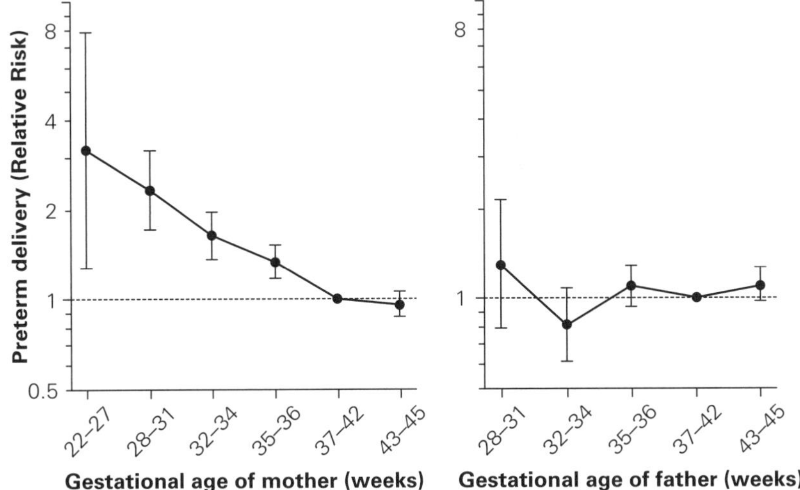

Figure 7-6. Risk of preterm delivery by gestational ages of the parents (Norway, 1967–2004) (bars indicate 95% confidence intervals) (Reprinted from Wilcox et al[18])

(Fig. 7-6).[18] The figure shows the relative risk of early delivery (defined here as less than 35 weeks of gestation) conditional on the gestational age of the mother and the father at birth. The more preterm the mother, the more likely she is to deliver her own baby early. No such pattern is seen for the father.

In the absence of any evidence for an association through the father, there is little to support fetal genes (from either parent) as a major contributor to preterm delivery. (An exception would be a contribution through imprinted fetal genes.)

For associations that pass entirely through the mother, it seems likely that heritable aspects of the mother's phenotype play a major role. For preterm delivery, relevant aspects of maternal phenotype might include genetic susceptibility to exposures (for example, infections) that increase preterm risk. It is also possible that shared environmental factors across generations could produce the association, although such a factor would have to be more strongly related to preterm delivery than any environmental causes yet discovered. A third possibility is that being born early in some way might make a woman less able to carry her own fetus to term (although such mechanisms are at this point speculative). In any event, for outcomes (such as preterm delivery) with largely unknown etiologies, patterns of generational inheritance may help point to promising research directions.

Other Uses of Recurrence Risk

Recurrence risk is also a tool for clinical studies. Observational studies had strongly suggested that folic acid reduces the risk of neural tube defects (NTDs).[19]

The Role of Linked Data

Estimates of perinatal recurrence risk require data that link related persons. Unfortunately, such data cannot be dependably reconstructed from vital statistics. Each birth certificate exists in isolation, without connection to the records of other births having the same mother or father.

It might seem simple to use vital statistics to link sibling birth certificates through the mother's name, birth date, etc., but in fact this effort is frustrated by the presence of common names, by spelling errors or inconsistencies, and by the mother's name changes. Furthermore, women who cannot be successfully linked are not a random sample of the population—they typically are from disadvantaged subgroups of the population. As a result, linked records based only on vital statistics are rarely representative of the whole population.

The most reliable linked data sets come from special registries in countries with unique personal identification numbers. There are a few countries in the world with population-based systems for using such linkages, mostly in Scandinavia. Linked data from Norway, Denmark, and Sweden provide much of what is known about recurrence risks of pregnancy.

A clinical trial was needed, but neural tube defects are a rare outcome—they occur in fewer than 3 per 1,000 births. An enormous sample size would be needed to demonstrate a protective effect. This problem was circumvented by recruiting women who had had a previous baby with an NTD. These women have a much higher risk of NTDs among their offspring (on the order of 3 per 100). With this higher birth prevalence, investigators were able to demonstrate the efficacy of folic acid supplements for the prevention of neural tube defects.[20,21]

After the clinical trials of NTDs, some skeptics argued that effects on recurrence risk could not necessarily be generalized to occurrence risk. For the generalization to fail, one would have to propose that highly susceptible people incur their risk through unique mechanisms unrelated to ordinary risk. This is theoretically possible, but for most diseases it seems likely that risk is a continuum, as in Figure 7-1, and that recurrence risk expresses the same basic underlying risk factors as occurrence risk. Thus, this strategy of studying previously affected mothers can be used to improve the power of almost any study of reproductive problems.

The predictive power of prior outcomes is also useful to clinicians who wish to identify high-risk women for closer surveillance. Women with a history of pregnancy problems are more likely to be referred to high-risk clinics. Such referral patterns can create problems for unwary epidemiologists. Specialty obstetric clinics often have higher rates of preterm birth or perinatal mortality. These referral centers can create misleading patterns of risk in surveillance data, for example, simply because women with previous poor outcomes have been referred to the centers. Control for measurable risk factors in the current pregnancy would not adequately adjust for this excess risk.

Adjustment for Prior Pregnancy Outcomes

A confusing dilemma of reproductive epidemiology is whether to adjust for previous pregnancy outcomes. A woman's history of one miscarriage strongly predicts the occurrence of another. At first glance, it may seem logical in a study of miscarriage risk to control for a prior miscarriage. If the purpose is prediction, then including prior outcomes in a multivariate adjustment may be appropriate. However, if the purpose is to understand causation, statistical adjustment for previous miscarriage is fraught with the possibility of bias, and there is no simple solution.[22,23] Some women may have changed their behaviors as the result of a previous poor pregnancy outcome. An analysis that adjusts for previous pregnancy outcome without having data on exposures for that pregnancy could be biased because of a dependency between current exposure and past pregnancy history.[24]

Heterogeneity of Risk and Selective Fertility

Chapter 3 discussed methods by which couples are able to control their fertility and achieve their desired family size. We now consider how this "selective" fertility (that is, the control of fertility to produce a certain number of children) can combine with risk heterogeneity to produce analytic trouble.

Miscarriage Risk and Gravidity

A woman's gravidity is the number of times she has ever been pregnant. Risk of miscarriage increases with gravidity.[24] This association is seen even after carefully controlling for maternal age and social class, and has led to speculations about biological pathways through which past pregnancies might increase the risk of miscarriage.

This association between miscarriage risk and gravidity turns out to be an artifact of selective fertility and heterogeneity of risk.[7,25] To understand this, consider an extreme situation in which every woman wants two children, and all women control their fertility perfectly so that no woman has more than two living children. In this setting, the only women who will have three pregnancies are women who lost one of their first two pregnancies. Thus, all women proceeding to a third pregnancy will be women selected as being at higher risk for pregnancy loss. This will produce an apparent increase in risk of loss among the third pregnancies. The same bias (on a milder scale) explains the observation of increasing risk of miscarriage with gravidity. Women who are at high risk are overrepresented among the higher gravidities.[7]

Birth Interval and Pregnancy Outcome

There is an extensive literature on pregnancies conceived only a short time after a previous pregnancy.[26] Such pregnancies are more likely to end in loss. Hypotheses have been developed about maternal depletion of essential nutrients with closely-spaced pregnancies. The more difficult questions are to what extent the short interval is a true cause of pregnancy loss, and to what extent the association is a function of selective fertility.

One reason women get pregnant again after a minimum delay is the loss of the baby in the earlier pregnancy. Thus, high-risk women are overrepresented among women with short pregnancy intervals.[27] Careful account must be taken of the outcome of the earlier pregnancy in order to rule out reverse causation (women at high risk having short pregnancy intervals, rather than short pregnancy interval producing higher risk in the second pregnancy). The presence of reverse causation has been cleverly shown in an analysis of babies born *before* a short pregnancy interval.[28] Those babies had an increased risk similar to the babies born after the short interval. Even so, if women with poor outcome at the previous pregnancy are excluded, the adverse effects of pregnancy interval are not eliminated.[27,29] Short pregnancy interval may in fact contribute to an increased risk of preterm delivery.

Birth Order and Perinatal Mortality

The association of birth order with perinatal mortality has been extensively researched (in part because of the easy availability of vital statistics data). Although the question may appear simple, the answer is not—for the same reason as in previous examples.

The usual pattern of birth order and perinatal mortality is shown in Figure 7-7. Based on birth records (cross-sectional data), there is a decrease in mortality from first to second births and then a gradual increase in mortality with subsequent

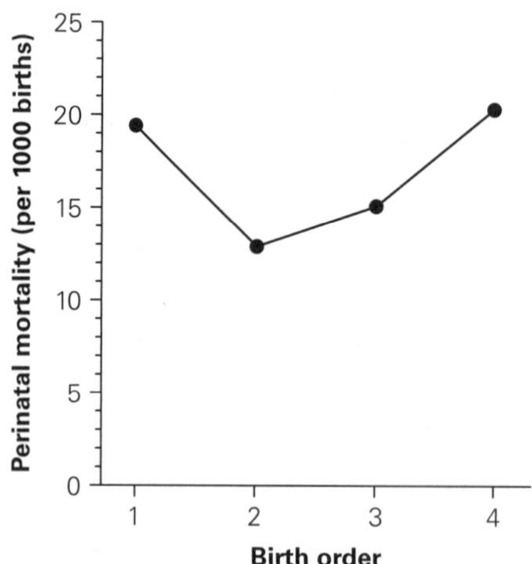

Figure 7-7. Perinatal mortality by birth order (Norway, 1967–84)[30]

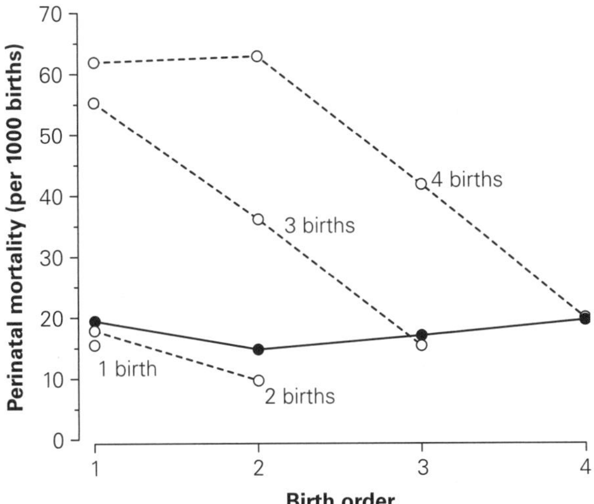

Figure 7-8. Perinatal mortality by birth order and total number of births (Norway, 1967–73)[31]

births. Investigators have proposed that cross-sectional data used for this purpose are misleading and in fact the pattern is strikingly different when considered within families[31] (Fig. 7-8). When data are stratified by completed family size, women with two pregnancies have a decline in mortality at the second pregnancy. For women with three pregnancies, mortality is higher in the first birth but again drops sharply from the first to second to third pregnancies. This pattern is repeated for women with four pregnancies, with perinatal risk falling at the later pregnancies. According to the investigators, these patterns show that mortality falls with increasing parity (parity being a woman's number of previous deliveries). The authors concluded that the increasing mortality with birth order in cross-sectional data must be an artifact.

Instead, the artefact lay in the authors' own analysis. Notice how much higher the mortality is for first pregnancies of women with four pregnancies compared with women with only two pregnancies. The explanation lies in the selection of women by total number of pregnancies. Women with four pregnancies include women who wanted only two or three children but lost babies on the way. By conditioning the analysis of first births on women's total number of pregnancies (in effect, conditioned the outcome of first birth on future events), the authors inadvertently conditioned on women's underlying risk for poor pregnancy outcome. The mortality by birth order, when stratified by total number of pregnancies, provides no information on the biological effects of birth order. (What this analysis does demonstrate is the tendency of women to stop their reproduction with a success, but this is not an effect of birth order.)

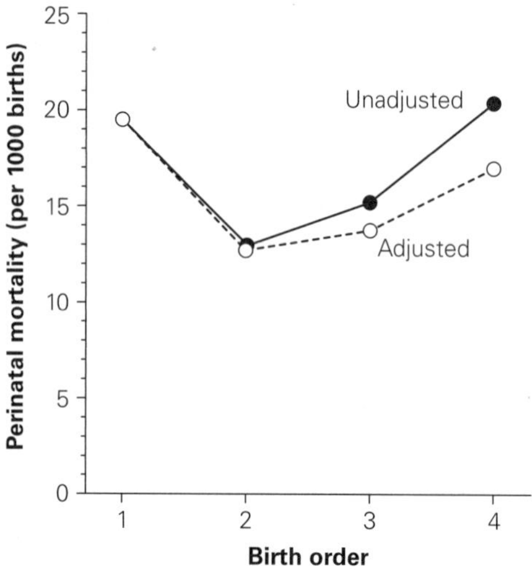

Figure 7-9. Perinatal mortality by birth order, before and after adjusting for the overrepresentation of high-risk women at higher birth orders (Norway, 1967–84)[30]

The naive cross-sectional analysis actually comes closer to describing the biological effects of birth order. One shortcoming of the cross-sectional data is that there is a modest inflation of risk at the higher birth orders with the overrepresentation of high-risk women (those with earlier perinatal deaths). Adjusting for this overrepresentation modifies the birth-order pattern slightly, without fully removing the higher mortality at higher birth orders[30] (Fig. 7-9). This increase in adjusted mortality at subsequent pregnancies may reflect residual confounding from unmeasured socioeconomic factors. In contrast, the higher mortality in first pregnancy compared with second is not explained by selection or confounding and may be a real biological difference between first and second births.

Stratification by completed family size in the analysis of parity (Fig. 7-8) is an easy error to make. (Indeed, the same mistake appears in 1999 in a report on reducing perinatal and neonatal mortality.[32]) George Santayana's caution about the fate of those who do not learn from the past is apt for epidemiologists. We have to understand the missteps of the past—including our own—if we are to avoid repeating them.

References

1. Gardiner EM, Yerushalmy J. Familial susceptibility to stillbirths and neonatal deaths. *Am J Hyg* 1939;30(1):11–31.
2. Oyen N, Skjaerven R, Irgens LM. Population-based recurrence risk of sudden infant death syndrome compared with other infant and fetal deaths. *Am J Epidemiol* 1996;144(3):300–5.

3. Van Naarden Braun K, Autry A, Boyle C. A population-based study of the recurrence of developmental disabilities—Metropolitan Atlanta Developmental Disabilities Surveillance Program, 1991–94. *Paediatr Perinat Epidemiol* 2005;19(1):69–79.
4. Lie RT, Wilcox AJ, Skjaerven R. A population-based study of the risk of recurrence of birth defects. *N Engl J Med* 1994;331(1):1–4.
5. Hathout H, Kasrawi R, Moussa MA, Saleh AK. Influence of pregnancy outcome on subsequent pregnancy. *Int J Gynaecol Obstet* 1982;20(2):145–7.
6. Regan L, Braude PR, Trembath PL. Influence of past reproductive performance on risk of spontaneous abortion. *BMJ* 1989;299(6698):541–5.
7. Wilcox AJ, Gladen BC. Spontaneous abortion: the role of heterogeneous risk and selective fertility. *Early Hum Dev* 1982;7(2):165–78.
8. Fogh-Andersen P. *Inheritance of Harelip and Cleft Palate.* Copenhagen: Arnold Busck, 1942.
9. Lie RT, Wilcox AJ, Taylor JA, et al. Maternal smoking and oral clefts : the role of detoxification pathway genes. *Epidemiology* 2008;19(4):606–15.
10. Wilcox AJ, Lie RT, Solvoll K, et al. Folic acid supplements and risk of facial clefts: national population based case-control study. *BMJ* 2007;334(7591):464.
11. Surkan PJ, Stephansson O, Dickman PW, Cnattingius S. Previous preterm and small-for-gestational-age births and the subsequent risk of stillbirth. *N Engl J Med* 2004;350(8):777–85.
12. Sivertsen A, Wilcox AJ, Skjaerven R, et al. Familial risk of oral clefts by morphological type and severity: population based cohort study of first degree relatives. *BMJ* 2008;336(7641):432–4.
13. Bakketeig LS, Bjerkedal T, Hoffman HJ. Small for gesational age births in successive pregnancy outcomes: results from a longitudinal study of births in Norway. *Early Hum Dev* 1986;14(3–4):187–200.
14. Klebanoff MA, Mills JL, Berendes HW. Mother's birth weight as a predictor of macrosomia. *Am J Obstet Gynecol* 1985;153(3):253–7.
15. Lie RT, Wilcox AJ, Skjaerven R. Maternal and paternal influences on length of pregnancy. *Obstet Gynecol* 2006;107(4):880–5.
16. Brooks AA, Johnson MR, Steer PJ, Pawson ME, Abdalla HI. Birth weight: nature or nurture? *Early Hum Dev* 1995;42(1):29–35.
17. Sorensen HT, Sabroe S, Rothman KJ, et al. Birth weight and length as predictors for adult height. *Am J Epidemiol* 1999;149(8):726–9.
18. Wilcox AJ, Skjaerven R, Lie RT. Familial patterns of preterm delivery: maternal and fetal contributions. *Am J Epidemiol* 2007;167:474–9.
19. Botto LD, Moore CA, Khoury MJ, Erickson JD. Neural-tube defects. *N Engl J Med* 1999;341(20):1509–19.
20. Hosseinzadeh S, Eley A, Pacey AA. Semen quality of men with asymptomatic chlamydial infection. *J Androl* 2004;25(1):104–9.
21. Prevention of neural tube defects: results of the Medical Research Council Vitamin Study. MRC Vitamin Study Research Group. *Lancet* 1991;338(8760):131–7.
22. Weinberg CR. Toward a clearer definition of confounding. *Am J Epidemiol* 1993;137(1):1–8.
23. Howards PP, Schisterman EF, Heagerty PJ. Potential confounding by exposure history and prior outcomes: an example from perinatal epidemiology. *Epidemiology* 2007;18(5):544–51.
24. Naylor AF, Warburton D. Sequential analysis of spontaneous abortion. II. Collaborative study data show that gravidity determines a very substantial rise in risk. *Fertil Steril* 1979:31(3):282–6.

25. Kline JI. An epidemiological review of the role of gravidity in spontaneous abortion. *Early Hum Dev* 1978;1(4):337–44.
26. Conde-Agudelo A, Rosas-Bermudez A, Kafury-Goeta AC. Birth spacing and risk of adverse perinatal outcomes: a meta-analysis. *JAMA* 2006;295(15):1809–23.
27. Smith GC, Pell JP, Dobbie R. Interpregnancy interval and risk of preterm birth and neonatal death: retrospective cohort study. *BMJ* 2003;327(7410):313.
28. Erickson JD, Bjerkedal T. Interpregnancy interval. Association with birth weight, still-birth, and neonatal death. *J Epidemiol Community Health* 1978;32(2):124–30.
29. Basso O, Olsen J, Knudsen LB, Christensen K. Low birth weight and preterm birth after short interpregnancy intervals. *Am J Obstet Gynecol* 1998;178(2):259–63.
30. Skjaerven R, Wilcox AJ, Lie RT, Irgens LM. Selective fertility and the distortion of perinatal mortality. *Am J Epidemiol* 1988;128(6):1352–63.
31. Bakketeig LS, Hoffman HJ. Perinatal mortality by birth order within cohorts based on sibship size. *Br Med J* 1979;2(6192):693–6.
32. Child Health Research Project Special Report Reducing Perinatal and Neonatal Mortality. *Report of a Meeting*. Vol 3 No. 1. Baltimore, MD, 1999.

8

Reproductive Epidemiology

Themes and Variations

Reproductive biology presents particular advantages—and also some challenges—for epidemiologists. As with other epidemiologic specialties, the particularities of reproductive epidemiology can shed light on the practice of epidemiology more generally.

Each specialized area of epidemiology adjusts to fit its subject matter. In turn, each epidemiologic specialty develops tools and insights that enrich epidemiology as a whole. Infectious disease epidemiologists led the way in integrating laboratory methods into field studies. Cancer epidemiologists contributed to the design and analysis of case-control studies. It may be too early to say what reproductive epidemiology will provide, but it is possible to describe some of its distinctive aspects.

Study Designs

All the standard epidemiologic study designs are useful for reproductive epidemiology, with some interesting twists. For case-control studies of rare outcomes (such as birth defects), the relatively brief time between exposure and outcome allows more accurate reconstruction or recall of exposure. The compressed time-window for reproductive outcomes also make cohort studies attractive for the study of frequent outcomes. Pregnancy cohort studies (usually of women recruited during pregnancy or at delivery) have provided a wealth of data on maternal exposures during pregnancy and the events of delivery and early infant development. Such cohort studies often become the foundation for continuing follow-up studies, sometimes long past the original plans.[1] More recent and larger birth cohort studies in Denmark,[2] Norway,[3] and the United States[4] provide ongoing research opportunities.

The fact that women typically have more than one pregnancy presents reproductive epidemiologists with further options. It is possible to study the effects of exposures that change within women from one pregnancy to the next. Women serve as their own controls, perfectly matched for genes and well matched for many background factors. An example is the effect of maternal smoking during pregnancy on cognitive function of the offspring. Several studies have suggested that mother's smoking is associated with mild deficits in her child. A problem in interpreting this association is the possibility of residual confounding by social class or other factors. Swedish researchers found that among women who smoked during one pregnancy but not the next, there was slightly reduced academic performance among both the exposed and unexposed children,[5] thus implicating factors besides smoking. This approach is attractive in principle but requires large linked data sets.

Challenges

Epidemiology is shaped not only by the questions that need to be addressed but by the obstacles that have to be overcome. None of the following problems is unique to reproduction, but taken as a whole, these conditions convey the distinctive flavor of reproductive epidemiology.

1. **Some reproductive outcomes lack a true denominator.** The *sine qua non* of epidemiology is the denominator. Even so, reproductive epidemiologists must cope with outcomes for which the denominator is unknown. The classic example is birth defects. We observe the *prevalence* of malformations at birth, but we cannot observe *incidence* at the time the embryo's organs are being formed. To the extent that malformations reduce the survival of the embryo and fetus during pregnancy, birth prevalence will be less than the incidence.
2. **We can observe only eligible segments of the population, not the whole.** To the extent that some people never attempt pregnancy, it is not possible to describe the prevalence of reproductive problems for a "whole population." We can observe outcomes only among the subset who participate in reproduction. For example, the prevalence of infertility cannot be known for an entire population but only for those who have unprotected intercourse. Those who (for whatever reason) never participate in unprotected intercourse are not a random sample of the population; this group can vary in size and characteristics among different populations.

3. **Couples who are trying to conceive at any given time are highly selected.** Most people are biologically capable of producing more children than they want. As a result, most people take measures to restrict their fertility during most of their reproductive lives. Such restrictions are not random—they depend on access to effective contraception, social and economic conditions, and the outcomes of previous pregnancies. Past outcomes can influence future behavior in particularly complex ways. If a couple's experience of a poor outcome alters their behavior (including decisions about future pregnancies), then their behaviors can become associated with risk in misleading and noncausal ways (see Chapter 7).
4. **The quality of data on reproductive outcomes varies from near-perfect to nonexistent.** At one end of the spectrum, variables such as infant mortality and birth weight are precisely measurable, recorded by law, and freely available online for whole populations. Data of more middling quality are recorded for miscarriages and birth defects in clinical and official records, with no single source capturing them all. At the low end of the data-quality spectrum are very early pregnancy losses (those occurring before 6 weeks). In the past 25 years, roughly 37 million early losses have occurred in the United States, of which 143 have been documented.[6–11]
5. **Pathologic conditions involve more than one person.** Unlike most diseases, reproductive problems usually involve several people. In studies of infertility, both the man and the woman must be considered. If the endpoint is preterm delivery, then studies must include at least the mother and her fetus. If birth defects are the topic, then father, mother, and fetus are all relevant contributors. In a study of the genetic aspects of reproductive problems, family relationships become even more important. For example, if both the fetus and the mother carry a gene variant that impairs the metabolism of folate, the risk of neural tube defects may be greater than if only one of them carries the variant.[12]
6. **Adverse events range from the extremely common to the extremely rare.** The incidence of reproductive endpoints spans four orders of magnitude. Homocystinuria (a genetic error of metabolism for which newborn babies are routinely screened) is found in 0.5 out of 10,000 births.[13] There are dozens of birth defects in the range of 5 to 10 per 10,000 births.[14] Stillbirth and infant mortality both fall in the range of 50 to 100 births per 10,000 in many developed countries. Preterm delivery occurs in about 500 to 1000 of 10,000 births, the risk of miscarriage is about 1,200 per 10,000 clinical pregnancies, and earlier loss (before clinical recognition) occurs in about 2,500 per 10,000 implantations.[6] For the relatively common outcomes (such as preterm delivery or miscarriage), the odds ratio does not provide an accurate estimate of the relative risk. This is a common mistake when interpreting the analysis of reproductive data.

7. **Time between exposure and outcome can be very short or very long.** An often-stated advantage of studying reproductive toxicants is the short time from exposure to outcome. Teratogens can produce a detectable birth defect within 9 months. A toxicant could in principle make a man azospermic in 9 weeks—the time it takes mature spermatozoa to develop from the spermatogonia. However, not all latencies are short. Exposures in pregnancy can also produce damage to the fetus that does not become apparent for decades. Diethylstilbestrol (DES) given to pregnant women caused changes in their female fetuses that, 50 years later, caused the daughters to have an increased risk of breast cancer.[15] The possibility of extremely long latency is a serious complication in studies of toxic exposures to the fetus (see Chapter 20).
8. **Reproductive endpoints do not occur in isolation.** Even though studies focus on particular endpoints (infertility or miscarriage risk or specific birth defects), these endpoints are all part of a continuum of development. If a reproductive toxicant has different effects on this continuum at different doses, a confusing dose-response pattern may result. For example, an exposure at low doses might increase the risk of a birth defect, whereas at high doses it may cause frank embryonic death. A study of the birth defect alone might suggest greater risk at low doses of the exposure than at high doses.[16]
9. **Reproductive data are a private matter.** Epidemiologic studies may require the collection of information on topics that are not ordinarily shared with strangers. These include sexual behaviors, sexual partners, sexual orientation, sexually transmitted diseases, methods of birth control, history of fetal or infant deaths, and induced abortions. The information people are willing to provide may not be complete or accurate.
10. **Not all domains of reproduction lie within the medical sphere.** Cases cannot necessarily be identified within a clinical setting. For example, not all infertile couples seek medical assistance. To do population-based studies of infertility or miscarriage risk may require data collection outside the medical system. It follows that the clinical validation of certain outcomes may be difficult.
11. **Reproductive endpoints can compete with one another.** An increase in one risk can decrease the risk of another. For example, if a pregnancy ends in miscarriage, the pregnancy cannot end in a preterm birth. A pregnancy that ends in preterm delivery is not at risk of stillbirth at term. Such trade-offs among competing outcomes could easily lead to mistaken causal inferences. To the extent possible, the events of reproduction should be considered comprehensively rather than as isolated outcomes.
12. **Different reproductive endpoints can be linked by shared causes.** Unmeasured factors can disrupt reproduction at several stages and, in so doing, create associations that link seemingly unrelated problems. For example, couples who are subfertile also have a higher risk of preeclampsia.[17] Such

associations can create further confusions in that treatment for the earlier outcome may be associated with the later outcome. Thus, fertility treatments might be blamed for preeclampsia when the association is a result of the relation of infertility with preeclampsia.

13. **Is the unit of analysis the mother or the pregnancy?** In exploring pregnancy risk, one can analyze pregnancies as individual events or as the total reproductive experience of a given mother. When the mother is the unit of analysis, the observed outcomes of her pregnancies provide a "sample" of her underlying risk. The choice of approach depends in part on the question being addressed. The assessment of individual pregnancies is appropriate when the risk factor varies by place or time. More stable risk factors (such as genes or persistent exposures) may be better approached by considering a woman's complete reproductive history. One unbiased approach is to restrict analysis to first pregnancies.[18] The options may also be limited by the data source. Vital statistics provide data for pregnancies in isolation, not linked by mother, and so pregnancies are of necessity the unit of analysis. The mother can be the unit of analysis when data come from studies that collect complete pregnancy histories (with the potential for recall errors) or from population registries that link all pregnancies of a given mother. Registries have beginning and ending dates, which complicate the assessment of "complete" pregnancy histories.
14. **Strong associations suggest reverse causation.** Large risks are generally considered evidence for causation, and reproductive studies are no exception—except that in reproductive epidemiology, reverse causation is also a source of strong associations. An example is prenatal care and preterm delivery. Mothers who have more frequent prenatal visits have a markedly reduced risk of preterm delivery.[19] At first, it was tempting to interpret this association as an argument in support of more prenatal visits. However, an association can arise because mothers with shorter pregnancies have less opportunity for prenatal visits. In this case, preterm birth causes the reduced number of prenatal visits, rather than vice versa. More subtle variations of reverse causation abound in reproductive epidemiology, in part because the events of reproduction occur in such a compressed time period.[20]

References

1. Hardy JB. The Collaborative Perinatal Project: lessons and legacy. *Ann Epidemiol* 2003;13(5):303–11.
2. Olsen J, Melbye M, Olsen SF, et al. The Danish National Birth Cohort—its background, structure and aim. *Scand J Public Health* 2001;29(4):300–7.
3. Magnus P, Irgens LM, Haug K, Nystad W, Skjaerven R, Stoltenberg C. Cohort profile: the Norwegian Mother and Child Cohort Study (MoBa). *Int J Epidemiol* 2006;35(5):1146–50.

4. Keim S. The National Children's Study of Children's Health and the Environment. *Children Youth Environ* 2005;15(1):240–56.
5. Lambe M, Hultman C, Torrang A, Maccabe J, Cnattingius S. Maternal smoking during pregnancy and school performance at age 15. *Epidemiology* 2006;17(5):524–30.
6. Wilcox AJ, Weinberg CR, O'Connor JF, et al. Incidence of early loss of pregnancy. *N Engl J Med* 1988;319(4):189–94.
7. Zinaman MJ, Clegg ED, Brown CC, O'Connor J, Selevan SG. Estimates of human fertility and pregnancy loss. *Fertil Steril* 1996;65(3):503–9.
8. Eskenazi B, Gold EB, Lasley BL, et al. Prospective monitoring of early fetal loss and clinical spontaneous abortion among female semiconductor workers. *Am J Ind Med* 1995;28(6):833–46.
9. Ellish NJ, Saboda K, O'Connor J, Nasca PC, Stanek EJ, Boyle C. A prospective study of early pregnancy loss. *Hum Reprod* 1996;11(2):406–12.
10. Taylor CA Jr, Overstreet JW, Samuels SJ, et al. Prospective assessment of early fetal loss using an immunoenzymometric screening assay for detection of urinary human chorionic gonadotropin. *Fertil Steril* 1992;57(6):1220–4.
11. Hakim RB, Gray RH, Zacur H. Infertility and early pregnancy loss. *Am J Obstet Gynecol* 1995;172(5):1510–7.
12. van der Put NMJ, van den Heuvel RP, Steegers-Theunissen RPM, et al. Decreased methylene tetra hydrofolate reductase activity due to the 677C-to-T mutation in families with spina bifida offspring. *J Molec Med* 1996;74(11):691–4.
13. Hellekson KL. NIH consensus statement on phenylketonuria. *Am Fam Physician* 2001;63(7):1430–2.
14. Lary JM, Paulozzi LJ. Sex differences in the prevalence of human birth defects: a population-based study. *Teratology* 2001;64(5):237–51.
15. Palmer JR, Wise LA, Hatch EE, et al. Prenatal diethylstilbestrol exposure and risk of breast cancer. *Cancer Epidemiol Biomarkers Prev* 2006;15(8):1509–14.
16. Selevan SG, Lemasters GK. The dose-response fallacy in human reproductive studies of toxic exposures. *J Occup Med* 1987;29(5):451–4.
17. Basso O, Weinberg CR, Baird DD, Wilcox AJ, Olsen J. Subfecundity as a correlate of preeclampsia: a study within the Danish National Birth Cohort. *Am J Epidemiol* 2003;157(3):195–202.
18. Olsen J. Options in making use of pregnancy history in planning and analysing studies of reproductive failure. *J Epidemiol Community Health* 1994;48(2):171–4.
19. Shwartz S. Prenatal care, prematurity, and neonatal mortality. A critical analysis of prenatal care statistics and associations. *Am J Obstet Gynecol* 1962;83:591–8.
20. Stein Z, Susser M. Miscarriage, caffeine, and the epiphenomena of pregnancy: the causal model. *Epidemiology* 1991;2(3):163–7.

II

OUTCOMES

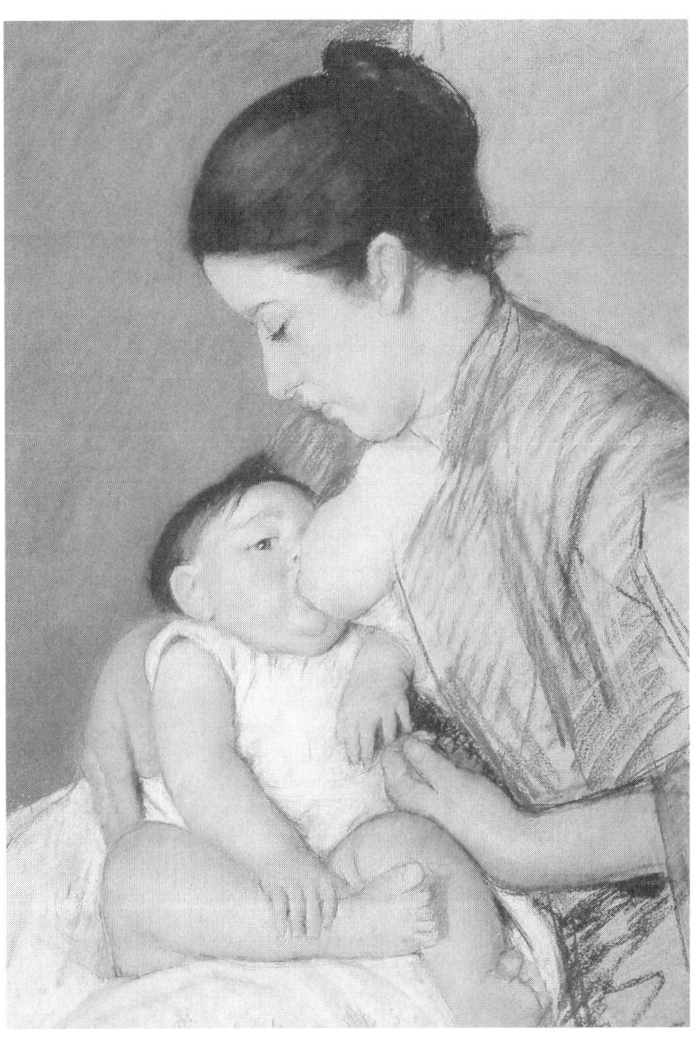

Maternite, Mary Cassatt, 1890

9

Fertility and Fecundability

The capacity to conceive is, for most couples, a valued part of their health. Despite its importance, there is no comprehensive way to assess this capacity before the couple actually attempts pregnancy. The assessment of fertile capacity at a population level is nearly as difficult.

Infertility is one of the most common health concerns among young adults. Ten to fifteen percent of couples report that they are unable to have the number of children they would like.[1] Behind this simple statistic lies a much more complex picture.

Fertility as a Continuum

At its essence, fertility is a matter of probability. A couple's chances of conceiving with unprotected intercourse on the most fertile days of a menstrual cycle can vary from zero to quite high. This underlying probability is expressed in the time (number of cycles) a couple requires to conceive. Couples with a high probability of conception are likely to conceive within one or two cycles. Couples with a low probability of conceiving may take many cycles of trying. These couples may be diagnosed as *subfertile* or *infertile*—that is, reduced in their chances compared with most couples. Couples with a zero chance of conceiving will not conceive naturally no matter how many cycles they try—they are *sterile.*

The fact that fertility is a continuous variable means that any definition of infertility is somewhat arbitrary. Infertility is usually defined clinically as a failure to conceive after 1 year (or sometimes 2 years) of trying.[2] Some clinicians regard even 6 months without pregnancy as evidence of subfertility and a basis for clinical treatment,[3] especially in older women whose window of opportunity is already diminished. In any group of couples having trouble conceiving, some will be sterile and others will not; indeed, some couples will conceive in their next cycle of trying. This capacity of "infertile" couples to conceive must be kept in mind when evaluating clinical interventions. (Conception by an "infertile" couple is not proof that a therapy is efficacious.)

Another difficulty with defining infertility is the fact that it is a characteristic of two people, not one. Two relatively infertile people may have difficulty conceiving with each other but be successful with other partners who are more fertile. Thus, an individual's apparent fertility may change (for better or for worse) with a change in partners.

Infertility is usually not diagnosed until the couple has actually attempted to conceive. Some couples may be aware of potential problems (for example, if the woman has had extremely irregular cycles, or the man has experienced mumps as an adult). However, for most healthy couples, the current tools of clinical examination and testing are unlikely to provide reliable information on the couple's capacity to conceive.[4] The best way for most couples to know their reproductive capacity is actually to try to become pregnant. This creates a dilemma for couples who might prefer to defer their childbearing but would not delay if they knew their fertility was already marginal.

Definitions

The definitions of fertility and infertility are further complicated by the fact that the terms are not always used consistently. *Fecundity* is generally accepted as a person's (or a couple's) capacity to produce a baby. *Fertility* is also commonly used in this way (as in this chapter so far). *Fertility* is also used in a completely different sense, as the actual production of a baby rather than the capacity to produce a baby. This definition is standard among demographers. (For example, the *total fertility rate* discussed in Chapter 3 uses fertility in this sense.) Epidemiologists follow the more colloquial (and medical) use of fertility as capacity to conceive.

Infertility is a term used to describe couples who are having difficulty conceiving but are not necessariliy unable to conceive. *Primary infertility* refers to couples who have been unable to conceive at any time in the past, and *secondary infertility* describes couples with at least one previous pregnancy who have problems subsequently. *Subfertility* is a loosely defined term that means "less fertile than normal."

The word *fecundability* is a less familiar term, but a useful one for epidemiologists. Fecundability is a quantitative measure of a couple's capacity to conceive, defined as the couple's probability of conceiving in one menstrual cycle (assuming the couple is having regular unprotected intercourse). We cannot know a given couple's fecundability, but we can calculate the mean fecundability for a group

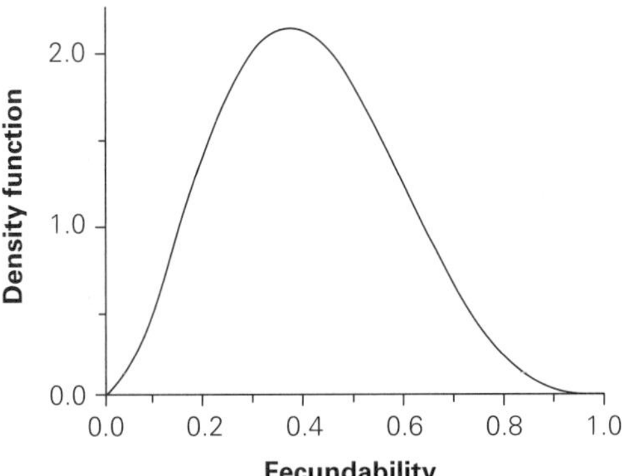

Figure 9-1. Estimated distribution of fecundability (calculated from time-to-pregnancy data for 486 nonsmoking women, Minnesota, 1983) (Adapted from Weinberg and Gladen[5])

of couples. Like any probability, fecundability cannot be less than zero or greater than 100%. Fecundability probably never actually reaches 100%, but we know there is a wide range among couples. Figure 9-1 shows an estimated distribution of fecundability.[5] Couples who are at the low end of the spectrum could expect to have to try for a while before they are able to achieve pregnancy. Couples who have high fecundability will, on average, conceive quickly.

Fertility as an Epidemiologic Endpoint

Epidemiologists have several options for the study of human fertility, all of them imperfect. One is the study of male semen characteristics. This can in principle be done among the general population, although the proportion of men who are willing to participate in such studies is limited. In women, one can study the menstrual cycle. Women with irregular cycles are at increased risk of infertility, although ordinary menstrual patterns are no guarantee of normal fertility. Yet another epidemiologic approach is the study of clinically diagnosed infertility, based on the selected couples who seek clinical treatment. A fourth option is the study of fecundability, based on measures of time to pregnancy.

Epidemiologic Measures of Male Fertility

A semen sample (usually obtained by masturbation) allows sperm characteristics to be assessed at a particular point in time. Semen analysis includes measures of semen volume and sperm concentration, motility, and morphology. (Sperm assays based on DNA integrity hold promise for epidemiologic studies, although these assays have not yet been as well characterized.[6]) Although semen analysis has the advantage of being a direct bioassay, the data are not simple to interpret. To begin with, the necessary laboratory methods are not simple. Large variations are found among laboratories, and quality control procedures are often lacking.[7]

Semen characteristics also vary for a given man. One very important consideration is time since last ejaculation: a man's sperm concentration can double as the time since previous ejaculation increases.[8] Other factors that affect semen parameters are conditions at collection, the way the specimen is stored and handled before analysis, and season of the year. Even controlling such factors does not remove individual variability. Figure 9-2 shows changes in sperm concentrations within men who collected monthly specimens under well-controlled conditions.[9] Because of this variability, semen specimens are sometimes collected from men at several points in time and averaged to get a more stable assessment of a man's baseline semen parameters.

As if these problems were not enough, epidemiologists must also cope with the fact that true population-based studies of sperm characteristics are virtually impossible. Many men are reluctant to take part in semen studies. Although participation can sometimes reach 50%, many published studies are based on data with participation rates less than 30%.[10,11] Low participation rates leave open the possibility of selection among participants—for example, men with prior evidence

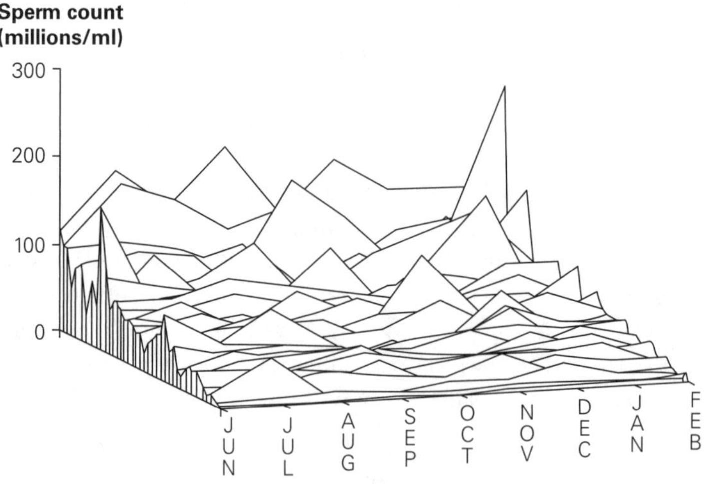

Figure 9-2. Individual variation in sperm concentration over time (monthly data from 45 young men for nine consecutive months, United States, 1986–87)[9] (Unpublished figure courtesy of Steven Schrader)

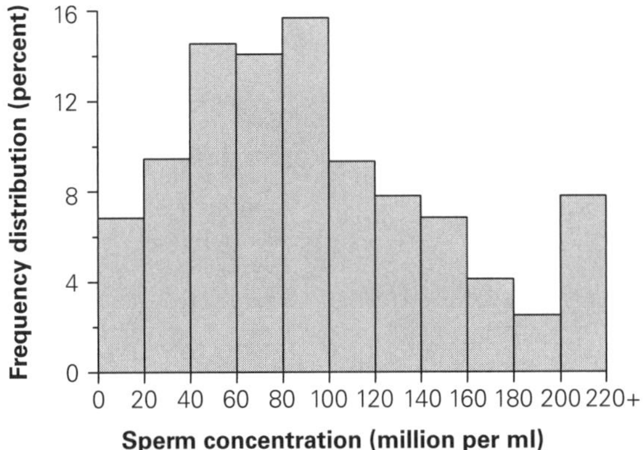

Figure 9-3. Variability in sperm concentration among fertile men at vasectomy (190 men, France, 1973–78) (Data from David et al[16])

of infertility problems are more likely to volunteer for semen studies.[12] Men with vasectomies cannot participate and are likely to be among the most fertile. Thus, even the most basic descriptive statements about "population-level" semen characteristics must be regarded with caution.

The Sorry Tale of DBCP

One of the most notorious exposures related to fertility is dibromochloropropane (DBCP), a highly effective fumigant used to eradicate plant pests. In 1977, a paper in *The Lancet* reported that of 25 men who worked in the manufacture of DBCP, 11 had either no sperm or sperm concentrations below 1 million per cc.[13] The U.S. EPA suspended most uses of DBCP immediately, and Dow Chemical Company halted all production of DBCP. However, Dow had some left over and sold 500,000 gallons of the fumigant to Dole Foods for their banana plantations in Central America. (DBCP increases banana harvests by 20%.) Subsequent exposures to thousands of plantation workers in Latin America have generated ongoing lawsuits.[14]

Given all these caveats, the most striking thing about human semen is its low quality compared with that of other mammals.[15] Even in "normal" men, most sperm have abnormal forms. Figure 9-3 shows a distribution of one of the most basic semen parameters, the concentration of sperm (in millions) per milliliter of semen (colloquially called the "sperm count"). These data come from 170 men who had fathered at least one child and who provided a semen sample at the time of vasectomy.[16] Although these data do not necessarily characterize the men at the time they fathered a child, the data suggest that sperm counts can vary widely even among fertile men—in this example, more than 10-fold.

Table 9-1 WHO reference values for "normal" semen parameters

Semen parameters	WHO normal value[17]
Volume	2 cc or more
Concentration	20 million per cc or more
Motility	50% or more
Viability	75% or more
Normal morphology	30% or more

What constitutes an "abnormal" semen finding? The World Health Organization has provided criteria for "normal" levels of various semen parameters (Table 9-1).[17] Given the wide variability across laboratories, WHO emphasizes that these numbers are only guidelines, although, in the absence of better alternatives, these criteria are widely cited. At the lowest extreme, there is no question that poor semen parameters predict poor fertility: men without sperm are sterile. Men whose sperm lacks normal motility or morphology are severely limited in their capacity to father children. But the true relationship of sperm measures to fertility is not well captured in dichotomies.

Figure 9-4 shows the estimated fecundability (the per-cycle probability of conception) across four standard semen parameters.[18] The semen parameters that best predict fertility are sperm concentration (in the lower range) and the proportion of nonmotile sperm. Semen volume has practically no association with fecundability.

LATENCY OF TOXIC EFFECTS ON SPERM. A few occupational exposures have been associated with effects on semen parameters, including DBCP (see Box on DBCP) and lead.[19] One factor that complicates the epidemiologic study of semen parameters is the fact that toxic effects can have latencies ranging from days to decades. An acute exposure that damages adult spermatozoa (perhaps impairing motility) could in principle be detected almost immediately. Damage to spermatogenesis would not be manifest in men until 9 weeks after exposure, at the time the exposed cohort of sperm reaches maturity. At the extreme, exposures may not be manifest until a generation later. Maternal smoking during pregnancy has been associated with lower sperm concentrations in their adult sons.[20]

Epidemiologic Measures of Female Fertility

The most easily observed aspect of a woman's reproductive function is her menstrual cycle. The absence of menses usually means a woman is not ovulating. Irregular menses are associated with reduced fecundability[21] and can be a sign of underlying pathology (such as polycystic ovary disease or thyroid dysfunction). However, even women with highly variable cycles can be fertile.

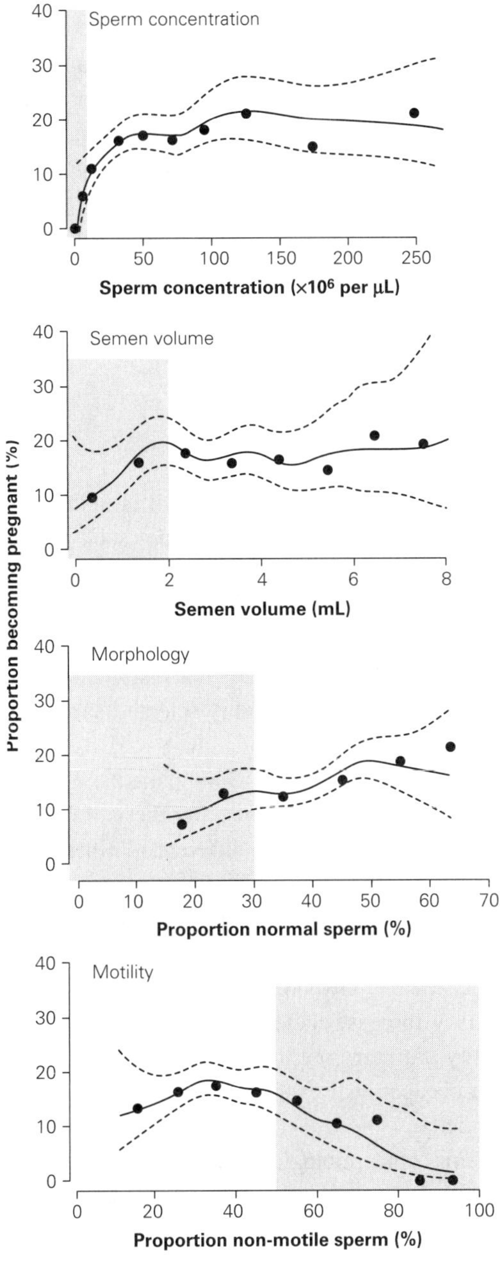

Figure 9-4. Mean fecundability by four standard semen parameters. Dashed lines are 95% confidence intervals (Shaded areas correspond to semen parameters outside the "normal" range according to WHO criteria.) (Reprinted from Bonde et al[18] © 1998, with permission from Elsevier)

Menstrual cycles can be studied at various levels of detail. Women can simply be asked their usual cycle length and how much their cycles usually vary. More exact information can be obtained from menstrual diaries, in which women prospectively record their bleeding days. The most detailed information comes from menstrual diaries combined with daily hormonal measures (usually in urine). Within the usual range of variation, even cycle-related hormones may have little value in predicting fertility.[22] Female hormone levels (follicle-stimulating hormone and estradiol) have some predictive value among infertile women being treated by assisted reproductive technology,[23] but it is not known how well these tests might generalize to an unselected population. Menstrual disruption may be useful as a marker of exposure to reproductive toxicants, but this remains a relatively unexplored area of epidemiologic research.[24]

Epidemiologic Study of Clinical Infertility

Infertility is an unusual "health problem" in that it is neither visible nor life threatening. Those who are affected may or may not seek medical care. Data from several countries suggest that among couples who meet the usual medical criterion of infertility (12 months of trying without pregnancy), only about half go to a doctor for advice.[25] Among those who see a doctor, fewer than half have diagnostic procedures and get treatment. Thus, studies of infertility based on diagnosed patients are likely to be a highly selected sample of all infertile couples.

There are further difficulties in studying clinic patients. There are a range of possible diagnostic procedures and treatments, and these are not conducted in a systematic order. Different clinics may have different routines, and the diagnosis given to a couple who has multiple problems may vary depending on the order in which tests are conducted. Even with complete workups, not every infertile couple has an obvious reason for their difficulty; 5%–15% of infertile couples are normal on every clinical test.[26,27] Given the effectiveness of in vitro fertilization for most types of infertility, there is becoming less reason to establish a firm cause of the couple's infertility. Furthermore, clinic patients are likely to offer small numbers of cases with occupational exposures or other exposures suspected of having reproductive toxicity.

Despite these problems, epidemiologic studies of clinic patients offer some advantages. The diagnostic tests performed as part of the clinical workup provide information about specific mechanisms of infertility (for example, anovulation or blocked tubes or low sperm count) that can help focus etiologic hypothesis. Also, couples who are already being seen in a clinical setting are often willing to undergo additional tests as part of a research protocol (for example, semen analyses or ultrasound procedures). Some of the more common clinical causes of infertility are discussed below.

CLINICAL REASONS FOR MALE INFERTILITY. Among the diagnoses that contribute to male infertility are adult mumps, birth defects of the male genitalia including undescended testicle (even after repair), Klinefelter syndrome, and microdeletions in the Y chromosome.[28] Even though varicocele (varicose veins of the testes) is often discussed as a "treatable" cause of infertility,[29] a Cochrane review of clinical trials has found no evidence that treatment improves fertility.[30] Obesity has recently been identified as a risk factor for male infertility, perhaps through endocrine dysregulation.[31]

CLINICAL REASONS FOR FEMALE INFERTILITY. A common condition underlying female infertility is polycystic ovary syndrome. Symptoms are irregularity or absence of ovulation (with resulting menstrual irregularity), obesity, and increased body hair caused by excess production of androgens. Women with polycystic ovary syndrome are often insulin resistant or frankly diabetic. The causes of polycystic ovary syndrome are unknown, and there is no known cure. There are several obstacles to the epidemiologic study of this condition: the pathology that gives this condition its name (cysts in the ovary) is not externally apparent, its symptoms are nonspecific, and the diagnostic criteria remain a matter of controversy.[32]

Other common causes of infertility are endometriosis and fibroids (see Chapter 18) and pelvic inflammatory disease (see Chapter 4). Women with Turner syndrome (a single X chromosome) are completely sterile. Low caloric intake and obesity are both associated with female infertility,[33] as is extreme exercise.[34]

Epidemiologic Study of Fecundability

Fecundability is a simple concept: it is the probability that a couple will conceive in a given menstrual cycle, given ordinary patterns of intercourse and no use of birth control. (By *conceive*, we usually mean a pregnancy that survives long enough to become clinically detectable; fecundability can also be defined as time to the conception of live births.) Fecundability integrates all the biological pathways that contribute to conception as well as factors that affect the survival of the fertilized conceptus to the time of clinical recognition or birth. Thus, fecundability provides a broad, non-specific fertility endpoint. It is impossible to determine fecundability directly, but it can be measured indirectly through the number of cycles a couple takes to become pregnant (time to pregnancy).

Time to pregnancy is only an approximation of a couple's fecundability. Two couples with equal fecundability (say, 20%) may have completely different experiences in trying to get pregnant simply because of chance. Twenty percent of such couples will conceive in their first cycle of trying, and 7% will still not be pregnant even after 12 cycles. If each couple could provide time-to-pregnancy data for 50 or 100 pregnancies, we could arrive at a good estimate of their fecundability.

Unfortunately for epidemiologists, this is not practical. The best we can do is to estimate the mean fecundability for groups of couples and then observe how this mean fecundability might differ across groups that differ by some key characteristic we are interested in studying.

Demographers developed the original concept of fecundability and, from studies of live births, determined that the average probability of conceiving in 1 month is around 25%.[35] This percentage is affected by how pregnancy is defined. The fecundability rate would be slightly higher when pregnancies that end in miscarriage are also included. The highest estimates of fecundability would include all detectable pregnancies, as observed for example in prospective studies that monitor conceptions among women who are trying to conceive.[36] A typical pattern of conception rates for clinical pregnancies is seen in Table 9-2.

This life-table presents a theoretical cohort of 1,000 couples who are discontinuing any methods of birth control in order to become pregnant. Fifty couples (5%) are designated as sterile, although they are not aware of this at the beginning of observation (5% is the estimated sterility rate for young couples.[37]). Each row represents a menstrual cycle. A certain proportion of women conceive in each cycle (column D) and are thus removed from further consideration (they are no longer eligible to become pregnant). The "survivors" are couples who do not conceive in a given cycle and are thus available to try again.

The proportion who conceive (fecundability) is highest in the first cycle and steadily declines thereafter (column E). This decline does not represent a true change in fecundability over a short time. Rather, it reflects the gradual accumulation of infertile and sterile couples among those who have not yet conceived. The couples who are most fertile conceive the most quickly (on average), leaving the less fertile to try again. Sterile couples comprise a steadily growing proportion of the surviving couples (column B as a proportion of column A). The increasing concentration of the less fertile and the sterile among the "survivors" produces the apparent drop in fecundability.

The numbers in this table are a fair summary of results seen in many studies. Typically, about 60% of couples conceive within 3 cycles, about 80% within 6 cycles, and about 90% within 12 cycles.[3,38] Even among the "infertile" (those who have not conceived after a year), about half will conceive in the next 3 years even without medical treatment. (In the life table example, 58 nonsterile couples still had not conceived after 12 cycles of trying, out of a total of 108 nonpregnant couples.) All these percentages can of course vary depending on age and other factors that affect the couple's fertility, as well as the proportion of sterile couples in the population.

The first cycle is not merely the cycle with the highest proportion of pregnancies—it is also the cycle that demonstrates the mean fecundability for the population. The proportion conceiving in the first cycle is an unbiased estimate of the true fecundability of the whole population (including the sterile couples) before any selection has taken place.

Table 9-2 A simulated pattern of monthly conception rates among 1,000 couples who have discontinued a nonhormonal method of birth control

Cycle	A Couples trying to conceive at the beginning of the cycle	B Sterile couples	C Fertile couples (A−B)	D Clinical pregnancies	E Percentage of couples who conceive (D/A)	F Cumulative percentage of couples who have conceived
1	1,000	50	950	285	29%	29%
2	715	50	665	180	25%	46%
3	535	50	485	121	23%	59%
4	414	50	364	87	21%	67%
5	327	50	277	61	19%	73%
6	266	50	216	43	16%	78%
7	223	50	173	33	15%	81%
8	190	50	140	25	13%	84%
9	165	50	115	19	12%	85%
10	145	50	95	15	10%	87%
11	130	50	80	12	9%	88%
12	118	50	68	10	8%	89%
13	108	50	58			

STUDYING TIME TO PREGNANCY. The crucial data required for Table 9-2 are times to pregnancy (number of cycles) for a cohort of couples. This information can be collected either prospectively or retrospectively and then used to calculate the underlying fecundability of the group. Intercourse frequency and timing can affect fecundability, especially if frequency is low.[39] Data on intercourse frequency should be included in fecundability analyses if possible.

As mentioned above, fecundability can be conveniently estimated by the proportion who conceive in the first cycle, although this does not take full advantage of the available information. A more powerful way to estimate fecundability is to model the underlying distribution of fecundability, for example, as a beta-geometric distribution.[40]

For comparing the fecundability of different groups, the usual approach is to use a discrete form of the Cox proportional hazard model.[41] This provides an estimated hazards ratio (in this case, a fecundability ratio) that lends itself to multivariate adjustment. Unlike hazards ratios for outcomes such as cancer or heart disease, in which a ratio less than 1.0 indicates a benefit, a fecundability ratio less than 1.0 indicates impairment. (Thus, a fecundability ratio of 0.5 means that couples are only half as likely to conceive in a given cycle as the reference group.) This approach allows adjustments for confounding and the capacity to adjust for exposures that change from cycle to cycle.

Collection of data. The gold standard for time to pregnancy is prospective data collection. Such studies have been conducted, although women who plan a pregnancy in advance may be a selected group (especially in the United States and other countries with a high proportion of unplanned pregnancies). Fortunately, women seem to be reasonably able to recall how many cycles they took to become pregnant (although perhaps not if the recall time is long[42]). Thus, time to (clinical) pregnancy can be a reasonable endpoint for retrospective studies. Also, couples may be more likely to cooperate in retrospective studies than in more intensive prospective studies, making it possible to generate fecundability estimates that are more nearly representative of the general population. For these reasons, fecundability has become an increasingly used tool in reproductive epidemiology.

Limitations to time-to-pregnancy studies. Although the measurement of time to pregnancy is simple in principle, the actual collection and analysis of data are fraught with pitfalls.[43] For example, the definition of cycle number needs to be handled carefully in questionnaires. Some couples who conceive immediately after stopping their birth control may say that they got pregnant in zero cycles, and others may say in one cycle. Such misclassification can create problems. Some women are unable to provide any number because they conceived accidentally. In that case, the correct time to pregnancy would be the total number of cycles in which the woman was at risk of accidental pregnancy, a number that is not straightforward to reconstruct.

Unplanned pregnancies are usually excluded from fecundability studies, but they leave behind selection problems in the remaining sample. Unplanned pregnancies tend to occur more often among the most fertile couples. (If two couples are using the same imperfect method of birth control, the couple more likely to conceive accidentally is the one that is more fertile.) Thus, where many pregnancies are unplanned, subfertile couples will be overrepresented among the remaining planned pregnancies. If unplanned pregnancies are more common among women with a particular exposure, this could bias an association between the exposure and reduced fecundability.

Another disadvantage of retrospective studies of time to pregnancy is that there is no simple way to include sterile couples. If an exposure were to cause sterility in a susceptible subgroup but had no effect on the fecundability of the remainder of the exposed, this effect could be missed in a study based only on couples who conceived.

Exposures would ideally be measured in every cycle, but this is seldom possible. The most relevant cycle is the first cycle of trying. Studies that measure exposure only in later cycles (for example, the cycle in which conception occurred) could be badly biased if the woman changed her behavior because she was having trouble conceiving.

Exposures that change over time can create other problems.[44] Suppose an exposure has become more prevalent with time (cell phones, for example). Women with the longest times to pregnancy will be the most likely to have begun their attempt when the exposure was less prevalent. Conversely, women with the shortest times to pregnancy will be more likely to have started their attempts later, when exposure prevalence had increased. An analysis that measures exposure only in the first cycle of trying (and fails to account for the changing prevalence of exposure over time) would conclude that cell phones improve fecundability. In the same manner, an exposure that has become less prevalent over time would appear to damage fecundability.

In spite of these difficulties of time-to-pregnancy studies, fecundability provides a fertility endpoint that integrates many possible biological mechanisms. One need have no specific mechanism in mind in order to explore factors that have an overall association with reduced fertility. One of the first applications of time-to-pregnancy was to show that cigarette smoking decreases women's fecundability.[45,46] The harmful effect of smoking on female fertility is widely accepted today, even though the specific pathways through which this occurs are still not established.[47] Other exposures that are emerging as possible factors that reduce fecundability include women's occupational exposures to solvents[48] and antineoplastic drugs,[49] and men's occupational exposure to pesticides.[50] Multivitamins with folic acid may reduce the risk of ovulatory infertility.[51]

Sterilization as Worker "Protection"

Companies can protect their workers from reproductive toxicants in several ways. One is to discontinue the use of the toxicant, as in DBCP (see Box on DBCP). Another is to improve industrial hygiene. This was the strategy taken with anesthetic gases. Initial studies had suggested that anesthetic gases may cause an increased risk of miscarriage.[52] More conclusive studies were never conducted because protections were so easily implemented. A third option is to ban fertile workers. This was the path chosen by a battery manufacturer known as Johnson Controls. Workers at Johnson Controls were exposed to such high levels of lead that it potentially endangered the fetuses of pregnant women. The company's response was to require women to certify that they were sterile before they were allowed to work in production jobs. Women who declined to be sterilized could lose their jobs. This policy was struck down by the U.S. Supreme Court in 1991 as discriminatory.[53]

RELATION OF FECUNDABILITY TO OTHER ADVERSE OUTCOMES. Infertile women appear more likely than other women to have a range of perinatal difficulties if they become pregnant. These include increased risks of preeclampsia,[54] preterm delivery,[55] and birth defects.[56] These correlations presumably reflect the presence of etiologic factors that contribute to both infertility and pregnancy problems. Although these problems may not be directly caused by fertility treatments, it is treatment that allows those perinatal risks to be expressed. The burden of those risks can fairly be regarded as part of the total public health burden associated with infertility and treatment.[57]

Is Human Fertility Declining over Time?

Why is the Birth Rate Constantly Declining?

Is there a general decline in fertility among Western civilized nations?... The one question which all must dread becomes apparent: not whether the birth rate is falling, but whether the fertility of our people is falling.

The New York Times, July 16, 1916[58]

Concerns about a possible decline in human fertility have been around for at least a century. One difference today is that the wide distribution of environmental pollutants provides reasonable hypotheses for possible causes of reduced fertility. Concern has been exacerbated by astonishingly low birth rates in some developed countries, often far below replacement levels (see Chapter 3). This has spurred speculation that we may be experiencing an actual biological decline in fecundability and not simply a reduction in desired family size.[59]

A decline in human fecundability would have profound consequences. Fiction writers have presented unsettling pictures of human societies dealing with mass infertility (*The Handmaid's Tale* by Margaret Atwood and *The Children of Men*, by P. D. James). The question is whether our fecundability is truly in decline and how soon we might be able to recognize it if it were.

Sperm Concentration over Time

In 1992, a meta-analysis was published showing an apparent decline in sperm concentration over the previous 50 years.[60] Data from this paper are shown in Figure 9-5. This report has been cited more than 1,000 times in the scientific literature, some dismissing the results, some supporting them, and some interpreting them differently. The weaknesses of the paper include all the problems with measuring semen analyses (discussed above) and more. As other authors have pointed out, when the data are restricted to studies from the last 20 years (the interval with most of the data), the figure shows an increase in sperm counts.[61]

Regardless of its validity, this paper has brought increased scientific attention to the epidemiology of semen parameters. There is some evidence that environmental pollutants such as polychlorinated biphenyls (PCBs) may affect aspects of semen, especially motility.[62]

"TESTICULAR DYSGENESIS SYNDROME." The hypothesis has been advanced that cryptorchidism, hypospadias, testicular cancer, and impaired semen parameters are all expressions of testicular toxicity that are increasing as a result of the presence of hormonally active environmental pollutants.[63] It is true that testicular

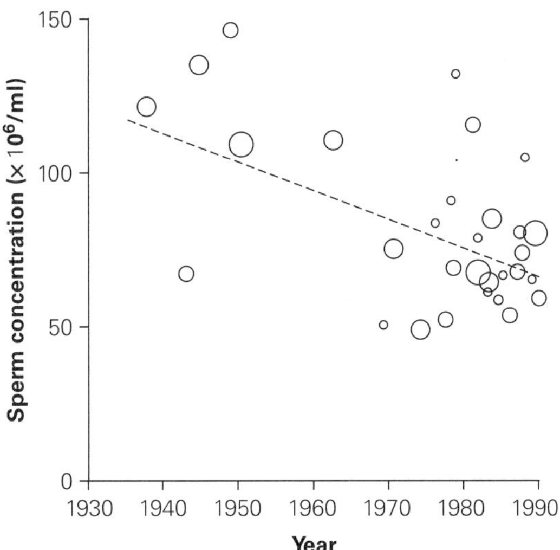

Figure 9-5. Mean sperm concentration over time as reported in 61 studies (Circles are proportional to the sample size of each study) (Reproduced from Carlsen et al[60] with permission from BMJ Publishing Group Ltd)

cancer rates are on the rise[64]—one of the few examples of cancer that is increasing. However, time trends for cryptorchidism and hypospadias (as well as sperm concentration) are much less clear.[65,66] The possibility that these several testicular conditions constitute an environmentally sensitive syndrome is intriguing (and one that its proponents are energetically pursuing), but it remains unproven.[67]

Fecundability over Time

A general decline in sperm quality would unquestionably be a matter of public health importance. However, even if such a trend were firmly established, it would not necessarily mean a detectable effect on human fecundability. A decline in mean sperm concentration could occur by a decrease in high sperm concentrations, for example, with no overall loss of fertility (Fig. 9-4).

Studies of time to pregnancy have attempted to reconstruct fecundability over recent decades, with mixed results. There have been vast social changes over the past five decades in the type and availability of birth control measures and in the availability of abortion. These social changes alter the mix of fecundability among the subset of couples who are trying to conceive, and this group is the only one that provides information on time to pregnancy. (These problems are less severe when various groups are compared within a given cultural context at a given point in time.) Assessing changes in fecundability during periods of social change raises daunting questions,[68] and studies of fecundability over time have shown little consistency.

There is no question that an extreme drop in fecundability would be detectable by current methods. The problem lies in the relative insensitivity of our methods and whether we would be able to recognize a more subtle decline in fecundability early enough to discover its cause and do something about it. For the meantime, the question of a possible decline in the human capacity to conceive remains unanswered.

References

1. Fertility, Family Planning, and Women's Health: New Data from the 1995 National Survey of Family Growth. In: Statistics USNCfH, ed. *Series 23: Data from the National Survey of Family Growth.* Hyattsville, MD, 1997.
2. Marchbanks PA, Peterson HB, Rubin GL, Wingo PA. Research on infertility: definition makes a difference. The Cancer and Steroid Hormone Study Group. *Am J Epidemiol* 1989;130(2):259–67.
3. Gnoth C, Godehardt E, Frank-Herrmann P, Friol K, Tigges J, Freundl G. Definition and prevalence of subfertility and infertility. *Hum Reprod* 2005;20(5):1144–7.
4. Maheshwari A, Bhattacharya S, Johnson NP. Predicting fertility. *Hum Fertil (Camb)* 2008;11(2):109–17.
5. Weinberg CR, Gladen BC. The beta-geometric distribution applied to comparative fecundability studies. *Biometrics* 1986;42(3):547–60.

6. Lewis SE, Agbaje I, Alvarez J. Sperm DNA tests as useful adjuncts to semen analysis. *Syst Biol Reprod Med* 2008;54(3):111–25.
7. Keel BA. How reliable are results from the semen analysis? *Fertil Steril* 2004;82(1):41–4.
8. Blackwell JM, Zaneveld LJ. Effect of abstinence on sperm acrosin, hypoosmotic swelling, and other semen variables. *Fertil Steril* 1992;58(4):798–802.
9. Schrader SM, Turner TW, Breitenstein MJ, Simon SD. Longitudinal study of semen quality of unexposed workers. I. Study overview. *Reprod Toxicol* 1988;2(3–4):183–90.
10. Giwercman A, Bonde JP. Declining male fertility and environmental factors. *Endocrinol Metab Clin North Am* 1998;27(4):807–30, viii.
11. Aggerholm AS, Thulstrup AM, Toft G, Ramlau-Hansen CH, Bonde JP. Is overweight a risk factor for reduced semen quality and altered serum sex hormone profile? *Fertil Steril* 2008;90(3):619–26.
12. Bonde JP, Giwercman A, Ernst E. Identifying environmental risk to male reproductive function by occupational sperm studies: logistics and design options. *Occup Environ Med* 1996;53(8):511–9.
13. Whorton D, Krauss RM, Marshall S, Milby TH. Infertility in male pesticide workers. *Lancet* 1977;2(8051):1259–61.
14. Spano J. Dole must pay farmworkers $3.2 million. Los Angeles Times, Los Angeles, 6 November 2007.
15. Aitken RJ, Sawyer D. The human spermatozoon--not waving but drowning. *Adv Exp Med Biol* 2003;518:85–98.
16. David G, Jouannet P, Martin-Boyce A, Spira A, Schwartz D. Sperm counts in fertile and infertile men. *Fertil Steril* 1979;31(4):453–5.
17. WHO. *WHO Laboratory Manual for the Examination of Human Semen and Sperm-Cervical Mucus Interactions*. 3rd ed. Cambridge: Cambridge University Press, 1992.
18. Bonde JP, Ernst E, Jensen TK, et al. Relation between semen quality and fertility: a population-based study of 430 first-pregnancy planners. *Lancet* 1998;352(9135):1172–7.
19. Winker R, Rudiger HW. Reproductive toxicology in occupational settings: an update. *Int Arch Occup Environ Health* 2006;79(1):1–10.
20. Ramlau-Hansen CH, Thulstrup AM, Storgaard L, Toft G, Olsen J, Bonde JP. Is prenatal exposure to tobacco smoking a cause of poor semen quality? A follow-up study. *Am J Epidemiol* 2007;165(12):1372–9.
21. Kolstad HA, Bonde JP, Hjollund NH, et al. Menstrual cycle pattern and fertility: a prospective follow-up study of pregnancy and early embryonal loss in 295 couples who were planning their first pregnancy. *Fertil Steril* 1999;71(3):490–6.
22. Baird DD, Wilcox AJ, Weinberg CR, et al. Preimplantation hormonal differences between the conception and non-conception menstrual cycles of 32 normal women. *Hum Reprod* 1997;12(12):2607–13.
23. Frazier LM, Grainger DA, Schieve LA, Toner JP. Follicle-stimulating hormone and estradiol levels independently predict the success of assisted reproductive technology treatment. *Fertil Steril* 2004;82(4):834–40.
24. Harlow SD, Ephross SA. Epidemiology of menstruation and its relevance to women's health. *Epidemiol Rev* 1995;17(2):265–86.
25. ESHRE Capri Workshop Group, Social determinants of human reproduction. *Hum Reprod* 2001;16:1518–26.

26. Adamson GD, Baker VL. Subfertility: causes, treatment and outcome. *Best Pract Res Clin Obstet Gynaecol* 2003;17(2):169–85.
27. de Boer EJ, den Tonkelaar I, Burger CW, van Leeuwen FE. Validity of self-reported causes of subfertility. *Am J Epidemiol* 2005;161(10):978–86.
28. Sadeghi-Nejad H, Farrokhi F. Genetics of azoospermia: current knowledge, clinical implications, and future directions. Part II: Y chromosome microdeletions. *Urol J* 2007;4(4):192–206.
29. Report on varicocele and infertility. *Fertil Steril* 2008;90(5 Suppl):S247–9.
30. Evers JH, Collins J, Clarke J. Surgery or embolisation for varicoceles in subfertile men. *Cochrane Database Syst Rev* 2008(3):CD000479.
31. Hammoud AO, Gibson M, Peterson CM, Meikle AW, Carrell DT. Impact of male obesity on infertility: a critical review of the current literature. *Fertil Steril* 2008;90(4):897–904.
32. Porter MB. Polycystic ovary syndrome: the controversy of diagnosis by ultrasound. *Semin Reprod Med* 2008;26(3):241–51.
33. Nutrition and reproduction in women. *Hum Reprod* Update 2006;12(3):193–207.
34. Redman LM, Loucks AB. Menstrual disorders in athletes. *Sports Med* 2005;35(9):747–55.
35. Leridon H. *Human Fertility: The Basic Components.* Chicago, IL: University of Chicago Press, 1977.
36. Wilcox AJ, Weinberg CR, O'Connor JF, et al. Incidence of early loss of pregnancy. *N Engl J Med* 1988;319(4):189–94.
37. Trussell J, WIlson, C. Sterility in a population with natural fertility. *Population Studies* 1985;39:269–86.
38. Tietze C, Guttmacher AF, Rubin S. Time required for conception in 1727 planned pregnancies. *Fertil Steril* 1950;1:338–46.
39. Stanford JB, Dunson DB. Effects of sexual intercourse patterns in time to pregnancy studies. *Am J Epidemiol* 2007;165(9):1088–95.
40. Sheps MC. On the time required for conception. *Population Studies* 1964;18:85–89.
41. Baird DD, Wilcox AJ, Weinberg CR. Use of time to pregnancy to study environmental exposures. *Am J Epidemiol* 1986;124(3):470–80.
42. Cooney MA, Louis GMB, Sundaram R, McGuiness BM, Lynch CD. Validity of self-reported time to pregnancy. *Epidemiology* 2009;20(1):56–9.
43. Weinberg CR, Wilcox AJ. *Modern Epidemiology.* 3rd ed. Philadelphia, PA: Wolters Kluwer/Lippincott Williams & Wilkins, 2008.
44. Weinberg CR, Baird DD, Wilcox AJ. Sources of bias in studies of time to pregnancy. *Stat Med* 1994;13(5–7):671–81.
45. Rachootin P, Olsen J. The risk of infertility and delayed conception associated with exposures in the Danish workplace. *J Occup Med* 1983;25(5):394–402.
46. Baird DD, Wilcox AJ. Cigarette smoking associated with delayed conception. *JAMA* 1985;253(20):2979–83.
47. Dorfman SF. Tobacco and fertility: our responsibilities. *Fertil Steril* 2008;89(3):502–4.
48. Sallmen M, Neto M, Mayan ON. Reduced fertility among shoe manufacturing workers. *Occup Environ Med* 2008:65(8):518–24.
49. Fransman W, Roeleveld N, Peelen S, de Kort W, Kromhout H, Heederik D. Nurses with dermal exposure to antineoplastic drugs: reproductive outcomes. *Epidemiology* 2007;18(1):112–9.

50. Bretveld R, Kik S, Hooiveld M, van Rooij I, Zielhuis G, Roeleveld N. Time-to-pregnancy among male greenhouse workers. *Occup Environ Med* 2008;65(3):185–90.
51. Chavarro JE, Rich-Edwards JW, Rosner BA, Willett WC. Use of multivitamins, intake of B vitamins, and risk of ovulatory infertility. *Fertil Steril* 2008;89(3):668–76.
52. Buring JE, Hennekens CH, Mayrent SL, Rosner B, Greenberg ER, Colton T. Health experiences of operating room personnel. *Anesthesiology* 1985;62(3):325–30.
53. *Automobile Workers v. Johnson Controls, Inc.*, 499 U.S. 187 (1991). The Oyez Project 1991.
54. Basso O, Weinberg CR, Baird DD, Wilcox AJ, Olsen J. Subfecundity as a correlate of preeclampsia: a study within the Danish National Birth Cohort. *Am J Epidemiol* 2003;157(3):195–202.
55. Basso O, Baird DD. Infertility and preterm delivery, birthweight, and Caesarean section: a study within the Danish National Birth Cohort. *Hum Reprod* 2003;18(11):2478–84.
56. Zhu JL, Basso O, Obel C, Bille C, Olsen J. Infertility, infertility treatment, and congenital malformations: Danish national birth cohort. *BMJ* 2006;333(7570):679.
57. Schieve LA, Cohen B, Nannini A, et al. A population-based study of maternal and perinatal outcomes associated with assisted reproductive technology in Massachusetts. *Matern Child Health J* 2007;11(6):517–25.
58. Carpenter B. Why is the birth rate constantly declining? *New York Times* July 16, 1916.
59. Skakkebaek NE, Jorgensen N, Main KM, et al. Is human fecundity declining? *Int J Androl* 2006;29(1):2–11.
60. Carlsen E, Giwercman A, Keiding N, Skakkebaek NE. Evidence for decreasing quality of semen during past 50 years. *BMJ* 1992;305(6854):609–13.
61. Olsen GW, Bodner KM, Ramlow JM, Ross CE, Lipshultz LI. Have sperm counts been reduced 50 percent in 50 years? A statistical model revisited. *Fertil Steril* 1995;63(4):887–93.
62. Hauser R. The environment and male fertility: recent research on emerging chemicals and semen quality. *Semin Reprod Med* 2006;24(3):156–67.
63. Sharpe RM, Skakkebaek NE. Testicular dysgenesis syndrome: mechanistic insights and potential new downstream effects. *Fertil Steril* 2008;89(2 Suppl):e33–8.
64. Bray F, Richiardi L, Ekbom A, Pukkala E, Cuninkova M, Moller H. Trends in testicular cancer incidence and mortality in 22 European countries: continuing increases in incidence and declines in mortality. *Int J Cancer* 2006;118(12):3099–111.
65. Safe SH. Endocrine disruptors and human health—is there a problem? An update. *Environ Health Perspect* 2000;108(6):487–93.
66. Barthold JS, Gonzalez R. The epidemiology of congenital cryptorchidism, testicular ascent and orchiopexy. *J Urol* 2003;170(6 Pt 1):2396–401.
67. Vidaeff AC, Sever LE. In utero exposure to environmental estrogens and male reproductive health: a systematic review of biological and epidemiologic evidence. *Reprod Toxicol* 2005;20(1):5–20.
68. Sallmen M, Weinberg CR, Baird DD, Lindbohm ML, Wilcox AJ. Has human fertility declined over time? Why we may never know. *Epidemiology* 2005;16(4):494–9.

10

Early Pregnancy Loss

The loss of a pregnancy between conception and the time a woman recognizes she is pregnant is, from one perspective, a component of infertility. If all of a woman's conceptions were to end in early loss, she would perceive herself as sterile. From another perspective, very early loss is part of a spectrum of pregnancy losses that extends to stillbirth.

There is no marker for the occurrence of a human conception. Fertilization can be observed in vitro under the rarified conditions of assisted reproductive technology, but fertilization of an egg in a woman's body produces no measurable signal. The subsequent voyage of the fertilized egg through the oviducts to the uterus remains cloaked in secrecy. Only as the blastocyst begins to implant and secrete hCG does the first hormonal signal of pregnancy become identifiable in mother's blood or urine. It is at least another week or two before a woman notices that her period is delayed. Soon after, she may begin to experience symptoms of pregnancy.

If the conceptus dies at any stage up to this point, the death will probably be unnoticed. The failed conceptus will be washed out in menstrual flow that is indistinguishable from ordinary menses. From a public health standpoint, such losses are of little or no importance. Still, they constitute a major portion of human reproductive wastage. Furthermore, to the degree that these losses are more likely to occur among damaged or defective conceptuses, the losses potentially affect the prevalence of every reproductive problem we observe among the survivors.

The Incidence of Early Pregnancy Loss

Estimating the Outer Bounds

Until the 1970s, the amount of early loss in humans was mostly a matter of speculation.[1] At the most, such loss could not exceed the upper bound set by the observed fecundability in human populations. If the mean probability of conceiving a clinically recognized pregnancy in one cycle is around 25%, then no more than 75% of all human conceptions could end in early loss (assuming a 100% conception rate in every cycle with unprotected intercourse). To the extent that the true conception rate is less than 100%, the amount of early loss would be less than 75%.

At the other extreme, early loss rate could in principle be zero, with every fertilized egg producing a clinical pregnancy. Although early losses had been documented in other primates, the first evidence of early pregnancy loss in humans was published in 1959.

Surgical Evidence

An extraordinary study was conducted in the 1940s and 1950s by Hertig and Rock (the same Rock who developed the birth control pill).[2] These researchers invited premenopausal women who were scheduled for hysterectomy to engage in unprotected intercourse before their surgery. After surgical removal, their reproductive organs were carefully inspected for fertilized ova. Over a 17-year period, 210 women ages 25 to 43 participated. Of these, 34 were carrying a fertilized conceptus at surgery; 24 conceptuses were judged to be normal under microscopic examination and 10 were judged to be abnormal. These unique data provided strong evidence of early pregnancy loss in humans, but without a reliable estimate of its extent.

Biochemical Evidence

The crucial advance in the measurement of early loss took place in the 1980s with the development of sensitive and specific assays for human chorionic gonadotropin (hCG). Produced by the conceptus, hCG is the cardinal hormonal signal of early pregnancy. The hormone quickly becomes detectable in maternal blood around the time of implantation and is excreted in urine. Human chorionic gonadotropin is a robust molecule and is highly stable in urine over time and under varying conditions of storage, a great advantage for field studies.

NONPREGNANCY HCG. Although hCG is highly specific to pregnancy, it can also be produced by the pituitary during the extreme transitions of menopause[3] and is made by most types of cancer cells.[4] (It is probably not coincidental that cancer cells imitate trophoblast cells in the production of hCG; both types of cells are characterized by extremely rapid proliferation, although cancer cells are far less organized.)

As increasingly sensitive hCG assays were developed, it became apparent that minute quantities of hCG can be found in healthy nonpregnant persons, including men.[5] All human cells carry the genetic instructions for the production of hCG, so it is not surprising that a few cells at any given time might have their molecular machinery accidentally activated for the production of hCG.

VARIETIES OF HCG. Human chorionic gonadotropin has many functions in early pregnancy, including enhancement of embryo implantation, stimulation of trophoblast invasion, and modulation of gene expression and enzyme production.[6] This versatility is enhanced by important structural variants of hCG, including a hyperglycosylated form that serves as a promoter of trophoblast invasion.[7] Assays to distinguish these varieties of hCG may eventually offer tools that allow epidemiologists to assess the viability of early conceptuses or the quality of placentation.

ASSAY-BASED STUDIES OF EARLY LOSS. Human chorionic gonadotropin has evolved to mimic LH (see Chapter 1). It is not surprising, therefore, that the early hCG immunoassays were not able to distinguish hCG from luteinizing hormone (LH). The first biochemical studies of early loss based on hCG were limited by the fact that ovulation could not be distinguished from a transient pregnancy.[8,9]

The development of a highly specific and sensitive assay for hCG (with virtually no cross-reaction to LH)[10] allowed the first direct measure of early pregnancy loss.[11] In a North Carolina study, 221 women who were planning a pregnancy were recruited from the community at the time they stopped using their method of birth control. Women collected daily urine samples for up to 6 months. Because hCG might be present at very low levels in nonpregnant women, a comparison group of women with tubal ligations was also enrolled. The criterion for a pregnancy was three consecutive days of hCG above a certain level not seen in the sterilized group. By this criterion, 199 pregnancies were detected among more than 700 cycles. Twenty-four percent of these pregnancies were lost very early, within the first 6 weeks after the last menstrual period.[11]

There is no gold standard against which to validate these losses—the evidence is entirely indirect. The putative losses occurred soon after ovulation among women who were trying to conceive, and there is a continuum of hCG profiles that extends from those meeting the minimum criteria for elevated hCG to those that resemble clinical miscarriages (Fig. 10-1).

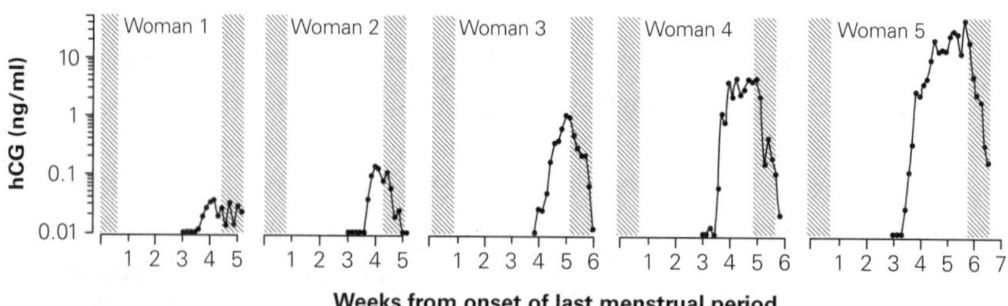

Figure 10-1. Spectrum of early pregnancy losses, as shown by hCG profiles from daily urine samples. Shaded bars indicate days of vaginal bleeding. (North Carolina, 1983–85) (Reprinted from Wilcox et al[11])

Women who volunteer for such intensive studies may not be representative of women in general, but similar estimates of early loss have been found with similar methods in a variety of settings.[12–15]

Estimating Total Pregnancy Loss

Studies of early pregnancy loss based on hCG can answer only one limited question: the extent to which pregnancies are lost after the time of implantation. The more complete question—the amount of loss after fertilization—remains tantalizingly beyond reach. One of the holy grails of reproductive biology has been a marker that would signal the fertilization of an ovum. Such markers have been claimed,[16] but none has so far proved valid.

The incidence of loss that occurs between conception and implantation could be substantial. In cycles being treated by advanced reproductive technologies (ART), more than half of embryos selected to be of good quality fail to implant.[17] If ART were carried out with all fertilized eggs instead of those selected to be good quality, the failure rate would presumably be even higher. However, the artificial conditions of ART make it difficult to extrapolate from these results to normally conceived pregnancies. Until there is a way to identify natural conception before implantation, this key chapter in the natural history of human pregnancy will remain incomplete.

Studies of Early Pregnancy Loss

Causes of Early Pregnancy Loss

In studies of early embryonic loss in domestic and laboratory animals, the risk of loss does not appear to be easily influenced by external exposures.[18] Among the handful of studies of early loss in humans, few external factors have been identified as possible causes, and none has been replicated.

Even the immediate biological causes of loss are not clear. It is plausible that many could be due to chromosomal abnormalities of the conceptus. Studies of later, clinically recognized miscarriages have found that about half carry chromosomal abnormalities.[19,20] Aneuploidy is also common among ART conceptions,[21] although the procedures of ART might contribute to this problem.

Conceptuses that take a longer time to implant after ovulation have a higher risk of early loss.[22] The direction of causality is not clear, however: do late-implanting conceptuses miss the window of optimum uterine readiness, or is their slowness a sign of their own frailty? As happens so often in reproductive epidemiology, both directions of cause and effect are plausible.

The Contribution of Early Loss to Time to Pregnancy

In principle, an increased risk of early loss will lengthen the time to clinical pregnancy. Thus, fecundability studies might provide an indirect way to detect an increase in early losses. As a simple example, assume a baseline mean fecundability of 30% for clinical pregnancies, and assume there is one undetected early loss for every three clinical pregnancies (25% loss). A doubling of the early loss rate (to 50%) would reduce the apparent clinical fecundability by one-third (from 30% to 20%). Thus, in interpreting a reduction in fecundability, one possible mechanism is increased early loss.

Does repeated early loss cause infertility in certain couples? There may be a subset of infertile women for whom repeated early losses are a factor.[14] However, for most women, an early loss appears to be relatively good news: early loss provides evidence that the woman is ovulating, the sperm are capable of reaching and fertilizing the egg, and the resulting conceptus is able to implant. Women who have an early loss appear to have relatively good fecundability in their subsequent cycle.[11,15]

Are Early Pregnancy Losses all "Unrecognized"?

There is a gray area of early loss in which it is difficult to distinguish between losses that occur without recognition and those that a woman recognizes. The bleeding that accompanies early losses provides no clue—bleeding with loss is like ordinary menses.[23] Whether the loss of an implanted conception is recognized depends on many things including a woman's attention to early symptoms, the regularity of her cycles (and the degree to which delayed menses might be apparent), and her access to pregnancy tests. A less subjective definition of early loss is loss within six weeks from the last menstrual period. This definition is easily replicated across studies, and 90% of the losses before this time occur without being specifically recognized by women.[11,24]

Bias in Studies of Early Pregnancy

An important potential bias in the estimation of early pregnancy loss comes from the hCG criterion chosen to define early pregnancy. Because trace hCG can come from nonpregnant sources, the definition of pregnancy usually requires hCG to persist above a certain level for a consecutive number of days. The more stringent this criterion, the more likely it is that small early losses might be missed. This lack of sensitivity will underestimate the proportion of pregnancy losses but without otherwise introducing bias.

In contrast, a lack of specificity in the definition of early loss will identify early losses in cycles where none exists. The problem with false positives is there are far more nonconception cycles (in which false positives might occur) than there are clinical conception cycles. Furthermore, nonconception cycles are not evenly distributed among women—they are more common in subfertile women. Thus, even a small false-positive error will lead to more apparent losses among less-fertile women, thus creating an association of early loss with factors associated with infertility.[25] The best protection against this bias is to set strict criteria that maximize specificity, even at the loss of some sensitivity.

The extent of loss among biochemically detected pregnancies is striking. Adding early losses to clinical miscarriages (discussed in the next chapter), we find that one-third of all implanted conceptions fail to survive beyond midpregnancy. For every two babies who are born, at least one is spontaneously lost along the way. (This estimate is surprisingly close to the original estimates of Hertig and Rock.[2]) The high mortality of early pregnancy (most of which occurs beyond the observation of ordinary epidemiologic studies) becomes an element in the interpretation of practically every pregnancy outcome that follows.

References

1. Roberts CJ, Lowe, C.R. Where have all the conceptions gone? *Lancet* 1975;305 (7905):498–9.
2. Hertig AT, Rock J, Adams EC, Menkin MC. Thirty-four fertilized human ova, good, bad and indifferent, recovered from 210 women of known fertility: a study of biologic wastage in early human pregnancy. *Pediatrics* 1959;23(1 Part 2):202–11.
3. Snyder JA, Haymond S, Parvin CA, Gronowski AM, Grenache DG. Diagnostic considerations in the measurement of human chorionic gonadotropin in aging women. *Clin Chem* 2005;51(10):1830–5.
4. Stenman UH, Alfthan H, Hotakainen K. Human chorionic gonadotropin in cancer. *Clin Biochem* 2004;37(7):549–61.
5. Griffin J, Odell WD. Ultrasensitive immunoradiometric assay for chorionic gonadotropin which does not cross-react with luteinizing hormone nor free beta chain of hCG and which detects hCG in blood of non-pregnant humans. *J Immunol Methods* 1987;103(2):275–83.
6. Ticconi C, Zicari A, Belmonte A, Realacci M, Rao ChV, Piccione E. Pregnancy-promoting actions of HCG in human myometrium and fetal membranes. *Placenta* 2007;28 Suppl A:S137–43.
7. Cole LA. Hyperglycosylated hCG. *Placenta* 2007;28(10):977–86.
8. Miller JF, Williamson E, Glue J, Gordon YB, Grudzinskas JG, Sykes A. Fetal loss after implantation. A prospective study. *Lancet* 1980;2(8194):554–6.
9. Edmonds DK, Lindsay KS, Miller JF, Williamson E, Wood PJ. Early embryonic mortality in women. *Fertil Steril* 1982;38(4):447–53.
10. Armstrong EG, Ehrlich PH, Birken S, et al. Use of a highly sensitive and specific immunoradiometric assay for detection of human chorionic gonadotropin in urine of normal, nonpregnant, and pregnant individuals. *J Clin Endocrinol Metab* 1984;59(5):867–74.
11. Wilcox AJ, Weinberg CR, O'Connor JF, et al. Incidence of early loss of pregnancy. *N Engl J Med* 1988;319(4):189–94.
12. Zinaman MJ, Clegg ED, Brown CC, O'Connor J, Selevan SG. Estimates of human fertility and pregnancy loss. *Fertil Steril* 1996;65(3):503–9.
13. Eskenazi B, Gold EB, Lasley BL, et al. Prospective monitoring of early fetal loss and clinical spontaneous abortion among female semiconductor workers. *Am J Ind Med* 1995;28(6):833–46.

14. Hakim RB, Gray RH, Zacur H. Infertility and early pregnancy loss. *Am J Obstet Gynecol* 1995;172(5):1510–7.
15. Wang X, Chen C, Wang L, Chen D, Guang W, French J. Conception, early pregnancy loss, and time to clinical pregnancy: a population-based prospective study. *Fertil Steril* 2003;79(3):577–84.
16. Clarke FM. Identification of molecules and mechanisms involved in the "early pregnancy factor" system. *Reprod Fertil Dev* 1992;4(4):423–33.
17. Scott L. Pronuclear scoring as a predictor of embryo development. *Reprod Biomed Online* 2003;6(2):201–14.
18. Angell R. Chromosome abnormalities in human preimplantation embryos. In: Yoshinaga K, Mori T, eds. *Development of Preimplantation Embryos and Their Environment.* New York: Alan R. Liss, Inc., 1989;181–7.
19. Goddijn M, Leschot NJ. Genetic aspects of miscarriage. *Baillieres Best Pract Res Clin Obstet Gynaecol* 2000;14(5):855–65.
20. Kline J, Stein Z, Susser M. *Conception to Birth: Epidemiology of Prenatal Development.* New York: Oxford University Press, 1989.
21. Wilton L. Preimplantation genetic diagnosis and chromosome analysis of blastomeres using comparative genomic hybridization. *Hum Reprod Update* 2005; 11(1):33–41.
22. Wilcox AJ, Baird DD, Weinberg CR. Time of implantation of the conceptus and loss of pregnancy. *N Engl J Med* 1999;340(23):1796–9.
23. Promislow JH, Baird DD, Wilcox AJ, Weinberg CR. Bleeding following pregnancy loss before 6 weeks' gestation. *Hum Reprod* 2007;22(3):853–7.
24. Wilcox AJ, Weinberg CR, Baird DD. Risk factors for early pregnancy loss. *Epidemiology* 1990;1(5):382–5.
25. Weinberg CR, Hertz-Picciotto I, Baird DD, Wilcox AJ. Efficiency and bias in studies of early pregnancy loss. *Epidemiology* 1992;3(1):17–22.

11

Miscarriage

The spontaneous death and expulsion of the fetus is the most frequent problem of clinical pregnancy. It is also one of the most erratically recorded, and least discussed.

In 1932, the Mexican muralist Diego Rivera was working on a magnificent series of murals at the Detroit Institute of Arts. The murals can still be seen today. The central figure in the first panel is a fetus in the bulb of a plant (Fig. 11-1). Diego's wife was pregnant at the time. His wife—Frida Kahlo—was a renowned artist in her own right.

Kahlo's pregnancy ended in a miscarriage (as did both of her other pregnancies). Kahlo created a harrowing portrait of her loss, with a fetus floating above

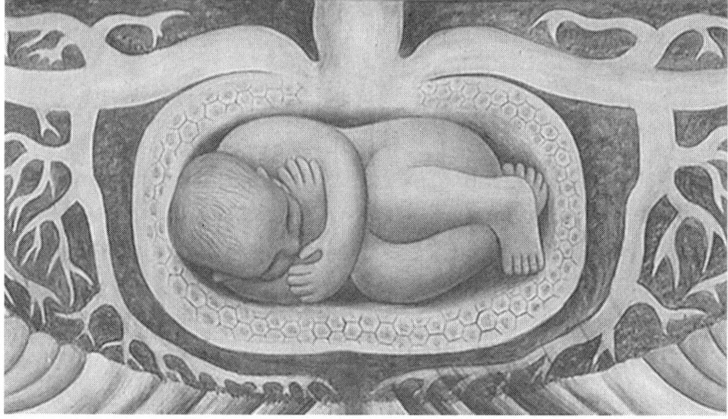

Figure 11-1. Fetus in the bulb of a plant (from mural by Diego Rivera) (Detroit Industry, East Wall [detail], Infant in the Bulb of a Plant. 1932–33. Diego M. Rivera, Gift of Edsel B. Ford, Photograph © 2001 The Detroit Institute of Arts, reprinted with permission)

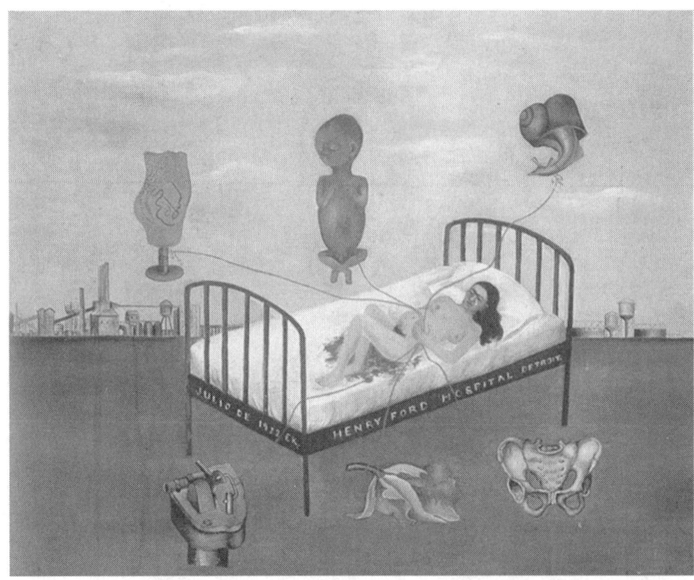

Figure 11-2. "Henry Ford Hospital, 1932" by Frida Kahlo (©2009 Banco de México Diego Rivera & Frida Kahlo Museums Trust, photo credit: Schalkwijk/ Art Resources NY, reprinted with permission)

Kahlo's blood-soaked bed (Fig. 11-2). This image is in stark contrast to the usual reserve with which miscarriage is treated in modern cultures.

Defining Miscarriage

Miscarriage (also called spontaneous abortion) is the expulsion of a fetus between the time a pregnancy is clinically recognized and the time it reaches a gestational age at which the fetus could presumably survive outside the uterus. (Fetal deaths after this point are defined as stillbirths.) For many years, the definition of miscarriage was a clinical loss before 28 weeks of gestation. However, the week used to separate miscarriage from stillbirth has moved to earlier gestational ages as more effective medical intervention has improved the survival of very preterm babies. The lower boundary of stillbirth (which is to say, the upper boundary of miscarriage) has shifted to 24 weeks, 22 weeks, or even 20 weeks, depending on the country.[1] Given the imprecision of gestational age (see Chapter 14), a criterion of fetal weight is often added to the definition (less than 350 g, or 500 g, or 1,000 g).[1,2]

The risk of miscarriage is expressed as the number of miscarriages divided by the total number of miscarriages and births (live and stillbirths). This proportion is usually expressed as a percentage and is typically 11% to 14% for women in their prime reproductive years.

About 40% to 50% of clinically recognized losses have some form of aneuploidy.[3,4] As discussed in Chapter 5, chromosomal abnormalities are usually lethal, with only a tiny fraction surviving to birth. A small portion of chromosomal abnormalities can be attributed to balanced chromosome translocation in one of the parents, but most chromosome errors are new events. The remaining miscarriages usually have no obvious pathology. There is little evidence that fetuses with malformations are at increased risk of miscarriage, independent of chromosomal abnormalities.[4 (Table 6-2)]

The clinical features of miscarriage vary depending on when during pregnancy the loss occurs. In early pregnancy, the bleeding can be similar to menses, sometimes with passage of clotted tissue. (On ultrasound examination, many of the pregnancies that end in early loss are empty amniotic sacs or severely disorganized embryos.) The earliest clinical losses may occur at home and not require medical attention. If miscarriage occurs later in pregnancy, the bleeding can be heavy and include the passage of recognizable fetal tissue. These late losses may require hospitalization, and surgery is sometimes performed to remove tissue retained in the uterus (a procedure known as dilatation and curettage, or D&C).

Measuring Miscarriage Risk

Retrospective Data

Unlike stillbirths, which are recorded by law, there is no requirement (and indeed, no practical mechanism) for the legal registration of miscarriages. Epidemiologic data can be extracted from medical records or based on women's self-report. Both tend to be incomplete. Miscarriage risk based on medical records has the advantage of using routinely collected data, but with underascertainment of the earliest recognized losses (which may be recognized by the mother but never medically recorded). Estimates based on women's own recall of their medical history also tend to miss the miscarriages that occur earlier in pregnancy.[5] Retrospectively recalled risk can be overestimated as well, for example in settings where induced abortions are illegal and past abortions are represented by women as miscarriages.

Prospective Data

Prospective data provide the most accurate estimates of miscarriage risk. Miscarriage data can be collected from women enrolled early in their pregnancy.

Although prospective data are the gold standard, such data are nonetheless sensitive to the stage at which the pregnancy comes under observation. The earlier a pregnancy is documented, the longer the surveillance time and the higher the cumulative risk of loss. Because few studies observe pregnancies from the beginning (and different pregnancies come under observation at different times), there is a problem with "left truncation." Partial observations of the earliest stages of clinical pregnancy can be dealt with through a life-table analysis and the calculation of week-by-week risk. When miscarriage risk is compared between exposed and unexposed groups, left truncation can be accommodated with Cox regression.[6] Right truncation can also be a problem in prospective data, for example, with women who choose to end their pregnancy with an induced abortion (see below).

Furthermore, life-table data are vulnerable to entry bias, in which women who are having symptoms of impending miscarriage may be more likely to seek medical care or to enroll early in a pregnancy study. This bias will inflate the apparent risk of loss in the first week of enrollment. For this reason, a careful life-table analysis requires the exclusion of the first few days of observation for each woman.[7]

The first life-table estimates of miscarriage risk were published in 1962 by French and Bierman.[8] Investigators conducted a 4-year study on the Hawaiian island of Kauai, in which all residents of the island were asked to report pregnancies within 1 month of their missed period. Only 10% of the 3,000 pregnancies in the study were registered within the first 2 months of pregnancy. Based on a life-table analysis, the total risk of pregnancy loss between 4 weeks and 20 weeks was calculated as 21%. Half of this risk was within the first time period of 4 to 7 weeks and may reflect the very high rates of early loss found before 6 weeks (see Chapter 10).

A more detailed life-table of fetal loss was published by Goldhaber and Fireman in 1991 (Fig. 11-3).[7] Their analysis was based on a retrospectively constructed cohort of nearly 10,000 California pregnancies registered in a comprehensive health care program. Follow-up began at the date of a woman's positive pregnancy test at the clinic or first prenatal visit, with a lag of 2 days to avoid entry bias. The calculated risk of loss from week 6 through week 20 was 11%. The California life-table data are very close to week-specific risks in the Danish Birth Cohort, which produced an estimate of 10% pregnancy loss between weeks 6 and 20.[9] A true gold standard would be the study of women who are enrolled before six weeks, with measurement of clinical miscarriage risk for all women starting at 6 weeks of gestation. Pooling data from four such prospective studies produces a miscarriage risk of 13% (95% confidence interval = 10% to 16%).[10-13]

Miscarriage risk reaches its highest levels at weeks 10 to 12 and then declines. Note that after week 20, the weekly risk is extremely low, around 1 per 1,000 per week (Fig. 11-3). For this reason, it makes little difference to the total risk of miscarriage whether the upper limit is set at 20 or 24 or 28 weeks. In contrast, variations in the lower bound of gestational age can have large consequences.

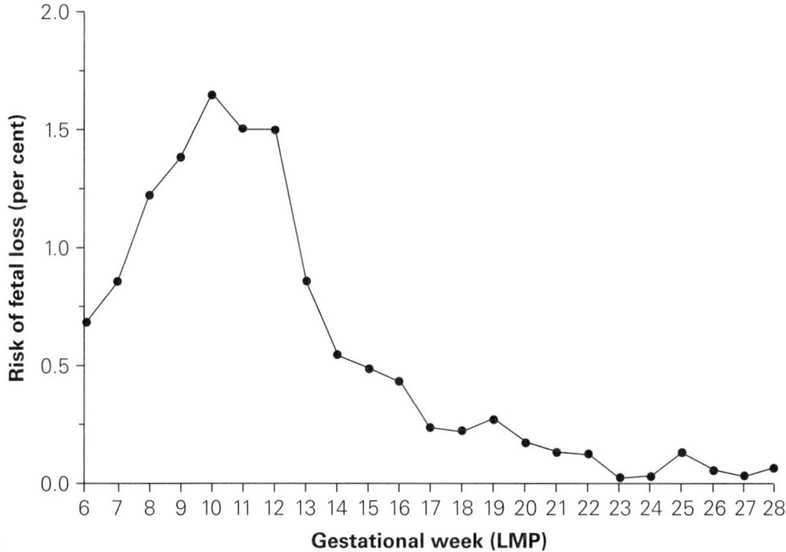

Figure 11-3. Rates of fetal loss, by week of pregnancy (California, 9055 singleton pregnancies, 1981–82)[7]

As described in the previous chapter, the risk of pregnancy loss is high before 6 weeks. If just a small portion of these earlier losses are included, the estimated total risk may be substantially increased (as in the Hawaii data above).

Date of Embryonic and Fetal Death

The date of a miscarriage is determined by the event of bleeding and expulsion of the products of conception. This is not necessarily the date of fetal death; in fact, the embryo may have died much earlier. The increasing use of ultrasound in early pregnancy detects many of these failed pregnancies before expulsion. A fetus that is apparently healthy on ultrasound (with a visible heartbeat) has a much lower risk of miscarrying than an unexamined pregnancy at the same gestational age: among ultrasound-normal fetuses, there is about a 3% risk of miscarriage starting at 8 weeks[14] compared with 10% for unexamined pregnancies.

Risk Factors for Miscarriage

For most reproductive endpoints, the best predictor of a poor outcome is a woman's previous experience of that outcome. Miscarriage risk is about 60% higher in women who have had a previous miscarriage.[4] This suggests that women (and perhaps couples) vary widely in their baseline risk of miscarriage.

Mother's Age

Another important factor determining miscarriage risk is the age of the mother. A typical pattern of age-related risk is shown in Figure 11-4.[4] The risk is fairly flat until women reach their mid-30s, at which time the risk begins to rise rapidly. The crude percentages in this figure include the influence of selective fertility. That is, women who have experienced miscarriages in the past will continue to attempt pregnancy in order to reach their desired family size and thus may be overrepresented at older ages. However, such bias explains only a small portion of the increasing risk with age.

What biological processes might explain the risk with maternal age? In broad terms, the problem could be in the egg or in the mother. The ova could deteriorate with age (perhaps becoming more susceptible to chromosomal errors in meiosis), or a woman's capacity to support and carry a pregnancy could decline with age.

Under ordinary circumstances, these two biological effects of aging would be inseparable (and for many decades, this question was unanswerable). However, pregnancies conceived through artificial means offer an opportunity to address this question. Schieve and colleagues provide revealing data from a U.S. registry of pregnancies conceived by artificial reproductive technologies. These data compare the risk of miscarriage among pregnancies conceived with the woman's own ova and among pregnancies conceived with ova from younger donors (in their 20s

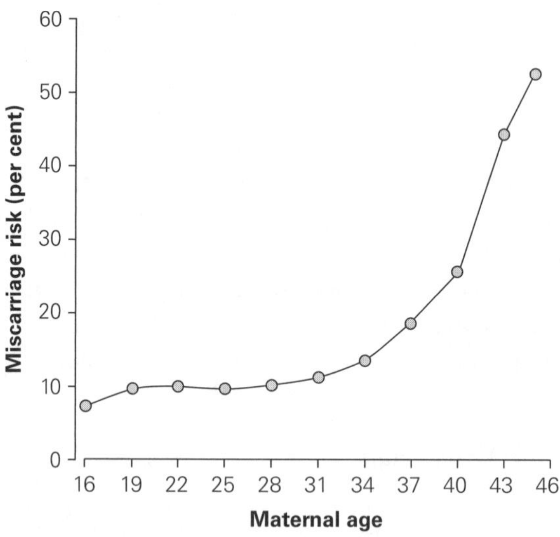

Figure 11-4. Risk of miscarriage by maternal age (Data provided by Jennie Kline from Fig. 17-2 of Kline, Stein, and Susser.[4] Includes all miscarriages regardless of whether the karyotype was known.)

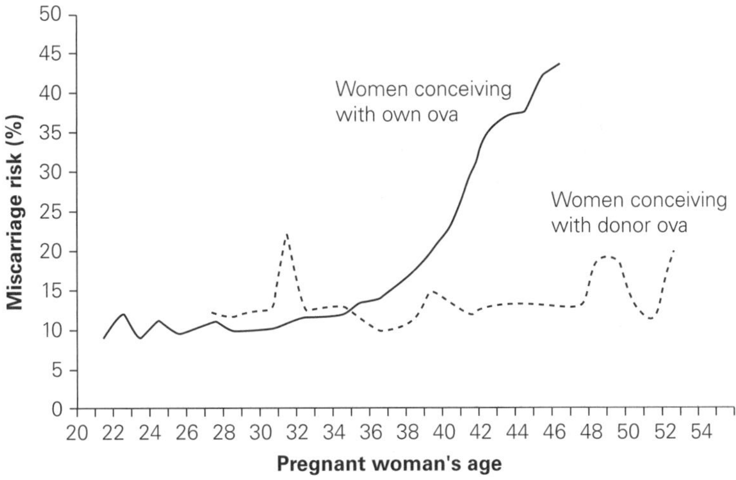

Figure 11-5. Miscarriage risk by pregnant woman's age, for ART pregnancies conceived with woman's own oocytes and by oocytes from young donors (United States, 1996–98) (Reprinted from Schieve et al[15])

or early 30s) (Fig. 11-5).[15] Risk rises rapidly with age for women who conceive with their own aging eggs (in a pattern very similar to the overall age effect in Fig. 11-4). In contrast, older women have low rates of miscarriage when the ova come from younger women. Thus, the main contributor to the increased risk of miscarriage with age is the decreasing quality of ova, whereas a woman's capacity to carry a pregnancy remains fairly stable.

Father's Age

A difficult problem in reproductive epidemiology is to separate the effects of an aging mother from the effects of an aging father, given that people tend to find partners near their own age. The decline of the ova with age is well established, but the contribution of aging sperm to reproductive failure is less clear. The hypothesis has been raised that male aging may lead to an accumulation of genetic mutations in the male germ cells (see Chapter 5). This could in principle increase the miscarriage risk among pregnancies fathered by older men. However, given the large effects of maternal age, huge sample sizes are required to avoid residual confounding by maternal age, even within small strata of maternal age. There is the further possibility of social confounding, in that the combinations of parental ages that are most informative (old fathers married to young mothers, and young mothers married to old fathers) are people who may be atypical in other ways as well. There have been few reports of effects of paternal age on miscarriage risk, and the evidence is limited.[16]

Medical Conditions

A few infectious diseases have been associated with miscarriages in humans, although evidence is weak (see Chapter 4). Maternal pathology such as malformed uterus, hypothyroidism, or poorly controlled diabetes may contribute a small proportion of miscarriages. There are also rare single-gene mutations of the fetus associated with miscarriage risk (PKU, G6PD deficiency).[17] Parentally shared human leukocyte antigen (HLA) genes and other immunologic problems have been proposed as contributors to miscarriage risk, but proof remains elusive.[18] When all conditions known or suspected to contribute to miscarriage risk are taken into account, these explain only a small fraction of chromosomally normal miscarriages. This has naturally led to a search for external causes.

Environmental and Lifestyle Exposures

The Love Canal is the poster child of toxic-waste dumps—a ditch in New York State where 12,000 tons of chemical waste was buried in the 1940s. The land was later sold for residential development.[19] In the 1970s, residents started noticing a foul sludge seeping into their basements, and the disaster was exposed. The health endpoint that first captured public attention was an apparent increase in miscarriages among women living closest to the waste dump.[19] Although this increase could not be confirmed, the observation raised scientific interest in the possibility that miscarriage might be an early sign of exposure to reproductive toxicants.[20]

Several decades of research have dampened this enthusiasm, in part because studies of miscarriage risk are so difficult and in part because few positive findings have held up. Women who smoke appear to have a modest increase in their risk of miscarriage, although this association is not entirely consistent across studies.[21] Other exposures such as caffeine[22] or alcohol[23] are even less consistent in their associations with miscarriage risk. There is no evidence that moderate stress or trauma in the mother affects the survival of pregnancy,[24] notwithstanding the drama of Scarlett O'Hara's tumble down the stairs and subsequent miscarriage.[25] Similarly, exercise appears to have no adverse effects.[26]

Concerns over environmental exposures and miscarriage have a long history. According to one biblical translation, the citizens of Jericho complained to the prophet Elisha that the pollution of their drinking water was causing miscarriages (2 Kings 2:19[27]). In the modern age, drinking water can contain solvents, disinfection byproducts, and other environmental contaminants with possible reproductive toxicity. Worrisome environmental exposures through other routes (air, food, etc.) include pesticides, phthalates, and persistent polychlorinated hydrocarbons (for example, dioxins). Despite these concerns, epidemiologic studies have provided little convincing data that environmental exposures contribute to miscarriage risk.[28] High levels of ionizing radiation and heavy metals (especially lead and mercury) can increase miscarriage risk, but evidence of effects from lower-level environmental toxicants is limited at best and absent for most.[29]

The fact that half of miscarriages are chromosomally abnormal has been proposed as a tool for etiologic inference.[4] In principle, causal factors should act differently on chromosomally normal and abnormal miscarriages. If so, the power to detect an effect by studying all miscarriages combined would be considerably weakened. A focus on the affected subgroup should in principle clarify associations that otherwise are ambiguous. One problem with implementing this approach is that most fetuses are not routinely karyotyped after miscarriage—especially miscarriages that occur earlier in gestation. Where karyotype information has been collected, the categorization of fetuses by chromosomal abnormalities has not advanced causal interpretation.

As with other reproductive problems, there is the possibility that a woman's exposures as a fetus or child could affect her risk. A preliminary report finds evidence that childhood passive exposure to parental smoking increases later risk of miscarriage in women who are conceiving by artificial technologies.[30]

Secular Trends: Contrast between Miscarriages and Stillbirths

As discussed above, the line between miscarriage and stillbirth is ill-defined (see Fig. 11-3). Even so, a striking difference emerges between these two types of fetal death when comparing populations. Miscarriage rates seem to be stable across populations and over time, whereas stillbirth rates vary greatly among populations and have fallen over time. The U.S. stillbirth rate (fetal deaths after 28 weeks of gestation) fell from 15 per 1,000 in 1950 to 3 per 1,000 in 2003.[31] Meanwhile, miscarriage rates have remained fairly constant, so far as we can tell.[32]

This contrast in time trends persists even within recorded vital statistics for early and late fetal deaths (20 to 27 weeks and 28 weeks or later). Figure 11-6 shows U.S. data over a recent 15-year period.[2] The occurrence of fetal deaths at 20–27 weeks (corresponding to what used to be called late miscarriage) has been virtually flat, while later fetal deaths have declined more than 40%. These trends reinforce the impression that early fetal mortality (miscarriage risk through 27 weeks) is more likely to reflect intrinsic biological processes than later fetal deaths. This suggests that miscarriage may not be a particularly sensitive endpoint for detection of environmental toxicants.

Problems in the Analysis of Miscarriage Risk

The Competing Risk of Induced Abortion

Induced abortions are not considered in the usual formula for miscarriage risk (miscarriages divided by the sum of miscarriages and births). This can create

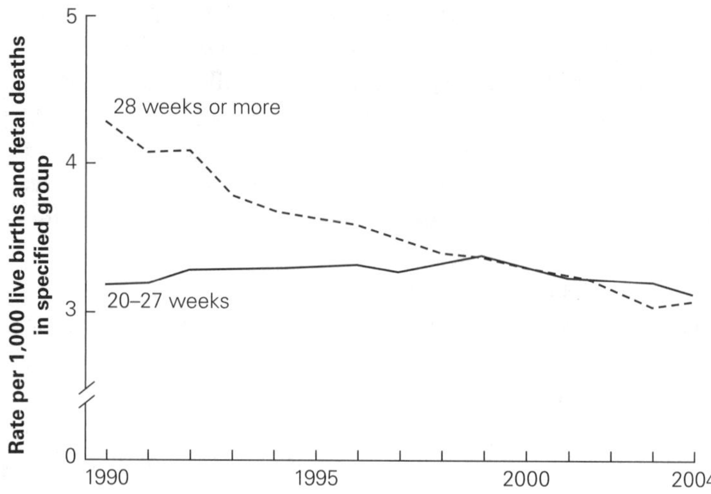

Figure 11-6. Changes over time for early and late stillbirths (United States, 1990–2004) (Reprinted from MacDorman et al[2]) (*Source*: CDC/NCHS, National Vital Statistics System)

analytic difficulties. Pregnancies destined for induced abortion can contribute miscarriages but not births and thus can distort the estimation of miscarriage risk. It follows that the larger the proportion of pregnancies scheduled for induced abortion in any given population, the higher the apparent risk of miscarriage. (Consider the extreme case: a population where every pregnant women gets an induced abortion would have a miscarriage risk of 100% by the standard definition.) To the extent that the prevalence of induced abortion varies among groups, the group with the higher prevalence of induced abortion will also appear to have the higher miscarriage risk.

This difficulty could be avoided by a careful life-table analysis. However, such analysis requires information on the gestational age at which induced abortions take place—information that is often not available. In the absence of such data, an approximate adjustment for induced abortions can be made by adding a number equal to half of the induced abortions to the denominator of miscarriage risk.[33]

Other Competing Risks

A small but occasionally vexing question of miscarriage analysis is what to do with other outcomes of pregnancy such as hydatidiform moles or tubal (ectopic) pregnancies. Should they be included in the denominator as part of the total population of pregnancies? Biologically, there is no simple answer, but pragmatically, the answer is easy. These outcomes are uncommon—tubal pregnancies occur in 1–2 per 100 pregnancies,[34] and molar pregnancies are less than 1 per 1,000.[35] Thus, to disregard them has little impact on the risk of miscarriage.

Selective Fertility

We have discussed how selective fertility can produce an artifactual association of miscarriage risk with gravidity (Chapter 7) and with maternal age (earlier in this chapter). Selective fertility can produce other distortions as well. In a cross-sectional study, the risk of miscarriage is likely to be lower in a woman's most recent pregnancy than in her earlier pregnancies. A naive analysis of such data might conclude that miscarriage rates are declining with age or over time. The correct explanation for this pattern is that women tend to stop their pregnancies with a success. Women with a miscarriage are more likely to become pregnant again soon, whereas a woman with a live birth may prefer not to get pregnant again for a while (and maybe not ever). This produces a time-length bias in which there is less time to observe that a woman's most recent pregnancy is a miscarriage than to observe that it is a live birth. Any study based on women's most recent pregnancies is vulnerable to biased estimates of miscarriage risk (or of any other adverse outcome of pregnancy).[36]

One analytic strategy for avoiding problems of selective fertility is to restrict analysis to first pregnancies.[37] Although such results have the advantage of being unbiased, they do not take full advantage of the data. An analysis of all pregnancies requires a careful consideration of the structure of the data collection and the goals of the analysis.

The "Unhealthy Worker" Effect

Epidemiologists familiar with occupational studies will recognize the phenomenon of the "healthy worker" effect, in which persons with health problems are generally less likely to remain in the workforce. As a result, the prevalent health in the workforce is usually better, and the incidence of new disease is lower, than in the general population. The opposite selection can occur with reproduction. Women who are fertile and achieve their desired family size are more likely to withdraw from the workforce to stay home with their children, whereas women who are infertile or otherwise impaired in their reproduction are more likely to remain employed. If control groups are not carefully selected for occupational studies, this selection can create an association between workplace exposures and poor reproductive performance.

The "Habitual Aborter"

There is a natural tendency for clinicians to dichotomize people into the sick and the well. However, when the underlying risk is continuous (as with miscarriage risk), dichotomies can be misleading. The "habitual aborter" is a clinical diagnosis based on the observation of repeated miscarriages. The label implies a pathologic condition when, in fact, this group includes some low-risk women who have just had bad luck. The mistaken notion that habitual aborters have little hope of successful pregnancy has led to uncontrolled studies of interventions in which success in subsequent pregnancies is presented as evidence of the efficacy of treatment.[38] Typically, 75% of women identified as having recurrent miscarriages will be successful with their next pregnancy in the absence of any treatment.[39]

Epidemiologists are not immune to the pitfalls of defining women as habitual aborters. Investigators sometimes assess the effects of an exposure for women with prior losses and those without. The inherent risks of abortion within the two categories (and the contrast between their observed risks in subsequent pregnancies) depend on such factors as the total number of past pregnancies and the extent to which women have controlled their fertility. Generally speaking, the categorization of women as habitual aborters should be avoided.[40]

Coffee and Miscarriage: The Problem of Reverse Causation

The association of coffee consumption and miscarriage is an example of the challenges of data interpretation in reproductive studies. Women who drink coffee in the first trimester are more likely to experience a miscarriage.[41] However, dietary patterns in early pregnancy are strongly related to the nausea and vomiting of early pregnancy, and such symptoms in turn are related to the health of the fetus. Although the presence of symptoms does not necessarily mean the conceptus is healthy, the absence of symptoms is associated with an increased risk of miscarriage.[42] (Pregnancies destined to end in miscarriage are less likely to produce the high hormone levels that trigger nausea.) Women who suffer symptoms tend to avoid coffee,[43] whereas women without pregnancy symptoms are likely to continue to drink coffee. The result is an association of coffee drinking with miscarriage that is difficult to interpret. Even carefully conducted prospective studies will not necessarily be able to disentangle cause and effect.[44] The coffee-and-miscarriage question remains unresolved.

Adjustment for Previous Pregnancy Outcome

A problem related to habitual aborters is whether—and how—to adjust for women's previous miscarriages. There is no single good answer to this question, and many wrong ones (see Chapter 7).

Clusters of Miscarriages

Because miscarriages are common, accidental clusters of miscarriages are also common. Clusters are especially likely to be observed in settings where women already have concerns about their health and are therefore more forthcoming in sharing information about their pregnancies. Miscarriages that otherwise might not have been openly discussed can suddenly appear to cluster when women become alarmed about a possible risk. Clusters have been reported in office buildings, trailer parks, public housing complexes, and the *USA Today* newsroom.[45] Such clusters sometimes lead to intensive epidemiologic studies but rarely (if ever) to the identification of a new reproductive hazard.

References

1. Gourbin C, Masuy-Stroobant G. Registration of vital data: are live births and stilbirths comparable all over Europe? *Bull WHO* 1995;73(4):449–60.
2. MacDorman MF, Munson ML, Kirmeyer S. Fetal and perinatal mortality, United States, 2004. *Natl Vital Stat Rep* 2007;56(3):1–19.
3. Goddijn M, Leschot NJ. Genetic aspects of miscarriage. *Baillieres Best Pract Res Clin Obstet Gynaecol* 2000;14(5):855–65.
4. Kline J, Stein Z, Susser M. *Conception to Birth: Epidemiology of Prenatal Development.* New York: Oxford University Press, 1989.
5. Wilcox AJ, Horney LF. Accuracy of spontaneous abortion recall. *Am J Epidemiol* 1984;120(5):727–33.
6. Howards PP, Hertz-Picciotto I, Poole C. Conditions for bias from differential left truncation. *Am J Epidemiol* 2007;165(4):444–52.
7. Goldhaber MK, Fireman BH. The fetal life table revisited: spontaneous abortion rates in three Kaiser Permanente cohorts. *Epidemiology* 1991;2(1):33–9.
8. French FE, Bierman JM. Probabilities of fetal mortality. *Public Health Rep* 1962;77:835–47.
9. Nybo Andersen AM. *Fetal Death—Epidemiologic Studies.* Copenhagen: University of Copenhagen, 2000.
10. Wilcox AJ, Weinberg CR, O'Connor JF, et al. Incidence of early loss of pregnancy. *N Engl J Med* 1988;319(4):189–94.
11. Miller JF, Williamson E, Glue J, Gordon YB, Grudzinskas JG, Sykes A. Fetal loss after implantation. A prospective study. *Lancet* 1980;2(8194):554–6.
12. Edmonds DK, Lindsay KS, Miller JF, Williamson E, Wood PJ. Early embryonic mortality in women. *Fertil Steril* 1982;38(4):447–53.
13. Whittaker PG, Taylor A, Lind T. Unsuspected pregnancy loss in healthy women. *Lancet* 1983;1(8334):1126–7.
14. Simpson JL, Mills JL, Holmes LB, et al. Low fetal loss rates after ultrasound-proved viability in early pregnancy. *JAMA* 1987;258(18):2555–7.
15. Schieve LA, Tatham L, Peterson HB, Toner J, Jeng G. Spontaneous abortion among pregnancies conceived using assisted reproductive technology in the United States. *Obstet Gynecol* 2003;101(5 Pt 1):959–67.
16. Slama R, Bouyer J, Windham G, Fenster L, Werwatz A, Swan SH. Influence of paternal age on the risk of spontaneous abortion. *Am J Epidemiol* 2005;161(9):816–23.
17. Cramer DW, Wise LA. The epidemiology of recurrent pregnancy loss. *Semin Reprod Med* 2000;18(4):331–9.
18. Porter TF, Scott JR. Alloimmune causes of recurrent pregnancy loss. *Semin Reprod Med* 2000;18(4):393–400.

19. Heath CW Jr. Field epidemiologic studies of populations exposed to waste dumps. *Environ Health Perspect* 1983;48:3–7.
20. Kline J, Levin B, Stein Z, Susser M, Warburton D. Epidemiologic detection of low dose effects on the developing fetus. *Environ Health Perspect* 1981;42:119–26.
21. US Surgeon General. *Women and Smoking*, 2001.
22. Signorello LB, McLaughlin JK. Maternal caffeine consumption and spontaneous abortion: a review of the epidemiologic evidence. *Epidemiology* 2004;15(2):229–39.
23. Henderson J, Kesmodel U, Gray R. Systematic review of the fetal effects of prenatal binge-drinking. *J Epidemiol Community Health* 2007;61(12):1069–73.
24. Baerga-Varela Y, Zietlow SP, Bannon MP, Harmsen WS, Ilstrup DM. Trauma in pregnancy. *Mayo Clin Proc* 2000;75(12):1243–8.
25. Mitchell M. *Gone with the Wind*. New York: Macmillan, 1936.
26. Latka M, Kline J, Hatch M. Exercise and spontaneous abortion of known karyotype. *Epidemiology* 1999;10(1):73–5.
27. (Various). *The New English Bible with the Apocrypha*. Oxford: Oxford University Press, 1970.
28. Weselak M, Arbuckle TE, Walker MC, Krewski D. The influence of the environment and other exogenous agents on spontaneous abortion risk. *J Toxicol Environ Health B Crit Rev* 2008;11(3–4):221–41.
29. Wigle DT, Arbuckle TE, Turner MC, et al. Epidemiologic evidence of relationships between reproductive and child health outcomes and environmental chemical contaminants. *J Toxicol Environ Health B Crit Rev* 2008;11(5–6):373–517.
30. Meeker JD, Missmer SA, Vitonis AF, Cramer DW, Hauser R. Risk of spontaneous abortion in women with childhood exposure to parental cigarette smoke. *Am J Epidemiol* 2007;166(5):571–5.
31. Health, United States, 2007, *With Chartbook on Trends in the Health of Americans*. Hyattsville MD: National Center for Health Statistics, 2007;Table 22.
32. Wilcox AJ, Treloar AE, Sandler DP. Spontaneous abortion over time: comparing occurrence in two cohorts of women a generation apart. *Amer J Epidemiol* 1981;114(4):548–53.
33. Susser E. Spontaneous abortion and induced abortion: an adjustment for the presence of induced abortion when estimating the rate of spontaneous abortion from cross-sectional studies. *Am J Epidemiol* 1983;117(3):305–8.
34. Lehner R, Kucera E, Jirecek S, Egarter C, Husslein P. Ectopic pregnancy. *Arch Gynecol Obstet* 2000;263(3):87–92.
35. Bracken MB, Brinton LA, Hayashi K. Epidemiology of hydatidiform mole and choriocarcinoma. *Epidemiol Rev* 1984;6:52–75.
36. Weinberg CR, Baird DD, Wilcox AJ. Bias in retrospective studies of spontaneous abortion based on the outcome of the most recent pregnancy. *Ann NY Acad Sci* 1994;709:280–6.
37. Olsen J. Options in making use of pregnancy history in planning and analysing studies of reproductive failure. *J Epidemiol Community Health* 1994;48(2):171–4.
38. Weil RJ, Tupper C. Personality, life situation, and communication: a study of habitual abortion. *Psychosom Med* 1960;22:448–55.
39. Brigham SA, Conlon C, Farquharson RG. A longitudinal study of pregnancy outcome following idiopathic recurrent miscarriage. *Hum Reprod* 1999;14(11):2868–71.
40. Gladen BC. On the role of "habitual aborters" in the analysis of spontaneous abortion. *Stat Med* 1986;5(6):557–64.

41. Leviton A, Cowan L. A review of the literature relating caffeine consumption by women to their risk of reproductive hazards. *Food Chem Toxicol* 2002;40(9):1271–310.
42. Klebanoff MA, Koslowe PA, Kaslow R, Rhoads GG. Epidemiology of vomiting in early pregnancy. *Obstet Gynecol* 1985;66(5):612–6.
43. Lawson CC, LeMasters GK, Wilson KA. Changes in caffeine consumption as a signal of pregnancy. *Reprod Toxicol* 2004;18(5):625–33.
44. Stein Z, Susser M. Miscarriage, caffeine, and the epiphenomena of pregnancy: the causal model. *Epidemiology* 1991;2(3):163–7.
45. Cohen J. *Coming to Term: Uncovering the Truth about Miscarriage*. New York: Houghton Mifflin, 2005.

12

Stillbirth and Infant Mortality

Birth is a dangerous passage. The baby's risk of dying is highest during labor and delivery and in the period immediately following birth. These deaths are registered by law in most countries, and mortality rates are used as an indicator of public health and economic development. Stillbirth and infant mortality rates have fallen dramatically around the world, demonstrating the strong influence of external factors. Even so, the specific reasons for the decline in mortality rate remain incompletely understood.

Birth is a time of perilous transition. Figure 12-1 shows the hourly rate of death around delivery. (Risk is on a log scale to accommodate the 2,000-fold range.) Although mortality at birth is low in absolute terms, the pattern is revealing. The risk of fetal death rises sharply as labor commences, reaches its maximum during the minutes around delivery, and then falls rapidly.

The extreme spike of mortality around delivery corresponds to the time in which the baby experiences high physical stress. The baby is extruded through an opening not quite large enough for its head and then undergoes an abrupt transition from complete life support to the first stages of independent living. The circulation of blood through the heart is rearranged, and the lungs experience air for the first time. The immediate causes of death during this time are often specifically related to labor, including birth trauma and asphyxia. The ordeal of delivery may be especially difficult if the fetus has been weakened by a hostile intrauterine environment (for example, intraamniotic infection). Once babies survive delivery, their risk of death rapidly falls and continues to decline in the months that follow.

The data in Figure 12-1 (from the British Perinatal Mortality Survey of 1958) offer a detailed look at the timing of fetal and infant death as it may naturally occur, before fetal monitoring and cesarean section were as widely used as they are today. However, technology appears not to have changed this pattern.

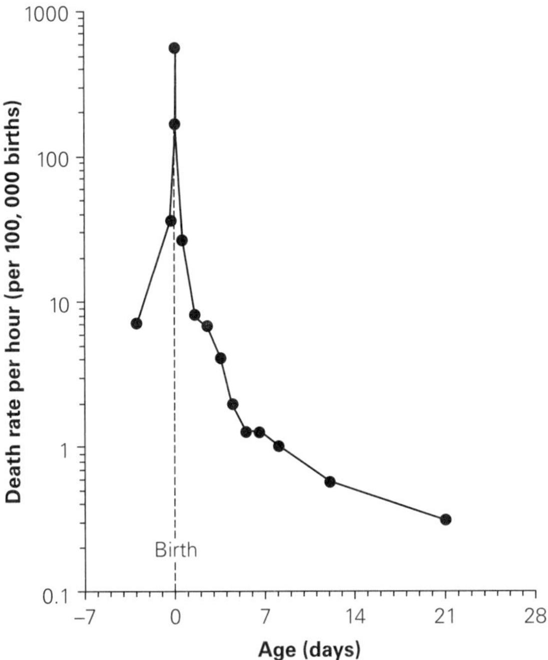

Figure 12-1. Hourly rates of babies' mortality around birth (British Perinatal Mortality Survey, 1958) (First data point assumes that stillbirths before the onset of labor are delivered within 1 week of death. Remaining data points are midpoints of varying time spans ending with deaths at 14 to 27 days of age.) (Data courtesy of Jon Johnson, Centre for Longitudinal Studies, Institute of Education, London)

Figure 12-2 shows similar data (although in cruder time categories) for deaths occurring to live births in the United States in 2003–2004. The 1958 British data are provided in the same categories for reference. Even though overall neonatal mortality is 75% lower in the more recent data, the pattern of extreme risk in the first hour after birth remains. (To some degree, modern technology may contribute to this pattern by intervening *because* a fetus is faltering and thus bringing delivery to the time of death rather than the delivery causing death.)

Definitions

Technically, the baby is a fetus until the completion of delivery, and an infant afterwards. By social convention, the spike of mortality at birth is split into two parts: stillbirth and infant mortality. Both stillbirths and infant deaths are recorded by law in most countries, although births in developing countries are

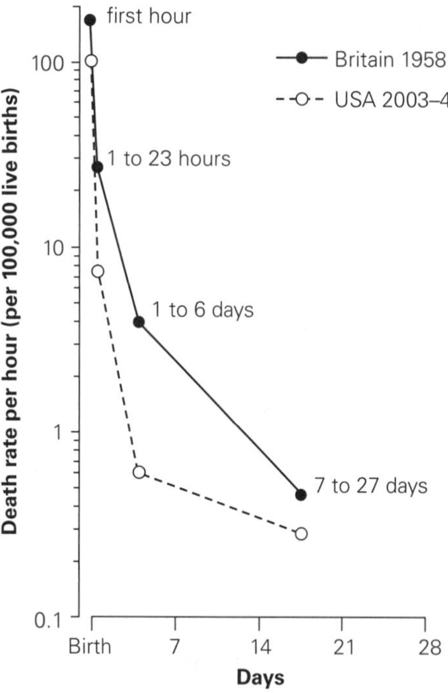

Figure 12-2. Neonatal mortality by time since birth, Britain 1958 and United States 2003–2004.

often unregistered.[1] (Examples of registration forms for fetal deaths, infant births, and infant deaths are provided in the Appendix.)

Stillbirth

Stillbirth is the death of a fetus mature enough to have survived outside the uterus. The concept is reasonable, but converting this idea into specific criteria is difficult. For many years, the gestational-age criterion for a stillbirth was a minimum of 28 weeks. As medical care for preterm babies has steadily improved, survival has become possible at earlier and earlier ages, and the criterion for stillbirth has had to change as well. In this era when survival at early gestations is steadily improving, there is no standard. Fetal deaths are reportable at 26 weeks in Belgium and at 16 weeks in Norway. Regardless of where the cutoff is set, stillbirths are usually underreported at the earliest legally required gestational age.[2] For fetuses born near the borderline, it is often easier administratively to dismiss the loss as a miscarriage than to give it legal status as a fetal death.

In order to sharpen the distinction between unregistered miscarriages and registered stillbirths, a birth weight criterion is sometimes added (e.g., 350 g, 500 g, or 1,000 g). With so many possible combinations of gestational age and birth weight, there are now a multitude of definitions of stillbirth among countries, and even among states within the United States.[3,4] Given that mortality is highest at these lower boundaries, boundary differences can have large effects on stillbirth mortality rates. For international comparisons, the WHO recommends that stillbirth be defined as a dead fetus of at least 28 weeks of gestation or at least 1,000 g birth weight.[5] The fuzzy distinction between miscarriage and stillbirth is further confused by terminology—both miscarriage and stillbirth are often referred to as "fetal death."

CALCULATIONS OF STILLBIRTH RISK. Stillbirth risk is defined as the proportion of all births ending in stillbirth. For vital statistics calculations, stillbirth risk is the number of stillbirths in a given year divided by the total number of live births and stillbirths in the same year. The definition of stillbirth as a proportion of all births is widely accepted as a summary measure, but its extension to gestational-age-specific risk of stillbirth is more contentious.

The argument has been made that stillbirth risk at a given gestational age should be expressed as a proportion of all continuing (in utero) pregnancies (the denominator from which the stillbirths arise) rather than as a proportion of only the deliveries at that gestational age.[6] This argument might reasonably apply to the stillbirths that occur before the onset of labor. For deaths that occur during labor and delivery, the population at risk might more logically be limited to those fetuses who experience the stresses of labor (i.e., birth). One problem in implementing this distinction between death before labor and death after the start of labor is that data on time of death for stillbirths are incomplete—in U.S. stillbirths, one-third of fetal death records lack this information.[7] Among those with recorded time of death, 83% were antepartum deaths (before onset of labor), and 17% were intrapartum deaths.

Some have argued that the use of all ongoing pregnancies as the denominator is an approach that should be extended to neonatal deaths and other birth outcomes.[8,9] Because much of neonatal death occurs very soon after delivery (and is presumably related to the ordeal of delivery), it is not obvious that fetuses who have not yet been put through this ordeal should be considered as at risk of its consequences.[10]

Infant Mortality

Infant mortality is simpler to define, although the definition is still not without problems. Infant mortality is the proportion of live births who die in the first year of life. For national statistics, this number is almost always estimated by the number of deaths among infants under the age of 1 year in a given calendar year, divided by the total number of live births in that calendar year. Thus, the numerator is not from the same cohort as the denominator, and the calculated infant mortality rate does not represent a specific cohort of births. Still, given that birth rates and death rates vary only slightly from year to year in most populations, this method provides a convenient approximation. (The same calendar approach is used to estimate neonatal and postneonatal mortality rates.)

The problem in defining live birth comes with the definition of "live." A fetus that dies in the few minutes before delivery is technically a stillbirth, whereas a baby who dies in the minutes just after delivery is a live birth that experiences neonatal death. The distinction between these two events can be subjective. How strong do the lingering signs of life in a dying baby have to be in order to declare that a baby was born alive?

As a general rule, splitting a distribution at its peak is a bad idea. This causes both parts to be maximally sensitive to small changes at the boundary. In this case, infant mortality is sensitive to any condition that affects the distinction between a stillbirth and an early neonatal death. For example, administrative convenience may matter. A fetal death creates less paperwork for a birth attendant because it requires the completion of only one legal form (a fetal death certificate), whereas a neonatal death requires both a birth certificate and a death certificate. In the middle of the night, these small things can make a difference.

To complicate matters, there may be legal criteria for "live birth" that override clinical signs. If a birth weight criterion is part of the definition of live birth, then a neonatal death that occurs to a live birth weighing less than the criterion will be regarded as a stillbirth.[3] There was a time in the Soviet Union when babies born very preterm were not counted as live births unless they survived the first week. This caused infant mortality to be underestimated by as much as 25%.[11]

Neonatal Mortality and Postneonatal Mortality

Infant mortality is often divided into subcategories as a way to accommodate the concentration of mortality during the first days and weeks of life. "Early neonatal mortality" describes deaths of live births during the first week after birth, and "neonatal mortality" describes deaths in the first month (28 days). Postneonatal mortality comprises deaths after the first month but in the first year.

Perinatal Mortality

"Perinatal mortality" is an alternative category of death designed to capture the whole peak of mortality around the time of birth. Perinatal mortality is the combination of stillbirths and deaths in the first week (or sometimes the first month). This summary measure is a useful epidemiologic endpoint in that it resolves problems arising from the indistinct boundary between stillbirths and early neonatal deaths.[12] In analyzing factors that affect both fetal and infant deaths, the use of perinatal mortality can improve power (for example, in the description of selective fertility[13]). However, to the degree that stillbirths and neonatal deaths have distinct etiologies, combining the two may confuse the picture.[14]

The Relative Distribution of Stillbirths and Infant Deaths

Figure 12-3 shows the categories of stillbirth and infant mortality in proportion to their numbers. As a rough rule of thumb, developed countries have about as many stillbirths as infant deaths. Perinatal mortality (through the first week of life) captures about three-quarters of all stillbirths and infant deaths. Among live births, one-half of all deaths in the first year occur in the first week (one-third in the first day, and 10% in the first hour[15]). Postneonatal mortality is a minor portion of all fetal and infant deaths. Although there is no reason to expect these relative proportions to remain fixed, the proportions have not changed much in developed countries during recent decades, even as the overall rates of stillbirth and infant mortality have continued to decline.[16]

In the poorest countries, the pattern is different. Infant deaths exceed stillbirths, and postneonatal deaths may equal or even exceed the number of neonatal deaths.[17] Poverty and infectious diseases undoubtedly contribute to the high rates of infant death after the neonatal period. Underreporting of stillbirths and very early neonatal deaths in the developing countries also contributes to these differences between developed and developing countries.

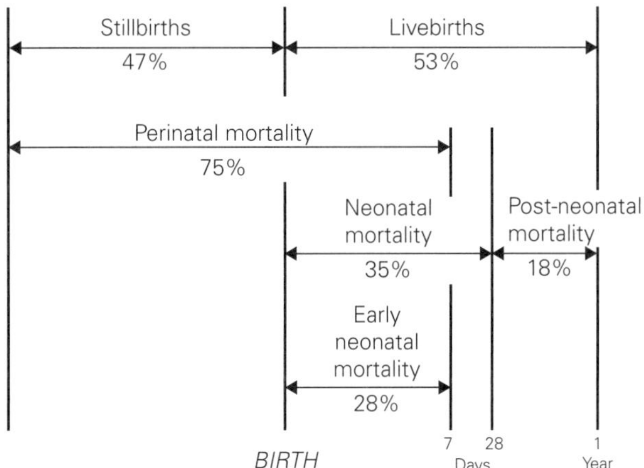

Figure 12-3. Definitions of the categories of fetal and infant mortality, with each category shown in proportion to its size (U.S., 2005)[4,18]

Trends over Time

Infant Mortality

The huge decline in infant mortality over the past century is one of the most remarkable phenomena in all of reproductive epidemiology. This decline has been linked to a host of improvements in medicine and public health, and no doubt many factors have contributed to this improvement. Still, our understanding of the forces that shape infant mortality is far from complete.

Figure 12-4 shows the decline of infant mortality in the United States since 1900. This picture is typical for developed countries. In 1900, infant mortality in the United States was 162 per 1,000 births—a rate higher than in any country today except war-torn Angola.[19] Within the first 25 years of the twentieth century, U.S. infant mortality fell by half. This huge decline took place before most of the important medical discoveries of the twentieth century, including antibiotics and vaccinations for whooping cough and diphtheria.

The downward trend of infant mortality over time has provided many tempting opportunities for interpretation. Credit for the decline has been given to virtually every emerging public health intervention, economic improvement, and medical advance. However, such "ecologic" correlations—in which two factors change together over time—is one of the weakest arguments for causation. It may be that medical or public health advances have played a role, but the analytic studies necessary to establish causation are rarely available.

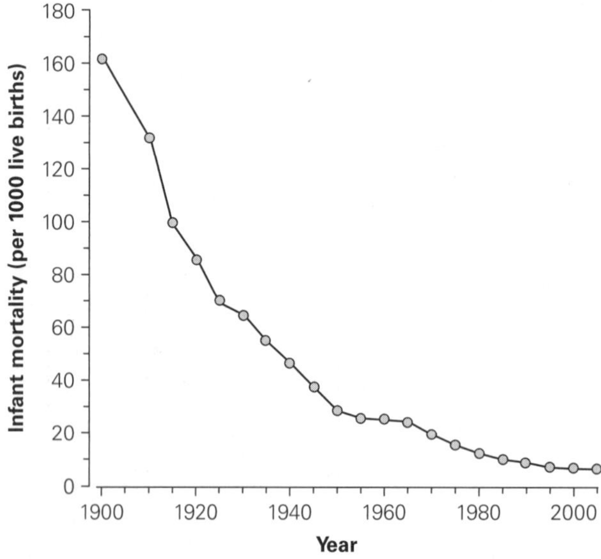

Figure 12-4. Decline of US infant mortality from 1900 to 2006 (US National Center for Health Statistics)

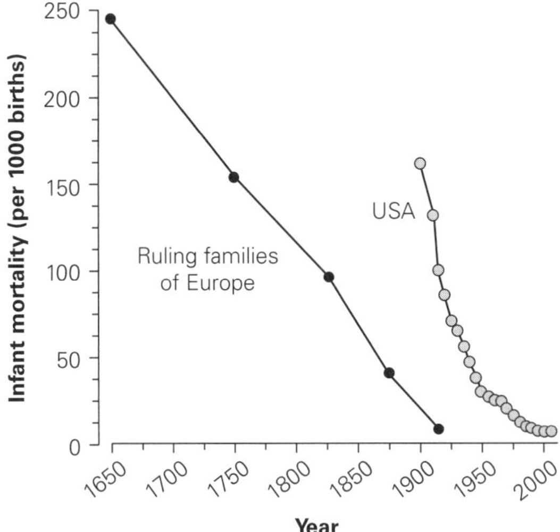

Figure 12-5. Infant mortality among the European aristocracy 1600–1930, compared with U.S.[20]

The importance of economic factors in infant mortality (in contrast to medical factors) is underscored by historical data assembled by Peller.[20,21] Peller used detailed historical records for families of the European aristocracy to reconstruct the mortality among live births across several centuries. In the 1600s, infant mortality in these families was around 25% (Fig. 12-5). This risk declined in the 1700s and continued to fall steadily. By the last half of the 1800s, infant mortality among the aristocracy had reached 40 per 1,000, a rate not achieved in the United States until the 1940s. In the first three decades of the 1900s, the infant mortality among the aristocracy was 8 per 1,000—equal to the U.S. rate in 1994.

The improvement among the aristocracy may reflect the advantages of adequate nutrition, hygiene, insulation from infectious diseases, and other comforts. It may be possible that factors such as good nutrition benefit infants cumulatively across generations, through mechanisms not yet well understood such as epigenetics.[22]

Neonatal and Postneonatal Mortality

Figure 12-6 separates the decline of U.S. infant mortality into two components: deaths within the first 4 weeks (neonatal) and subsequent deaths in the first year (postneonatal).[23] These two mortality curves are presented on a logarithmic scale to highlight the ratio between the two. (A constant distance on a log scale indicates a constant ratio.) Between 1915 and the late 1940s, postneonatal mortality went from being greater than neonatal mortality to being about half of neonatal

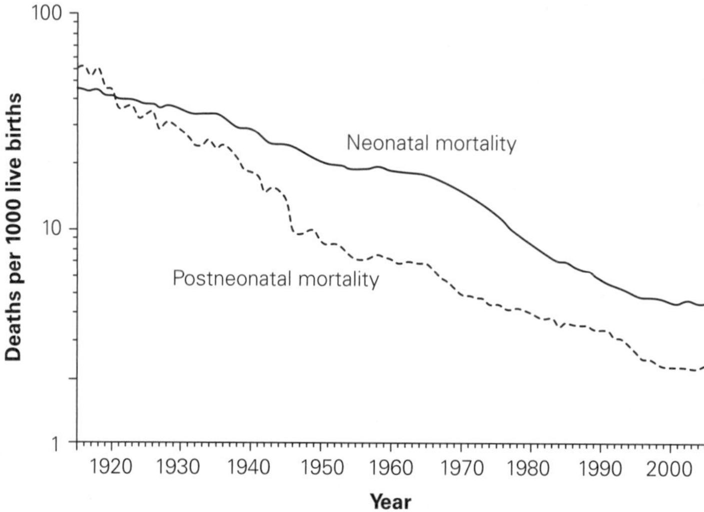

Figure 12-6. Neonatal and postneonatal mortality over time (U.S., 1915–2005) (US National Center for Health Statistics)

mortality. This general relationship has continued with the exception of the period from the mid-1970s to the mid-1990s (see Box on SIDS).

SIDS: "Back to Sleep"

Sudden infant death syndrome (SIDS) is the unexpected and unexplained death of an infant between the ages of 3 weeks and 9 months.[24] By definition, SIDS is mostly a postneonatal death. Through the 1980s and 1990s SIDS was a chief cause of postneonatal mortality in developed countries. In the early 1990s, epidemiologic and clinical data strongly suggested that SIDS could be averted by placing infants to sleep on their backs. Public health campaigns led to the decline in SIDS deaths by at least a third in the United States and other countries.[25,26]

What is sometimes lost in the telling of this public health success story is the tragedy of its origins. Putting children to sleep on their backs was once customary practice. In the 1970s, physicians began to recommend that babies be put to sleep on their stomachs, among other reasons to avoid the theoretical possibility of aspiration of regurgitated food.[26] In the absence of supporting data (but with a seemingly self-evident rationale), parents were encouraged to place babies to sleep on their stomachs. In Sweden, this led to a nearly fourfold increase of SIDS deaths between 1973 and 1990.[26] Rates returned to their previously low levels only after the "back-to-sleep" campaigns of the 1990s.

Stillbirth Mortality

Stillbirth mortality has also declined over recent decades.[27,28] As noted in the previous chapter, most of the decline has been among fetuses that survive to at least 28 weeks, with little change among earlier fetal deaths (see Fig. 11-6). This pattern implies that external risk factors are more likely to contribute to stillbirths occurring after 28 weeks than before.

Infant Mortality and Life Expectancy

Infant mortality and life expectancy are among the world's most widely cited health statistics. Infant mortality is a prime indicator of general health and economic development. The annual release of new statistics on infant mortality is reported in the media, and regions take pride (or suffer embarrassment) on its account. Similarly, life expectancy statistics provide a universal measure of the well-being of a population.

The close links between infant mortality and life expectancy are seldom appreciated. Mortality risk in the first year of life is often the highest that people experience at any age until late adulthood. In the United States, the death rate does not exceed the risk of death in the first year until a person reaches their late fifties.[29] In developing countries, people typically do not reach the newborn risk until their 70s.[30] It follows that improvements in infant mortality can contribute strongly to improvements in life expectancy.

Life expectancy is a widely misunderstood statistic. Consider the following newspaper quote: "When [U.S.] Social Security was enacted in 1935, with full benefits kicking in at 65, the average life expectancy in America was 63. [Thus]...the average American worked nearly until he (or she) died."[31] The author mistakenly concludes that because the U.S. life expectancy was 63, people did not have much chance of making it to age 65.

Life expectancy is the average number of years of life remaining for persons who have reached a given age, assuming a given set of age-specific death rates.[29] Life expectancy is most commonly estimated at birth and thus includes the relatively high mortality around birth. One common misunderstanding is that life expectancy defines the age at death. It does not—it is an average, with some people dying sooner and some dying later.

Another misunderstanding is that the life expectancy at birth is the age an adult can expect to reach. Not so—adults have the advantage of having survived the high death rates of infancy, and so their life expectancy is longer. In 1900, the U.S. life expectancy was 48 years, but this does not mean that most adults never made it to age 50. Indeed, people who reached age 48 in 1900 had a life expectancy of 23 more years, to age 71. Going back to the newspaper article about Social Security, U.S. men of working age in 1935 had a life expectancy of age 70, with half of them living even longer. Nearly two-thirds of U.S. men who were 40 in 1935 could expect to live past age 65 and collect Social Security benefits.

The major contributor to improved life expectancy over the past century has not been better treatment of the diseases of old age (although that has surely helped), but rather the enormous decline in infant mortality. Since 1900, the life expectancy at birth in the United States has increased by 30 years, but the life expectancy of a 48-year-old has increased by only 10 years.

International Comparisons

The World Health Organization estimates that less than 15% of the world's births are recorded, despite the fact that most countries have laws requiring the registration of births.[32] Stillbirths are especially prone to underreporting, and international comparisons are therefore sketchy. The best available estimates suggest a sixfold range of stillbirth rates across nations (ranging from 5 to 32 per 1,000).[33]

In contrast, there is more than a 60-fold difference in infant mortality rates around the world. Differences among nations today are as striking as the decline in infant mortality experienced in the rich nations during the last century. In 2008, the median infant mortality for the nations of the world was 19 deaths per 1,000 births[19] (equivalent to the rate in the United Kingdom around 1965). In the worst-off nations, where poor nutrition and infectious diseases are rampant, infant mortality is eight times higher than the median. At the other end of the spectrum, infant mortality in the most privileged countries is one-eighth the median. The explanation for the extremely low rates is not as obvious as the reasons for the high rates.

There is a strong association between infant mortality and a nation's economic development. Figure 12-7 shows the infant mortality of 200 nations of the world, plotted according to their per capita gross domestic product.[19] When both values are logged, the relation is remarkably linear.

Just as we have little understanding of what specifically has driven the decline of infant mortality over time, neither do we know how low the mortality can go.

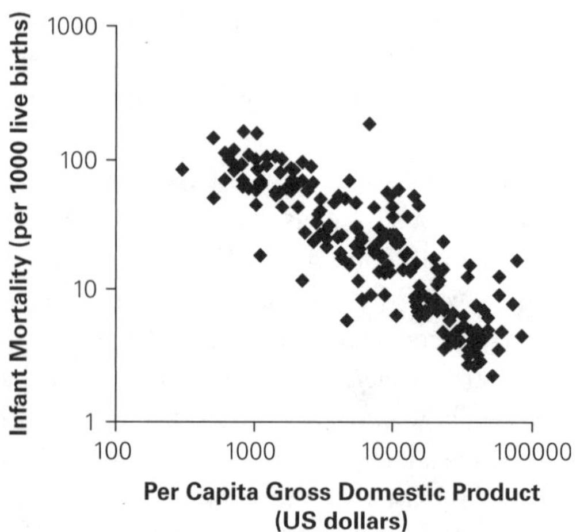

Figure 12-7. Relation between national infant mortality rates and per capita gross domestic products (GDP) (2007) (World Factbook[19])

It is always easy to explain patterns after the fact—it is our predictions that reveal our ignorance. A few decades ago, infant mortality in several countries was approaching the previously unimagined level of 10 per 1,000. Experts declared that the risk of infant mortality would soon plateau at an irreducible minimum[34] and that ongoing improvements in the less-developed countries would proceed to narrow the gap among nations.

The Apgar Score

The most widely used clinical scale for assessing newborn vitality is the Apgar score. *Apgar* may sound like an acronym, but Virginia Apgar (1909–74) was a real person.[35] She was an anesthesiologist who studied the use of anesthesia in childbirth. At a time when most concerns about the side effects of anesthesia were focused on the mother, Apgar was worried about effects on the newborn. She developed her score as a simple and structured way to assess the newborn. The score comprises five easily observed aspects of the neonate, and assigns each aspect a score of zero (absent) to 2 (normal). The aspects are skin color (pink is 2, pale is 0), heart rate (over 100 per minute is 2, none is 0), reflex irritability (withdrawal from uncomfortable stimulus is 2, no response is 0), muscle tone (active movement is 2, no movement is 0), and breathing (strong is 2, none is 0). The score is usually tallied twice, once at 1 minute and once at 5 minutes of life. Confusion over the origins of the name Apgar is compounded by the fact that her score can be expressed in words that actually do spell her name (Appearance, Pulse, Grimace, Activity, and Respiration).

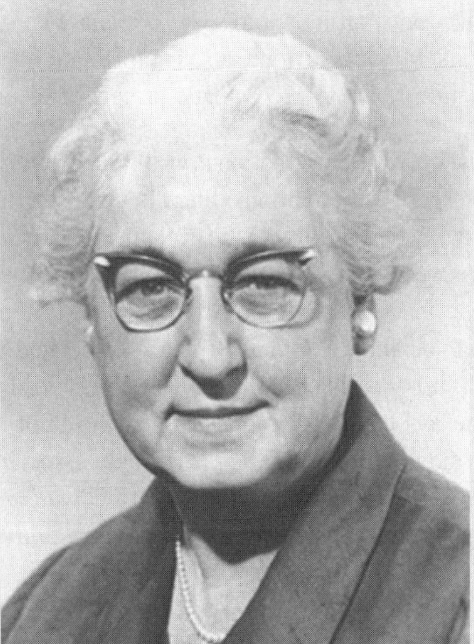

Virginia Apgar, 1909–74. Reprinted Courtesy of the U.S. National Library of Medicine[36]

The predictions were wrong. Infant mortality has continued to decline in all countries of the world, even faster in the wealthy nations (on a percentage basis) than in the rest of the world. The lowest rates of infant mortality today are in Asia and the Nordic countries, with four countries in 2008 having fewer than 3 infant deaths per 1,000 births (Sweden, Singapore, Japan, and Hong Kong). The burden of infant mortality continues to fall most heavily on the poor countries. Figure 12-8 compares world maps with nations shown in proportion to their land area, their population, and their number of infant deaths. Relatively few infant deaths occur in Europe or in North or South America. The vast majority of infant deaths occur in Africa and South Asia.

Risk Factors

Infant Mortality

It is a truism of epidemiology that where problems are greatest, the quality of data is the worst. Ninety-nine percent of deaths in the first month of life take place in low-income and middle-income countries where registration is often incomplete, and data on cause of death are unreliable or absent. Meanwhile, most research focuses on the 1% of deaths occurring in the richest countries.[37] Global estimates of infant mortality and its causes are therefore limited. In developing countries, tetanus and diarrhea are estimated to account for 10% of neonatal deaths, with sepsis and pneumonia contributing another 25%.[37] These causes of death are rare in developed countries. Major contributors to infant death in all countries include congenital malformations, birth asphyxia, and preterm delivery.

SOCIAL FACTORS. The correlation of national wealth and infant mortality between nations has its counterpart within nations: there is a consistent correlation of economic well-being and infant mortality within even the richest societies. In the United Kingdom, the link between social class and infant mortality was not altered when nationalized medicine made medical care free to all.[38] In the egalitarian Nordic countries, markers of social class remain strongly associated with infant mortality.[39] To some degree, it is possible that poor health may lead to reduced income, thus confounding the association of social class with infant mortality. However, the same cannot be said of ethnicity, which is strongly associated with social class in many countries and shows similar associations with infant mortality.[40] In the United States, blacks have more than twice the infant mortality of whites.

MATERNAL AND INFANT CHARACTERISTICS. Certain maternal characteristics are consistently related to infant mortality risk. A mother's first birth has a 15% higher risk of infant death than later births, for reasons that remain unclear. The extremes of young and old maternal age are associated with moderately raised

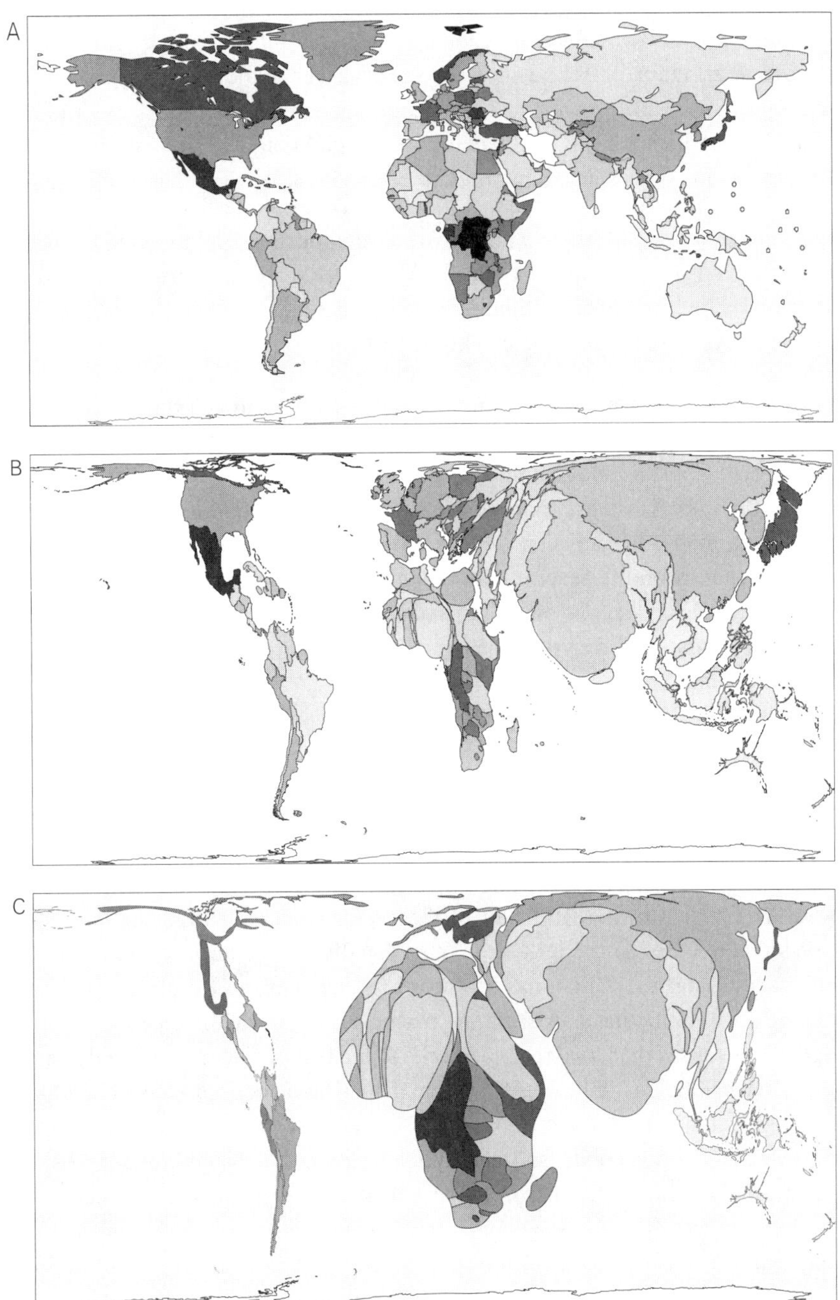

Figure 12-8. The nations of the world, shown in proportion to their (A) land area, (B) population, and (C) number of infant deaths. © Copyright 2006 SASI Group (University of Sheffield) and Mark Newman (University of Michigan)

risks,[18] which to some degree reflect a concentration of higher-risk women at the extremes of age. Boy babies have about 20% higher mortality than girl babies in the first year, again for unknown reasons. This excess male risk is so reliably seen that, where it is absent, one must suspect an unequal treatment of boys and girls at birth (see Chapter 17). Twins have about a fivefold higher risk of mortality than singletons, and triplets about a 10-fold increased risk.[41]

TOXIC EXPOSURES. Mothers who smoke have about a 40% increased chance of losing their babies in the first year.[42] Although cigarette packages around the world provide numerous specific warnings,[43] it seems that none explicitly tells pregnant women that smoking can kill their babies.

DIABETES AND OBESITY. Preexisting diabetes mellitus (either Type 1 or Type 2) is associated with perinatal problems including preeclampsia, stillbirth, and neonatal mortality.[44] Careful medical management of pregnant women with diabetes can reduce this risk. Obstetric management has become more complicated in recent years with the rising prevalence of obesity. Obesity by itself increases stillbirth and neonatal mortality severalfold[45] and also is associated with other conditions that increase risk, such as preeclampsia and gestational diabetes.[46] Even modest increases in maternal weight among nonobese women may adversely affect pregnancy outcome.[47]

RH FACTOR. Most people carry a protein on the surface of their red blood cells known as Rh factor. The Rh factor is inherited as an autosomal dominant trait. Nearly all people are "Rh-positive" except for those of European descent, among whom about one in six lacks the protein ("Rh-negative"). Rh factor has only one known health consequence, and it has to do with pregnancy. Rh-negative women who are exposed to the Rh factor of their fetus (inherited from the father) can develop antibodies to the Rh factor. This usually causes no problem in the first pregnancy, but if the mother has another pregnancy with an Rh-positive fetus, the mother's Rh antibodies can cross the placenta and attack the blood cells of the fetus. This causes the fetus' red blood cells to break down, leading to fetal anemia. Also, the metabolism of hemoglobin from the red blood cells produces bilirubin as a by-product, and high levels of bilirubin can damage the central nervous system. In severe cases, this condition (hemolytic disease or erythroblastosis fetalis) can be life-threatening to the baby. The problem can be prevented by injection of the mother with Rh immunoglobulin, which suppresses her development of Rh antibodies. Such injections are routinely given to Rh-negative mothers within 72 hours of delivering an Rh-positive baby, thus protecting future offspring.

Stillbirths

The study of risk factors for stillbirths is hampered by inconsistencies of definition and incompleteness of registration. Especially in developing countries, data on stillbirths may be virtually nonexistent.[33] Cause of death is often not recorded for stillbirths in vital statistics or population-based registries. Some increase in risk occurs with advanced maternal age,[48] although the extent to which selective fertility and recurrence risk might contribute to this association has not been fully explored (see Chapter 7). Most of the factors that affect infant mortality (smoking, obesity, diabetes) also affect stillbirth risk.[49]

Information on the time of stillbirth death is often lacking in vital statistics. Still, there appear to be distinct etiologic patterns for stillbirths depending on whether death occurs before onset of labor or during the ordeal of labor. Older maternal age and low education are more strongly associated with stillbirth before labor. Stillbirths before the onset of labor may trace their origins to events early in pregnancy.[50]

Preventing Stillbirth and Infant Mortality

There have been successes in the search for preventable causes of fetal and infant mortality. One is the discovery that immunizing a pregnant woman against neonatal tetanus also immunizes her fetus, thus protecting the baby from one of the major causes of infant mortality in developing countries.[51] Another is the discovery that folic acid supplementation reduces the risk of neural tube defects, a severe and often lethal birth defect.[52] A third is the recognition that sudden infant death syndrome (SIDS) is related to sleep position (although as discussed above, this victory is bittersweet). Educational campaigns instructing parents to place their babies to sleep on their backs have reduced SIDS by 50% or more.[53]

These successes demonstrate the main challenge in discovering further preventable causes of infant mortality. Infant mortality comprises deaths from many different causes. Each cause is likely to have its own distinct etiology and its own intervention. Notwithstanding the global trend of reductions in infant mortality from all causes, research efforts often focus on more narrowly defined conditions or diseases of the fetus and infant that contribute to infant mortality. Some examples of specific endpoints (such as preterm delivery and birth defects) are discussed in subsequent chapters.

References

1. UNICEF. *The State of the World's Children 2006: Excluded and Invisible.* Geneva: UNICEF, 2006.
2. Greb AE, Pauli RM, Kirby RS. Accuracy of fetal death reports: comparison with data from an independent stillbirth assessment program. *Am J Public Health* 1987;77(9):1202–6.
3. Gourbin C, Masuy-Stroobant G. Registration of vital data: are live births and stilbirths comparable all over Europe? *Bull WHO* 1995;73(4):449–60.

4. MacDorman MF, Munson ML, Kirmeyer S. Fetal and perinatal mortality, United States, 2004. *Natl Vital Stat Rep* 2007;56(3):1–19.
5. WHO. *International Classification of Diseases and Related Health Problems, Tenth Revision*. Geneva: WHO, 1993.
6. Yudkin PL, Wood L, Redman CW. Risk of unexplained stillbirth at different gestational ages. *Lancet* 1987;1(8543):1192–4.
7. Little RE, Weinberg CR. Risk factors for antepartum and intrapartum stillbirth. *Am J Epidemiol* 1993;137(11):1177–89.
8. Platt RW, Joseph KS, Ananth CV, Grondines J, Abrahamowicz M, Kramer MS. A proportional hazards model with time-dependent covariates and time-varying effects for analysis of fetal and infant death. *Am J Epidemiol* 2004;160(3): 199–206.
9. Joseph KS. Incidence-based measures of birth, growth restriction, and death can free perinatal epidemiology from erroneous concepts of risk. *J Clin Epidemiol* 2004;57(9):889–97.
10. Wilcox AJ, Weinberg CR. Invited commentary: analysis of gestational-age-specific mortality—on what biologic foundations? *Am J Epidemiol* 2004;160(3):213–4; discussion 215–6.
11. Anderson BA, Silver, BD. Infant mortality in the Soviet Union: regional differences and measurement issues. *Population Dev Rev* 1986;12(4):705–38.
12. Peller S. Mortality, past and future. *Population Stud* 1948;1(4):405–56.
13. Skjaerven R, Wilcox AJ, Lie RT, Irgens LM. Selective fertility and the distortion of perinatal mortality. *Am J Epidemiol* 1988;128(6):1352–63.
14. Kramer MS, Liu S, Luo Z, Yuan H, Platt RW, Joseph KS. Analysis of perinatal mortality and its components: time for a change? *Am J Epidemiol* 2002;156(6):493–7.
15. Linked Birth/Infant Death Records 2003–2004 on CDC WONDER On-line Database. *National Center for Health Statistics, Office of Analysis and Epidemiology*, Atlanta: CDC, 2008.
16. Wegman ME. Infant mortality in the 20th century, dramatic but uneven progress. *J Nutr* 2001;131(2):401S-8S.
17. Rutstein SO. Factors associated with trends in infant and child mortality in developing countries during the 1990s. *Bull WHO* 2000;78(10):1256–70.
18. Mathews TJ, MacDorman MF. Infant mortality statistics from the 2005 Period Linked Birth/Infant Death Data Set. *Natl Vital Stat Rep* 2008;57(2):1–32.
19. US CIA. *The World Factbook*. 2008.
20. Peller S. Studies on mortality since the Renaissance. *Bull Hist Med* 1943;13:427–41.
21. Wilcox AJ. Infant mortality revisited. *Paediatr Perinat Epidemiol* 1993;7(4):347–8.
22. Pembrey ME, Bygren LO, Kaati G, et al. Sex-specific, male-line transgenerational responses in humans. *Eur J Hum Genet* 2006;14(2):159–66.
23. NCHS. *Vital Statistics of the United States, 1993. Vol. II, Mortality, Part A*. Hyattsville, MD: National Center for Health Statistics, 2002.
24. Krous HF, Beckwith JB, Byard RW, et al. Sudden infant death syndrome and unclassified sudden infant deaths: a definitional and diagnostic approach. *Pediatrics* 2004;114(1):234–8.
25. Malloy MH, Freeman DH Jr. Birth weight- and gestational age-specific sudden infant death syndrome mortality: United States, 1991 versus 1995. *Pediatrics* 2000;105(6):1227–31.
26. Hogberg U, Bergstrom E. Suffocated prone: the iatrogenic tragedy of SIDS. *Am J Public Health* 2000;90(4):527–31.

27. *Health, United States, 2007, With Chartbook on Trends in the Health of Americans.* Hyattsville MD: National Center for Health Statistics, 2007, Table 22.
28. Kalter H. Five-decade international trends in the relation of perinatal mortality and congenital malformations: stillbirth and neonatal death compared. *Int J Epidemiol* 1991;20(1):173–9.
29. Arias E. United States life tables, 2004. *Natl Vital Stat Rep* 2007;56(9):1–39.
30. Lopez AD, Ahmad OB, Guillot M, et al. *World Mortality in 2000: Life Tables for 191 Countries.* Geneva: WHO, 2002.
31. Yarrow AL. "Retiring early? How selfish." *The Baltimore Sun.* Baltimore, 9 April 2008.
32. WHO. *The World Health Report 2005: Make Every Mother and Child Count.* Geneva: WHO, 2005.
33. Stanton C, Lawn JE, Rahman H, Wilczynska-Ketende K, Hill K. Stillbirth rates: delivering estimates in 190 countries. *Lancet* 2006;367(9521):1487–94.
34. Vallin J. [World trends in infant mortality since 1950]. *World Health Stat Rep* 1976;29(11):646–74.
35. Apgar V. A proposal for a new method of evaluation of the newborn infant. *Curr Res Anesth Analg* 1953;32(4):260–7. Available at http://www.nlm.nih.gov/changing the face of medicine/physicians/biography_12.html, last accessed October 27, 2009.
36. NLM. *Viriginia Apgar: Changing the Face of Medicine.* Washington, DC: US National Library of Medicine. Available at http://www.nlm.nih.gov/changingthe faceofmedicine/physicians/biography_12.html, last accessed October 27, 2009.
37. Lawn JE, Cousens S, Zupan J. 4 million neonatal deaths: when? where? why? *Lancet* 2005;365(9462):891–900.
38. Pamuk ER. Social-class inequality in infant mortality in England and Wales from 1921 to 1980. *Eur J Population* 1988;4:1–21.
39. Arntzen A, Mortensen L, Schnor O, Cnattingius S, Gissler M, Andersen AM. Neonatal and postneonatal mortality by maternal education—a population-based study of trends in the Nordic countries, 1981–2000. *Eur J Public Health* 2008;18(3):245–51.
40. Villadsen SF, Mortensen LH, Nybo Andersen AM. Ethnic disparity in stillbirth and infant mortality in Denmark 1981–2003. *J Epidemiol Community Health* 2008.
41. Mathews TJ, Menacker F, MacDorman MF. Infant mortality statistics from the 2002 period: linked birth/infant death data set. *Natl Vital Stat Rep* 2004;53(10):1–29.
42. Salihu HM, Wilson RE. Epidemiology of prenatal smoking and perinatal outcomes. *Early Hum Dev* 2007;83(11):713–20.
43. Wikipedia. Tobacco packaging warning messages. 2008.
44. Kapoor N, Sankaran S, Hyer S, Shehata H. Diabetes in pregnancy: a review of current evidence. *Curr Opin Obstet Gynecol* 2007;19(6):586–90.
45. Kristensen J, Vestergaard M, Wisborg K, Kesmodel U, Secher NJ. Pre-pregnancy weight and the risk of stillbirth and neonatal death. *Br J Obstet Gynaecol* 2005;112(4):403–8.
46. Rosenn B. Obesity and diabetes: a recipe for obstetric complications. *J Matern Fetal Neonatal Med* 2008;21(3):159–64.
47. Villamor E, Cnattingius S. Interpregnancy weight change and risk of adverse pregnancy outcomes: a population-based study. *Lancet* 2006;368(9542):1164–70.
48. Fretts RC, Schmittdiel J, McLean FH, Usher RH, Goldman MB. Increased maternal age and the risk of fetal death. *N Engl J Med* 1995;333(15):953–7.
49. Cnattingius S, Stephansson O. The epidemiology of stillbirth. *Semin Perinatol* 2002;26(1):25–30.

50. Smith GC, Crossley JA, Aitken DA, et al. First-trimester placentation and the risk of antepartum stillbirth. *JAMA* 2004;292(18):2249–54.
51. Vandelaer J, Birmingham M, Gasse F, Kurian M, Shaw C, Garnier S. Tetanus in developing countries: an update on the Maternal and Neonatal Tetanus Elimination Initiative. *Vaccine* 2003;21(24):3442–5.
52. Botto LD, Moore CA, Khoury MJ, Erickson JD. Neural-tube defects. *N Engl J Med* 1999;341(20):1509–19.
53. Moon RY, Horne RS, Hauck FR. Sudden infant death syndrome. *Lancet* 2007;370(9598):1578–87.

13

Twins and More

Twins and other multiple births are a tiny percentage of all births and differ in many ways from singletons. Although multiple births are often excluded from perinatal analyses, they are a worthy topic of study in their own right.

Multiple births are the step-children of reproductive epidemiology. Even though they are a natural variant of human pregnancy, twins and other multiple births are routinely excluded from perinatal analyses because they are few, and they are different. Multiple births have smaller birth weights, shorter gestational ages, and higher rates of birth defects and perinatal mortality. The frequency of multiple births varies somewhat, but a good rule of thumb is that about 1 in 100 naturally conceived pregnancies will be twins, 1 in 100^2 will be triplets, and 1 in 100^3 will be quadruplets. Thus, among all multiple births, about 99% are twins—the focus of this chapter. Most statements about twins apply even more strongly to higher-order multiple births.

The Biology of Twinning

Dizygotic Twins

There are two well-known types of twins: fraternal (or dizygous) and identical (or monozygous). Dizygous twins arise when two eggs are released at ovulation and both are fertilized. Such twins are genetically similar in the way that any two siblings are similar, sharing 50% of their genes. In addition, dizygotic twins share a common uterine environment during the same stages of development. To the extent that this shared fetal environment affects later development, dizygotic twins may be slightly more similar than siblings conceived in different pregnancies.

Monozygous Twins

Monozygous twins arise from a single fertilized egg that separates into two parts (for reasons not understood) after conception. Each of the resulting conceptuses carries the same set of genes and thus are "identical" in their genetic inheritance (Fig. 13-1). In practice, monozygous twins may not be completely identical. Genetic errors that occur after separation but during early development would affect the two twins differently. In identical twins that are female, the random inactivation of one of the two X chromosomes during the embryonic development may cause different X chromosomes to predominate by chance in the two girls. More subtle genetic differences can emerge through life as twins experience differential epigenetic activation of specific genes (see Chapter 5).

Monozygotic twinning is relatively rare among animal species. (A curious exception is the nine-banded armadillo, which regularly produces litters of four identical offspring.[1]) In humans, the rate of monozygous twinning is steady at about 3.5 to 4 per 1,000 deliveries.[2] This constancy suggests that monozygous twinning is more or less random and independent of outside influences. Some biologists have proposed that monozygous twins arise from conditions that also produce birth defects; that is, the separation of the conceptus into two parts occurs because of an irregularity or disruption at the early stages of development.[3] Supporting this notion is the observation that congenital malformations are twice as common in monozygotic twins as in singletons, whereas dizygotic twins have no increased risk.[2] However, it is also possible that the peculiar biology of monozygotic twins itself contributes to an increased risk of malformations. The rare but dramatic anomaly of conjoined twins ("Siamese" twins) occurs only among monozygotic twins, presumably as a result of incomplete separation of the conceptuses at a relatively late stage of embryonic development.

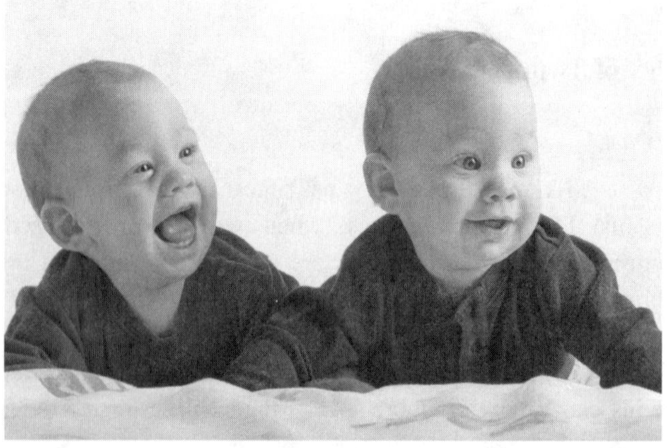

Figure 13-1. Monozygotic twins (*Source*: www.shutterstock.com)

"Vanishing Twins"

The widespread use of prenatal ultrasound examination has shown that in twin pregnancies, one embryo can suffer early death and resorption while the other embryo survives.[4] This loss may be accompanied by vaginal bleeding, or it may occur without clinical signs or symptoms. The loss of a twin is not rare; by one estimate, only 60% of twin pregnancies identified by ultrasound in the first trimester end in twin births.[4] If this is an accurate estimate, as many as 1% of singleton births might have started as twins.

A less frequent and more surprising reason for twins to disappear is the phenomenon of chimerism. In Greek mythology, a chimera was a monster made from the parts of different animals. In genetics, a chimera is a single creature composed of cell lines from two or more genetically distinct zygotes. Chimerism in humans can occur when dizygotic twins at a very early stage merge to make one conceptus. Chimerism is compatible with healthy development and may be discovered only by accident. A woman whose children were receiving genetic testing was told by her doctors that two of her children were not actually hers.[5] The woman assured the doctors they were wrong. It was subsequently discovered that the mother was chimeric, with different genetic cell lines having produced her ovaries and her blood. Although exceedingly rare, undiscovered chimerism could contribute to errors in paternity or to errors in criminal convictions based on DNA.

Twin Placentation

Placentation is complicated for twins. If monozygotic twins are formed late enough (after around day 5), they may remain connected to a single placenta. With only one placenta, connections can develop between the blood circulation of the two fetuses, leading to imbalanced blood supply ("transfusion syndrome") and increased risk of death for the undersupplied fetus.[6] At the other extreme, two fetuses can each be contained in its own chorionic sac, each with its own placenta. There are many possible variations of shared membranes and shared placentation.[7] The degree to which these variations affect the health of twins is unknown, in part because the placental anatomy is not always easy to decipher at birth.

The Epidemiology of Twinning

A key to the epidemiologic study of twins is to distinguish monozygous from dizygous twins. Molecular genetic data provide this information definitively, but such data are seldom available on a population basis. All unlike-sex twins are dizygotic, but same-sex twins can be either dizygotic or monozygotic. Indirect methods for identifying the type of same-sex twins have been developed. The examination of placental membranes at delivery is useful but not necessarily definitive. Physical similarity of the twins is the most common method, although even this is not infallible. Simple questions asked of parents ("are your twins as alike as two drops of water?")

are correct in about 96% of cases.[8] Parents who think their twins are monozygous are more often wrong than parents who identify their twins as dizygous.

Weinberg's Method

On the population level, the proportion of twins that are dizygous can be determined by a simple rule proposed more than a century ago by Weinberg.[9] The logic is as follows. If the distribution of sex among dizygous twins is random (and assuming the sex ratio is 50:50), then 50% of the twins will be female-male, 25% male-male, and 25% female-female. For every unlike-sex set of twins (which must be dizygous) there is also a dizygous set of twins that is same-sex. Therefore, doubling the proportion of unlike-sex twins provides the total proportion of dizygous twins. The remaining twins will be monozygous.

Weinberg's method is useful for the analysis of data from vital statistics or birth registries. The Weinberg method also allows epidemiologists to estimate the proportion of monozygous and dizygous twins in any stratum that includes infant sex. (The fact that the true sex ratio is closer to 51:49 than to 50:50 is too trivial to make a difference.[10])

Monozygous versus Dizygous Twinning

From an epidemiologic standpoint, monozygotic and dizygotic twins are strikingly different conditions. Very few epidemiologic variables are associated with monozygotic twinning, whereas many are associated with dizygotic twinning. For example, consider the relation of twinning to maternal age (Fig. 13-2).[11] The prevalence of monozygotic twins at birth rises only slightly (by no more than 20%) with age of the mother. In contrast, dizygotic twinning rises eightfold and then rapidly declines.

Parity is often regarded as an independent risk factor for dizygotic twinning.[12] However, there is no explicit biologic mechanism by which parity might affect twinning, and this association is more likely to be an artefact of confounding by fertility (see below) and residual confounding by maternal age. Strong differences in dizygous twinning are seen among ethnic groups, with women of African descent having more than twice the risk of Europeans, and women of Asian descent having less than half the risk.[2] Taken together, these data suggest strong heterogeneity among women in the risk of dizygotic twins but little heterogeneity in the risk of monozygotic twins. Consistent with these observations, the risk that a woman with one set of dizygotic twins will have another is increased by fourfold, with no evidence of increased recurrence of monozygotic twins.[2]

What physiologic characteristics of the woman might increase her chances of bearing dizygotic twins? Some clue may come from the increased risk with aging. As women age, there is a gradual rise in basal levels of follicle-stimulating hormone (FSH). This may occur as a result of a gradual decline in ovarian function (and decreased negative feedback to the pituitary). FSH is an effective stimulus of

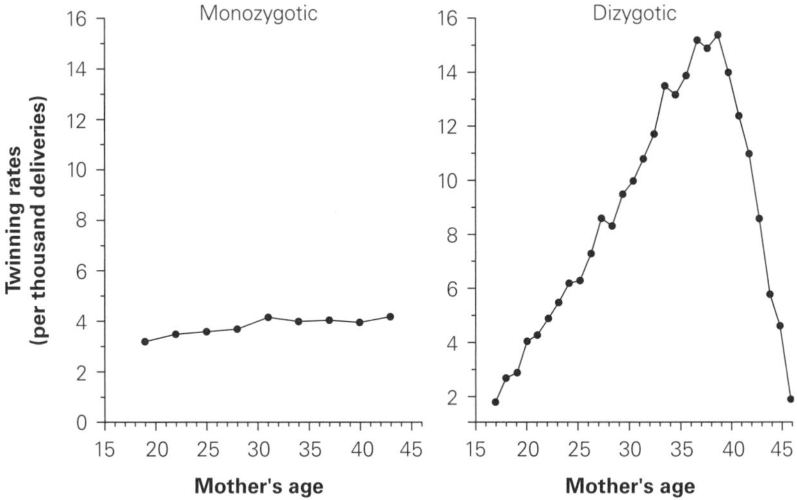

Figure 13-2. Twinning rates by mother's age, for monozygotic and dizygotic twins (Italy, 1949–54)[11]

ovulation (and multiple ovulation), and older women are more likely to produce two mature ovarian follicles in a single cycle.[13] Other factors associated with dizygotic twinning may also act through the hormonal milieu of the mother.

The Inheritance of Twinning

The ethnic differences in dizygotic twinning and the recurrence risk of dizygotic twins suggest that dizygous twinning may have a heritable component. Family data suggest that the sisters of mothers who deliver dizygotic twins themselves have twice the risk of dizygotic twins.[12] (Remarkably, some of the best family data on this topic come from the same 1901 paper in which Weinberg proposed a method for estimating the proportions of dizygotic and monozygotic twins.[9])

Secular Trends

Time-trend data are not usually calculated separately for dizygous and monozygous twins. Given the general stability of monozygous twinning, it is assumed that any trends over time reflect changes in dizygotic twinning. The prevalence of twins in industrialized countries was generally stable during the first half of the twentieth century, with twins comprising about 1.0% to 1.6% of births.[14] However, starting around 1950, twinning rates declined in most countries. By the late 1970s, twinning rates were in the range of 0.8% to 1.0%. Rates began to rise around 1980 and have risen to historic high levels. By the early 2000s, twinning in most countries was in the range of 1.2% to 2%.

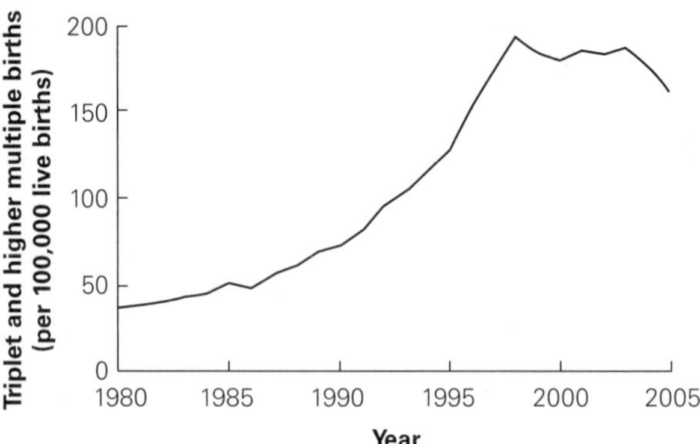

Figure 13-3. Triplet and higher multiple births over time (United States, 1980 to 2005) (Reprinted from Martin et al[16])

At least part of the recent increase has been caused by the rising number of pregnancies conceived through infertility treatments and assisted reproductive techniques.[14] Most infertility treatments include stimulation of ovulation, which often results in multiple eggs and twin or higher-order pregnancies. Furthermore, multiple embryos are usually transferred to the uterus with in vitro fertilization in order to increase the possibility of a successful conception. Triplet pregnancies increased fourfold in the United States at the beginning of the ART era[15] and then plateaued as the risks of bearing multiple fetuses became more widely appreciated (Fig. 13-3).[16] Even so, after taking into account ART and the trend toward older maternal ages, there may still be an increase in twinning rates.[17]

Dizygotic Twinning as a Marker of Reproductive Health

Natural dizygotic twinning has been proposed as an indicator of reproductive health, with a decline of twinning over recent decades interpreted as possible evidence of reproductive toxicants in the environment.[18] This argument is based on the link between twinning and high fecundability, for which there is good evidence. Women who conceive more quickly are more likely to have dizygotic twins,[19] and women who are subfertile have a low prevalence of twins among their pregnancies.[20] (The tendency of dizygotic twinning to increase with mother's age does not fit this pattern and has been described as a "paradox."[13]

However, it is not clear that increased dizygotic twinning rates are a marker of reproductive health. There is no direct evidence that reproductive toxicants reduce dizygotic twinning. In fact, maternal smoking (one of the most prevalent and well-established reproductive toxicants) seems to increase dizygotic twinning.[21] This observation, together with the increase in dizygotic twinning rates with age, might suggest that increased twinning rates are more likely to be a sign of impaired ovarian function.

"Quintland"

In an age when fertility drugs have made pregnancies of six or seven babies barely worth a news story, it is hard to appreciate the novelty of the Dionne quintuplets. Not only were they born at a time when quintuplets much more rare, but these girls were identical—the first set of identical quintuplets known to have survived birth. Marie, Cécile, Yvonne, Emilie, and Annette were born to a poor family in Ontario, Canada in 1935, in the depths of the Great Depression. The babies became international celebrities. A special nursery was built in which tourists could watch the sisters from an observation gallery. For a time, the sisters were Ontario's biggest tourist attraction, surpassing Niagara Falls. The girls were kept this way until age 9, without formal schooling or social contacts other than their caregivers. Annette and Cécile are still living.

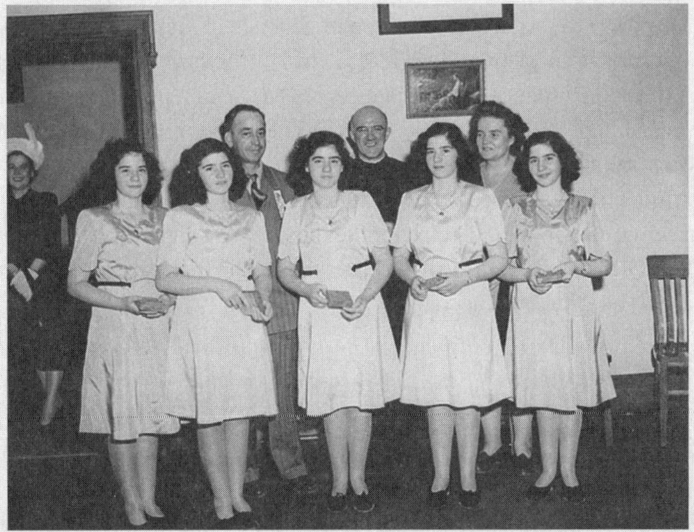

The Dionne quintuplets—Reprinted Courtesy of the National Film Board of Canada/Library and Archives Canada

Hazards of Twinning

Twins are born about 3 weeks earlier than singleton babies on average and have smaller birth weights at a given gestational age.[22] Infant mortality for twins is five times that of singletons.[23] In addition, twins are at increased risk for complications of pregnancy and delivery, such as breech birth. The second-born twin is at higher risk of perinatal death than the first. Twins are at higher risk later in life for mental retardation and cerebral palsy. There is further risk for the smaller twin if the two twins have a large difference in birth weights.[24] Historically, twins have had worse academic performance than singletons, although in more recent cohorts, this disadvantage of twins has disappeared.[25]

Disease Concordance and Genetic Inference

One intensely studied aspect of twins has nothing to do with twinning itself but with the use of twins as a window on genetic causes of disease. Francis Galton proposed this approach in 1875, and researchers continue to explore its possibilities. Galton's approach has great intuitive appeal. Monozygotic twins share the same intrauterine environment and (virtually) all their genes, whereas dizygotic twins share the uterine environment but only half their genes. To the degree that a disease is directly caused by genes, the disease will be more likely to be shared by monozygous twins than by dizygous twins. For example, if one monozygotic twin has a facial cleft, the chances are around 60% that its twin will also be affected. In contrast, the concordance between dizygotic twins is no more than 10%.[26] This difference points to the strong influence of genetics in facial clefts.

The interpretation of twin data is less straightforward for childhood or adult diseases. The concordance for prostate cancer has been reported as 19% in monozygotic twins and 4% in dizygotic twins.[27] The higher concordance in monozygotic twins might suggest a genetic contribution to the risk of prostate cancer. However, identical twins could also be more likely than other twins to choose the same environmental and behavioral exposures throughout their lifetimes. As in any family-based studies of recurrence, the possible effects of shared environment have to be taken into account.

References

1. Enders AC. Implantation in the nine-banded armadillo: how does a single blastocyst form four embryos? *Placenta* 2002;23(1):71–85.
2. Bulmer MG. *The Biology of Twinning in Man*. Oxford: Clarendon Press, 1970.
3. Hall JG. Twinning. *Lancet* 2003;362(9385):735–43.
4. Landy HJ, Keith LG. The vanishing twin: a review. *Hum Reprod* Update 1998;4(2):177–83.
5. Yu N, Kruskall MS, Yunis JJ, et al. Disputed maternity leading to identification of tetragametic chimerism. *N Engl J Med* 2002;346(20):1545–52.
6. Duncan KR. Twin-to-twin transfusion: update on management options and outcomes. *Curr Opin Obstet Gynecol* 2005;17(6):618–22.
7. Benirschke K. The placenta in twin gestation. *Clin Obstet Gynecol* 1990;33(1):18–31.
8. Christiansen L, Frederiksen H, Schousboe K, et al. Age- and sex-differences in the validity of questionnaire-based zygosity in twins. *Twin Res* 2003;6(4):275–8.
9. Weinberg W. Beitraege zur Physiologie und Patholgoie der Mehrlingsgeburten beim Menschen. *Pfluegers Arch ges Physiol* 1901;88:346–430.
10. Fellman J, Eriksson AW. Weinberg's differential rule reconsidered. *Hum Biol* 2006;78(3):253–75.
11. Bulmer MG. The effect of parental age, parity and duration of marriage on the twinning rate. *Ann Hum Genet* 1959;23:454–8.

12. Hoekstra C, Zhao ZZ, Lambalk CB, et al. Dizygotic twinning. *Hum Reprod* Update 2008;14(1):37–47.
13. Beemsterboer SN, Homburg R, Gorter NA, Schats R, Hompes PG, Lambalk CB. The paradox of declining fertility but increasing twinning rates with advancing maternal age. *Hum Reprod* 2006;21(6):1531–2.
14. D'Addato AV. Secular trends in twinning rates. *J Biosoc Sci* 2007;39(1):147–51.
15. Blickstein I, Keith LG. The decreased rates of triplet births: temporal trends and biologic speculations. *Am J Obstet Gynecol* 2005;193(2):327–31.
16. Martin JA, Hamilton BE, Sutton PD, et al. Births: Final data for 2005. *Natl Vital Stat Rep* 2007;56(6).
17. Herskind AM, Basso O, Olsen J, Skytthe A, Christensen K. Is the natural twinning rate still declining? *Epidemiology* 2005;16(4):591–2.
18. James WH. Monitoring reproductive health in Europe: what are the best indicators? *Hum Reprod* 2007;22(5):1197–9.
19. Basso O, Christensen K, Olsen J. Fecundity and twinning. A study within the Danish National Birth Cohort. *Hum Reprod* 2004;19(10):2222–6.
20. Zhu JL, Basso O, Obel C, Christensen K, Olsen J. Infertility, infertility treatment and twinning: the Danish National Birth Cohort. *Hum Reprod* 2007;22(4):1086–90.
21. Olsen J, Bonnelykke B, Nielsen J. Tobacco smoking and twinning. *Acta Med Scand* 1988;224(5):491–4.
22. Kleinman JC, Fowler MG, Kessel SS. Comparison of infant mortality among twins and singletons: United States 1960 and 1983. *Am J Epidemiol* 1991;133(2):133–43.
23. Mathews TJ, MacDorman MF. Infant Mortality Statistics from the 2005 Period Linked Birth/Infant Death Data Set. In: Statistics NCH, 2008;57:1–32.
24. Garite TJ, Clark RH, Elliott JP, Thorp JA. Twins and triplets: the effect of plurality and growth on neonatal outcome compared with singleton infants. *Am J Obstet Gynecol* 2004;191(3):700–7.
25. Christensen K, McGue M. Academic achievement in twins. *BMJ* 2008;337:a651.
26. Christensen K. The 20th century Danish facial cleft population—epidemiological and genetic-epidemiological studies. *Cleft Palate Craniofac J* 1999;36(2):96–104.
27. Gronberg H, Damber L, Damber JE. Studies of genetic factors in prostate cancer in a twin population. *J Urol* 1994;152(5 Pt 1):1484–7; discussion 1487–9.

14

Gestational Age and Preterm Delivery

Gestational age is arguably the most important measurement in reproductive epidemiology. Gestational age is what separates miscarriages from stillbirths and preterm from term births. Given its central importance, it is remarkable that gestational age can be estimated only approximately. This imprecision has consequences for virtually every aspect of pregnancy research.

It is a truism that normal pregnancies last 9 months. The early Christian Church set The Feast of the Annunciation (marking the conception of Jesus) as March 25—exactly 9 months before Christmas. Although 9 months provides women with a useful due date, this date is only an approximation. Observers as far back as Aristotle recognized that the length of pregnancy varies widely among women.[1] The probability that a woman will deliver on her due date is less than 5%[2] (or, as a Sicilian proverb puts it, "only the Virgin Mary actually delivered at 9 months").

Determining Gestational Age

The ideal measure of gestational age would be from the day of conception (which takes place less than a day after ovulation). Conception is not detectable, but ovulation is. Ovulation can be identified by the surge of luteinizing hormone that triggers ovulation or by the abrupt changes in estrogen and progesterone that follow ovulation.[3,4] These hormonal markers of ovulation are reasonably accurate when compared with ultrasound-documented ovarian follicle rupture.[5] Unfortunately, epidemiologists rarely have the benefit of data on ovulation, and must rely on less direct estimates of the time of pregnancy onset.

The Last Menstrual Period

The standard clinical benchmark for onset of pregnancy is the first day of a woman's last menstrual period (LMP). The due-date is calculated as 280 days (40 weeks) after the LMP. The use of 280 days goes back to at least 1709,[6] and was chosen not on the basis of data but because 10 menstrual cycles (of 28 days each) seemed a harmonious number. As it turns out, this was not a bad guess. A century later, Naegele provided a convenient way to estimate 280 days by adding 9 months and 1 week to the LMP.[6] This is still known today as Naegele's Rule.

LIMITATIONS OF LMP. The basic problem with LMP as the benchmark for conception is that LMP is only a surrogate. Conception takes place immediately after ovulation, which in turn occurs at a variable time after LMP. The assumption with LMP is that women ovulate an average of 2 weeks after the onset of their last menses. If the time interval from LMP to ovulation were always 2 weeks (or any other constant length of time), LMP would be a fine marker. However, this interval is far from constant. Figure 14-1 shows data (also provided in Fig. 1-10) for the distribution of follicular-phase length (time from onset of LMP to ovulation). The mode is 14 days, the mean is 17 days, and the tail to the right extends as far as 8 weeks.

A second source of error in LMP is women's recall. Women are routinely asked at their first prenatal visit for the date of their most recent menstrual period. The accuracy of their recall depends on the regularity of their cycles and how much time has elapsed since the LMP. Most women can recall their LMP within 1–2 days,[7] but for a few the error is much greater. Pregnant women who cannot

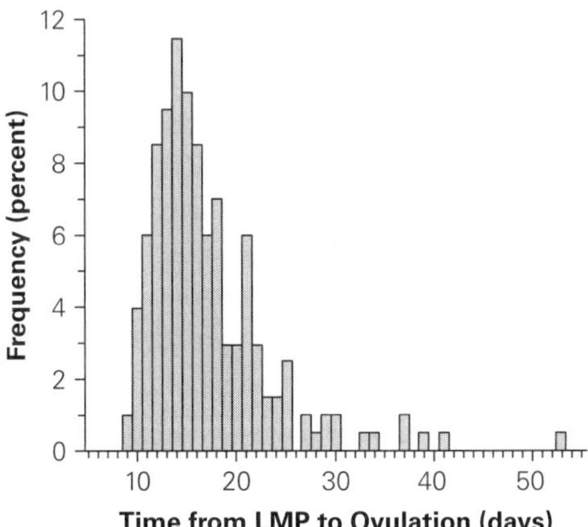

Figure 14-1. Variability in time from last menstrual period to conception (at ovulation) (estimated by distribution of follicular-phase lengths, 217 women, North Carolina, 1983–85)[3]

recall any date for their LMP are likely to have less education and in other ways be unrepresentative of the general population.[8] A few pregnant women have no LMP to recall. This can happen, for example, if conception has occurred with the first ovulation after a previous pregnancy (and before the first menses can occur).

Long follicular phases are as fertile as shorter ones. If we assume that the distribution of follicular-phase lengths in Figure 14-1 represents the distribution of ovulation times in conception cycles, then 15% of pregnancies would have a true gestational age at least 1 week shorter than their LMP prediction (follicular phase lasting at least 3 weeks), and 5% of pregnancies would have a true gestational age at least 3 weeks shorter (follicular phase lasting at least 5 weeks). In contrast, few pregnancies would have a true gestational age more than 1 week longer than the LMP-based prediction (follicular phase lasting less than 1 week). Thus, LMP introduces an asymmetric error in gestational age, producing more false "late" deliveries than false "early" deliveries.

Ultrasound-Based Dates

Fetal size in early pregnancy is another way to estimate gestational age. This assumes that the size of a fetus in the first half of pregnancy is a function of age alone, not of rate of growth. This assumption is not strictly true, but ultrasound measurements have nonetheless been widely used for this purpose. In most developed countries, ultrasound measurements of the fetus are routinely made during LMP weeks 16–20, with fetal age based on length of the femur or width of the fetal head (biparietal diameter). Before 13 weeks, gestational age can be estimated from the crown-rump length.

Ultrasound dimensions of the fetus are converted to an estimated gestational age (in terms of weeks from LMP). If there is a large enough discrepancy between the ultrasound- and LMP-based estimates, the age based on ultrasound measurement takes precedence; otherwise the LMP is kept as the best estimate of gestational age The amount of tolerable discrepancy varies—clinical guidelines are typically 7, 10, or 14 days difference between the LMP and ultrasound dates.[9]

Fetal size could in principle be used more directly to predict delivery date, without conversion to an LMP-based date. Norwegian researchers have provided estimates of the time from a given fetal size to natural delivery using data from a large number of pregnancies with ultrasound measures and delivery dates.[10] This approach provides a substantially tighter (i.e., more precise) distribution of delivery dates than LMP, with 87% of births occurring within plus or minus 14 days. This more direct approach has not yet become widely used.

The more usual ultrasound adjustment of LMP does improve the estimation of gestational age. Ultrasound-based adjustment substantially reduces the percentage of babies born postterm (presumably by replacing many of the LMPs that had included long follicular phases). Consequences for the percentage preterm are less consistent. Where LMP data are of good quality, ultrasound adjustment tends to increase the number of preterm births,[9] primarily among those born at 35 and 36 weeks. However, vital statistics data have more extensive errors in LMP, and the percentage preterm may actually be reduced after ultrasound adjustment.[11] Errors in vital statistics LMPs seem especially common among deliveries less than 32 weeks by LMP.[12]

LIMITATIONS OF ULTRASOUND DATES. Ultrasound measures are not a gold standard. Measurement error is inevitable. (Viewing a few blurry ultrasound images on the Internet will give you an idea of the difficulty of such measurements.) A difference of just 2 mm in head diameter or femur length can affect the estimated fetal age by half a week.[10]

Furthermore, any natural variations in the rate of fetal growth are automatically translated into variations in fetal age. Given two fetuses conceived on the same date, the one that grows more rapidly will be assigned an older gestational age by ultrasound than the one growing more slowly. Natural variation in fetal growth in the first half of pregnancy adds error to the ultrasound estimate of fetal age.[13] This error is probably of minor importance for most pregnancies but may complicate the interpretation of risk for fetuses with pathologically slowed growth. An exposure that damages the growth of fetuses but has no effect on length of pregnancy could, on the basis of ultrasound-assigned age, appear to increase the risk of preterm delivery.

Another problem with ultrasound dating is the potential for selection bias. If a substantial portion of the population does not have access to ultrasound or chooses not to have the examination, the advantages of adjusting dates by ultrasound will not apply equally across the population. Such selection could potentially confound the epidemiologic analyses of gestational-age-related outcomes.

Other approaches to the assessment of a newborn infant's gestational maturity have been proposed using clinical criteria of the baby's appearance at birth (developmental morphology, neurologic features), bone maturation (as assessed by x-ray), and others. These methods are extremely imprecise and have not proved useful for epidemiologic purposes.[14]

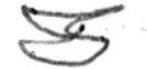

The Use of "Completed" Weeks

It is standard clinical practice to express the length of pregnancy in completed weeks rather than ordinal weeks. This approach is analogous to how we measure human age: a woman is not 20 years old until she completes her twentieth year of life. When applied to delivery dates, for example, week 40 starts on day 280, the beginning of the forty-first week. This numbering convention can be more confusing when extended to the earlier stages of pregnancy. The onset of the last

Table 14-1. Numbering convention for gestational age (completed weeks), in which day zero is the first day of the last menstrual period[a]

	LMP ⇩		Ovulation ⇩			
Obstetric days	0 1 2 3 4 5 6	7…13	14…20	…	273…279	280…286
Obstetric weeks	0	1	2	…	39	40
Embryo weeks	—	—	1st	…	38th	39th
Ordinal weeks	1st	2nd	3rd	…	40th	41st

[a] For comparison, the table also shows the numbering convention for embryologic age and the ordinal numbering of weeks from LMP.

menstrual period is *day 0*, and the first week after LMP is *week 0* (Table 14-1). Ovulation occurs (on average) around the beginning of obstetric week 2, which is the third week after LMP.

To muddle the picture further, embryologists use ordinal weeks to date fetal development. The first week of life after conception is week 1. If conception takes place on day 14 after LMP, then what embryologists call "week 1" is "week 2" by obstetric convention, and the third week from LMP by ordinary counting (Table 14-1). Embryologists often assume their numbering system is 2 weeks different from the LMP-based date (because of the 2 weeks that precede ovulation). In fact, their time-scales differ by only one week. A well-known embryology textbook has printed an illustration with incorrect obstetric dates through eight editions.[15]

The Frequency Distribution of Pregnancy Length

Even with all its limitations, the last menstrual period remains a widely used benchmark for gestational age (with or without corrections by ultrasound). Based on last menstrual period, gestational age at birth is shown in Figure 14-2 for 11.5 million U.S. singleton births (2000–2002).

The standard deviation of the main distribution of gestational ages for term births (37 to 42 weeks) is about 10 days. This variability has many sources, including errors in the recall of LMP and the variability of follicular-phase length. If we could remove all these extraneous sources of variation, how much natural variability would remain in the true length of gestation? In a prospective study of 126 naturally conceived babies born at term,[16] the mean time from ovulation to delivery was 263 days. The range of gestational ages (counting from ovulation) spanned more than 5 weeks, with a standard deviation of 6 days. These data suggest that, even with

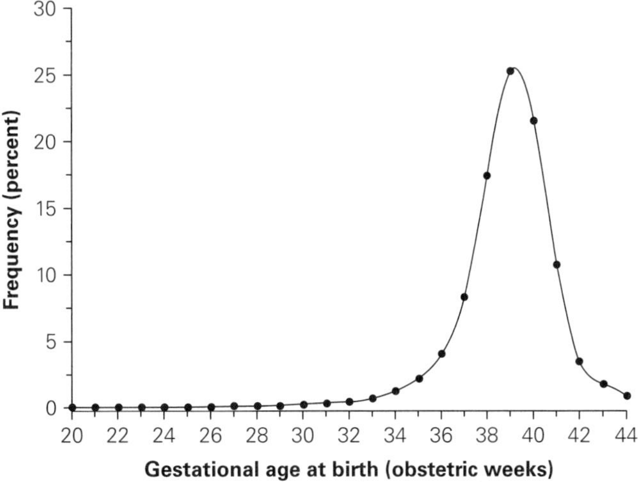

Figure 14-2. Distribution of the length of pregnancy (from last menstrual period) (11.5 million singleton live births, United States, 2000–2002) (*Source:* U.S. National Center for Health Statistics)

optimum measurement of conception, the duration of healthy term pregnancies has considerable biological variation.

Such variation may reflect differences in the pace of fetal maturation and also differences in the mother's capacity to carry the fetus as she approaches term. Twins are born much earlier than singletons on average, probably because of the effects of increased physical load in the uterus. Still, we know surprisingly little about the factors that determine when labor and delivery will take place.

The Enigma of Gestational Age

Conception is invisible,
but what triggers it is known to all.
Delivery is known to all,
but what triggers it is invisible.
—A.J.W.

Changes over Time

One of the striking aspects of the U.S. gestational age distribution in the last few decades is its shift to earlier gestational ages. For many years, the distribution of gestational age was regarded as relatively resistant to external influences. Unlike birth weight, which is relatively sensitive to such factors as sex of the baby or parity or maternal smoking, gestational age is relatively constant across these variables.[17] (The exception is ethnicity; African-Americans have pregnancies about 1 week shorter than women of European descent.[18]) The recent shift in gestational age in the United States has no precedent. From 1980 to 2004, the whole gestational age distribution shifted downward by more than a week, from a median of 282 days to 274 days.[19,20] This shift to earlier deliveries is presumed to reflect an increase in obstetric interventions.[20]

Influence of Clinical Interventions

Obstetricians increasingly intervene to provoke labor and delivery before it occurs naturally. This complicates epidemiologic studies of gestational length or gestation-specific outcomes. Labor is induced in 20% of U.S. deliveries, usually for medical reasons.[21,22] Indications include preeclampsia, fetal distress, and placental abruption.[23] Risks and benefits of this intervention are not well studied.

Cesarean section is a more invasive intervention than induction and usually requires a more definite medical indication. Fetal distress, prolonged or difficult labor, breech presentation, and previous cesarean section are common reasons. However, there is also an increasing trend toward offering cesarean section to women as an elective option.[24] In the United States, the rate of cesarean section is 30% and rising.[25] Private hospitals in Latin America have cesarean rates of 50%, with some hospitals as high as 80%.[26,27] As with induction, there are few data to allow full assessment of the risks and benefits of this intervention.

Preterm Delivery

Infants born too soon are less likely to be developmentally prepared for life outside the uterus. This self-evident fact is acknowledged in obstetrics textbooks since at least the mid-1800s, when prematurity was mentioned as a debilitating condition of the infant born after 6 months but before "term."[28] The pioneering epidemiologist William Farr added prematurity to the official causes of death in the British system of vital statistics in 1858.[29]

Figure 14-3 shows neonatal mortality among births at each gestational age. There is a steady increase in risk among deliveries at each week earlier than 40 weeks. (Note that mortality is shown on a logarithmic scale to accommodate the steep gradient.) Survival among babies born before 23 weeks remains uncommon.

Our current definition of prematurity is birth before 37 weeks. This definition was proposed in 1902[30] and initially won wide acceptance.[31] Then came the unfortunate detour of 1919–61.

"Prematurity" and Low Birth Weight

In 1919, an influential Finnish pediatrician named Arvo Ylppö suggested that a birth weight criterion of 2,500 g would be a useful way to identify premature

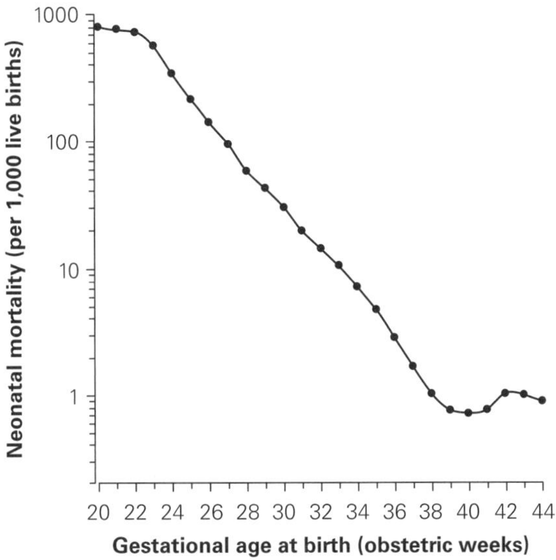

Figure 14-3. Neonatal mortality rates by gestational age at birth (11.5 million singleton live births, United States, 2000–2002) (*Source:* US National Center for Health Statistics)

infants.[32] Even though Ylppö cautioned that birth weight is an imperfect measure of maturity, his warning was quickly forgotten. The convenience of weight as a criterion led the 2,500-g definition of prematurity to usurp all others. Small size was equated with early delivery, and for decades, 2,500 g became the standard definition of prematurity in both the clinical and epidemiologic literature.

It was not until the 1950s that epidemiologists began to come to grips with the considerable error introduced by the 2,500-g definition of prematurity.[33] Data emerging from population-based birth studies showed that less than half of babies under 2,500 g were actually premature by reported gestational age, and less than half of babies preterm by gestational age were smaller than 2,500 g. In 1961, the World Health Organization recommended that babies less than 2,500 g no longer be referred to as "premature" but as "low birth weight."

Usage did not change overnight: a book published in 1977 with the title *The Epidemiology of Prematurity* is entirely about low birth weight.[34] The term *prematurity* remained so strongly connected with low birth weight that researchers gave up trying to redefine it and abandoned the word altogether.[35] Babies who are immature by gestational age came to be referred to as *preterm*, a usage that continues to this day. Prematurity remains a useful concept, and when enough years have passed, perhaps the word can be restored to use in its original sense, to describe a baby born before its time.

Occurrence of Preterm Delivery

The proportion of births delivered preterm (including stillbirths) ranges from 5% to 9% in most developed countries.[36] Data from developing countries are less reliable, and in many cases are unavailable. Even within developed countries, the risk of preterm can vary severalfold. The proportion of preterm is 5%–6% in the Nordic countries,[37] 7% in Hong Kong Chinese,[38] and 13% in the United States. Within the United States, rates are 12% in whites and 18% in blacks.[20] Factors that may contribute to these differences include regional differences in the criteria for registration of stillbirths and live births, differences in the extent of medical interventions (such as induction and cesarean section), and differences in the estimation of gestational age.

The proportion of preterm babies in the United States has been steadily rising.[20] This increase has been almost entirely among the relatively more mature preterm deliveries (35 and 36 weeks); very early preterm births have increased only slightly over recent decades.[39]

Subtypes of Preterm Birth

Preterm birth is the final common pathway for many different factors that can produce early delivery.[36] In an effort to clarify the causes of preterm birth, various attempts have been made to create more homogeneous subcategories. One approach is to categorize preterm births by gestational ages, for example, "very preterm" (before 32 weeks) and "extremely preterm" (before 28 weeks) (Fig. 14-4). (Definitions of these subgroups vary among studies.) Although the earliest preterm births carry the highest mortality risk, they are also rare. Among all U.S. live births, 0.5% are born extremely preterm (before 28 weeks), and another 1% are born very preterm (between 28 and 31 weeks). There is some evidence that the gestational-age subgroups of preterm may be etiologically distinct. A few risk factors (cigarette smoking,[40] race[20]) have relatively stronger effects on earlier preterm births than on later preterm.

The category of live births before 28 weeks is remarkable in that it exists at all. Only a few decades ago, births before 28 weeks did not even qualify as stillbirths because they were regarded as having no hope of survival. By 1995, 44% of infants born at 25 weeks in the United Kingdom were surviving to hospital discharge.[41]

Preterm births can also be categorized by their clinical presentation (idiopathic preterm labor, preterm premature rupture of the membranes, and induced labor or cesarean section for medical complications) or by their presumed etiologic pathway (infection, vascular pathology, specific complications, uterine overdistension).[40] Examples of all of these subcategories can be found in the epidemiologic literature, although these are not consistently defined or widely used.

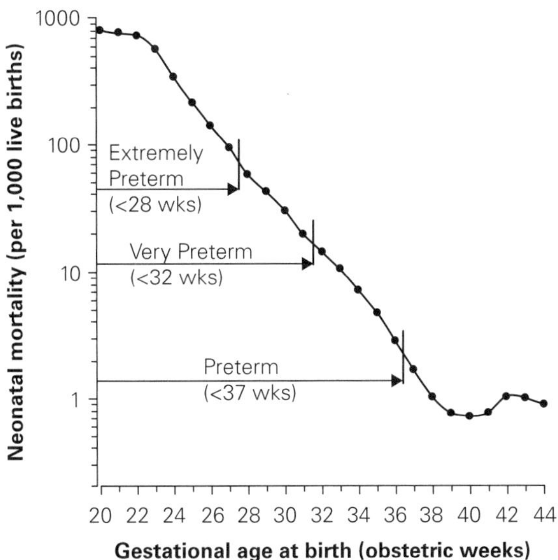

Figure 14-4. Categories of "preterm," "very preterm," and "extremely preterm" births

Direction of Causation?

Preterm delivery is often described as the leading cause of infant mortality in developed countries. This is based on the fact that the number of infant deaths among preterm babies far exceeds the number of deaths among babies born at term. It does not necessarily follow, however, that had all those preterm babies been born at term, their mortality would be as low as other term births. The mortality associated with preterm delivery is not simply a matter of the baby being delivered before it is ready. Pathological conditions that predispose the baby to preterm delivery (e.g., maternal diabetes or congenital malformations) can also contribute directly to the morbidity of the baby.

The fact that babies born preterm are smaller on average than the fetuses that continue in utero is further evidence that these babies are struggling even before they are delivered.[42] To the degree that impaired fetal development or fetal distress can cause preterm delivery, those conditions also contribute to the mortality and morbidity observed in association with preterm delivery. Thus, effective intervention must include prevention of the causes of preterm delivery, not simply interventions on early labor. Early delivery may be preferable to continuation if delivery allows an ailing fetus to escape adverse intrauterine conditions. (This is one rationale for physician-initiated deliveries.)

It follows from this argument that the risk with immaturity may be less than the observed rates of gestation-specific mortality would suggest. Evidence for

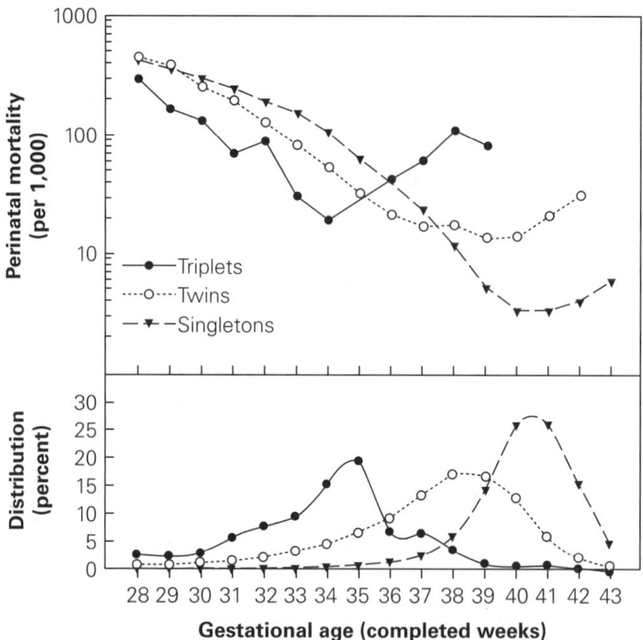

Figure 14-5. Gestational-age-specific mortality for singletons, twins, and triplets (Norway, 1967–98) (Reprinted from Lie[43])

this comes from a comparison of the perinatal mortality curves for singletons, twins, and triplets (Fig. 14-5).[43] Multiple births tend to deliver early for reasons related to their plurality rather than to any specific pathology. This could explain the lower mortality seen among twins—and especially among triplets—at early gestational ages compared with singletons. Put another way, the mortality of singletons at the same gestational age may be higher because singletons born at early gestational ages are more likely to have some predisposing problem that has triggered their preterm delivery. Delivery at an early gestational age could be less dangerous than suggested by the mortality rate of all babies born at that gestational age.

Causes of Preterm Delivery

PROXIMAL CAUSES OF PRETERM DELIVERY. Infections of the reproductive tract have been widely studied as a factor in preterm delivery. There are plausible biological pathways for this effect,[44] and extensive circumstantial evidence to support the hypothesis. For example, very preterm newborns are much more likely to have blood infections at birth.[45] The important question is whether outcome of pregnancy can be improved with antibiotic treatment. Although results are not conclusive, clinical trials suggest possible benefits with antibiotic treatment during pregnancy.[46,47]

IATROGENIC CAUSES. Medical procedures increase the proportion of preterm babies both directly and indirectly. A direct cause is the increased use of interventions to deliver babies early, usually for reasons of the mother's or baby's health. For example, preeclamptic pregnancies are more often being interrupted before the condition can advance to the point of endangering the mother. Although such interventions may increase the proportion of preterm deliveries, the purpose is to reduce mortality and morbidity, and there is some evidence that this is succeeding.[48]

Less directly, the increase in conceptions by assisted reproductive technology has contributed to an increase of preterm delivery. This happens in at least two ways. First, singleton babies conceived by ART have twice the preterm risk of other singletons.[49] (Some of this excess risk is probably caused by the underlying condition of the mother rather than by her treatment.[50] Even so, to the degree ART pregnancies would not otherwise occur, they contribute risk.) Second, ART pregnancies comprise about 17% of twins in the United States and about 40% of triplets.[51] Pregnancies with multiple fetuses are much more likely to deliver preterm and suffer the associated mortality.

SOCIAL AND BEHAVIORAL CAUSES. The strong contrast in U.S. preterm rates by maternal race suggests that socioeconomic and behavioral factors play an important role. Even in egalitarian societies such as the Nordic countries, mothers with less education have higher risk of preterm birth.[37] The epidemiologic search for factors underlying these associations has had limited success. Smoking increases the risk of preterm birth (especially early preterm birth).[40] This explains only a small part of the social-class association.[52] Other maternal characteristics associated with preterm delivery include thinness[53] and diabetes,[54] but these are weakly associated with social class. There is little evidence for an alcohol effect on preterm risk, except perhaps with very high levels of consumption. Illicit drug use (including opiates and cocaine) is difficult to study but may increase the risk of preterm birth.[40] Although observational studies suggest benefits from prenatal folic acid and iron supplements, these have not been confirmed in clinical trials.[55] Many studies have looked at the physical and psychological demands of employment as well as effects of leisure physical activities; no obvious patterns of association have emerged.[40]

ENVIRONMENTAL CAUSES. Many studies of environmental contaminants have considered effects on preterm birth; however, there is at best limited evidence for associations with a few exposures (lead, DDT, air pollution, and occupational exposure to PCBs).[56] For a host of other exposures, the evidence of association is regarded as inadequate.

Given the limited understanding of causes of preterm delivery, there is little that can be said about the time windows during which exposures might affect risk. Some causes may be proximal to delivery, whereas others undoubtedly act earlier (leading to reduced fetal growth, for example). Some factors may act long before women conceive. For example, women who had been exposed as fetuses to diethylstilbestrol (DES) are at two to three times the usual risk of preterm delivery in their own pregnancies.[57]

Markers of Preterm Risk

The previous delivery of a preterm infant is a strong predictor of preterm delivery in the next pregnancy. Genetics may play a role: mothers who are born preterm are at increased risk of delivering preterm themselves.[58] Pregnancies with vaginal bleeding during the first or second trimester are at increased risk of delivering early. With bleeding in both trimesters, the risk of preterm delivery is increased fourfold.[59] A more proximal marker of risk is fetal fibronectin in the vaginal fluid. If no fibronectin is present, the risk of impending delivery is very low, regardless of other clinical signs. If fibronectin is present, the risk of imminent delivery is modestly increased.[60]

The Treatment of Preterm Labor

Tocolytic agents are drugs intended to delay or arrest progression of preterm labor. In principle, such delay may defer birth long enough to permit other treatments (such as administration of steroids to accelerate lung maturation) that improve the baby's chances of survival. Many tocolytic treatments have been developed, but none has been demonstrated to improve the outcome of pregnancy.[61] Progesterone (the hormone that "supports pregnancy") appears to decrease the risk of early preterm delivery in some clinical trials, especially in women with previous preterm deliveries. More trials are in progress to help resolve this question.[62] Cervical cerclage (sewing the cervix shut) is a surgical procedure with a long history but little evidence of benefit.[61]

Long-term Sequelae of Preterm Delivery

Among the infants who survive preterm delivery, there is increased risk of developmental problems including epilepsy,[63] cerebral palsy, mental retardation, and autism.[64] The risks are highest among those born very early, with at least a 10-fold increase among babies born before 28 weeks compared with term babies.[64] As discussed earlier, it is not obvious to what extent these sequelae might stem from preterm delivery itself, and to what extent they might be associated with the factors that triggered preterm delivery. Those who survive preterm birth without major disabilities have good prospects of normal function.[64]

Postterm Delivery

Postterm delivery is defined as pregnancies that reach 42 completed weeks or more.[65] Gestational-age-specific mortality reaches its lowest levels during weeks 39 to 41 and rises at week 42 and thereafter (Fig. 14-3). Because mortality data are cross-sectional, the direction of cause and effect is unclear: Does longer pregnancy increase the risk of fetal problems, or do fetuses with problems fail to trigger delivery at the usual time?

About 5% of well-dated pregnancies end in postterm delivery.[66] This percentage can easily vary with the extent of LMP correction and the practice of induction of labor. Few risk factors are known to be associated with postterm delivery. Postterm may be increased for women who are pregnant for the first time or for women with lower social class or education, but these associations are not consistent.[66]

Errors in gestational age are a major contributor to postterm births, especially when due dates are based solely on the last menstrual period. A long follicular phase in the cycle of conception will cause an overestimation of true gestational age by adding time to the interval between LMP and conception. Correction of LMP-based gestational age by ultrasound reduces the number of "postterm" births by at least half.[66]

The higher risk with ongoing pregnancy after 40 weeks is a matter of clinical concern, especially with regard to stillbirths. Regardless of the direction of cause and effect, late stillbirths could in principle be averted with earlier delivery. With this rationale, induction of labor is commonly carried out in the United States after 41 weeks, even though clinical trials have shown little if any benefit from induced labor to prevent postterm births.[67] Admittedly, the low absolute levels of perinatal risk late in pregnancy make it difficult to perform clinical trials with power to detect a benefit.

Analytic Problems of Gestational Age

Gestational Age as a Time Variable

Gestational age is both a time scale and an epidemiologic endpoint, and therein lies a world of trouble. Consider the question of seasonal effects on preterm risk. A simple analysis might look at the percentage of preterm births by month. However, this would assume that conceptions (which create the denominator) are evenly distributed across the calendar, which they are not. An analysis of births at one point in time compares preterm births from one conception cohort with term births from another. If those two conception cohorts are different sizes (e.g., because of seasonal differences in conception), then preterm risk could appear different by season, even if season has no effect on preterm risk. The solution would be to compare preterm rates within cohorts of pregnancies defined by conception date, rather than by birth date.

Gestational time can be confused with exposure. Consider a reported association between maternal low blood pressure and high perinatal mortality.[68] The authors found that low blood pressure was associated with increased fetal risk. The authors hypothesized that low blood pressure could produce poor placental perfusion and poor fetal outcome. The mechanism is plausible, but the observation was actually caused by an analytic error. Blood pressure naturally increases during pregnancy. Women in the study were enrolled at various times during pregnancy. The earlier the enrolment, the lower the blood pressure and the greater the opportunity for women to deliver early (with consequent risk of perinatal mortality). Blood pressure measurements taken later in pregnancy were higher, and (all else being equal) those women had less opportunity to deliver early. Thus, although there was an "association" between low blood pressure and perinatal mortality, it was an artefact of the timing of blood pressure measurements. When stage of pregnancy was controlled for, the association of low blood pressure with perinatal mortality disappeared.[69]

Similar problems might occur with any exposure that systematically varies with gestational age. For example, maternal blood volume expands during pregnancy and can dilute the mother's blood concentration of micronutrients or environmental contaminants. Thus, biomarker concentrations may decline with advancing gestational age. An analysis of births stratified by blood concentration at delivery could show higher concentrations of an environmental contaminant with preterm birth, even when no direct causal association exists. Similarly, the longer a woman's pregnancy, the more prenatal visits she accumulates. An analysis of preterm risk stratified by total number of prenatal visits could suggest that prenatal visits protect against preterm delivery.

The Analysis of Gestational-Age-Specific Mortality

As discussed in Chapter 12, there are conflicting views on the way gestational-age-specific risk should be expressed.[70,71] The usual approach is shown in Figure 14-3, with deaths as a proportion of all births at a given week of pregnancy. An alternative is to express risk as a proportion of births plus all ongoing pregnancies (that is, the total number of fetuses at risk at a given gestational age).[72] With this approach used for stillbirth risk, for example, stillbirths delivered at week 29 would be expressed as a proportion of all births at 29 weeks plus all fetuses continuing in utero. This increases the denominator greatly, producing a much lower estimate of risk at most gestational ages.

Both methods provide a number that describes risk. The "fetuses at risk" approach seems most justified for stillbirths that occur before the onset of labor[73] and less justified for deaths that occur during delivery or after birth. Furthermore, when a risk factor shortens gestational age, the assessment of gestational-age-specific mortality can be problematic. If there are unmeasured factors that increase mortality and also cause early delivery, such factors can distort the comparison of gestational-age specific mortality rates.[74] For all these reasons, the analysis of gestational-age specific mortality remains a controversial issue.

References

1. Dunn PM. Aristotle (384–322 BC): philosopher and scientist of ancient Greece. *Arch Dis Child Fetal Neonatal Ed* 2006;91(1):F75–7.
2. Kloosterman GJ. Prolonged pregnancy. *Gynaecologia* 1956;142(6):372–88.
3. Baird DD, Weinberg CR, Wilcox AJ, McConnaughey DR, Musey PI. Using the ratio of urinary oestrogen and progesterone metabolites to estimate day of ovulation. *Stat Med* 1991;10(2):255–66.
4. Kesner JS, Knecht EA, Krieg EF, Jr, Wilcox AJ, O'Connor JF. Detecting pre-ovulatory luteinizing hormone surges in urine. *Hum Reprod* 1998;13(1):15–21.
5. Ecochard R, Boehringer H, Rabilloud M, Marret H. Chronological aspects of ultrasonic, hormonal, and other indirect indices of ovulation. *Br J Obstet Gynaecol* 2001;108(8):822–9.
6. Saunders N, Paterson C. Can we abandon Naegele's rule? *Lancet* 1991; 337(8741): 600–1.
7. Wegienka G, Baird DD. A comparison of recalled date of last menstrual period with prospectively recorded dates. *J Womens Health (Larchmt)* 2005;14(3):248–52.
8. Buekens P, Delvoye P, Wollast E, Robyn C. Epidemiology of pregnancies with unknown last menstrual period. *J Epidemiol Community Health* 1984;38(1):79–80.
9. Blondel B, Morin I, Platt RW, Kramer MS, Usher R, Breart G. Algorithms for combining menstrual and ultrasound estimates of gestational age: consequences for rates of preterm and postterm birth. *Br J Obstet Gynaecol* 2002;109(6):718–20.
10. Gjessing HK, Grottum P, Eik-Nes SH. A direct method for ultrasound prediction of day of delivery: a new, population-based approach. *Ultrasound Obstet Gynecol* 2007;30(1):19–27.
11. Joseph KS, Huang L, Liu S, et al. Reconciling the high rates of preterm and postterm birth in the United States. *Obstet Gynecol* 2007;109(4):813–22.
12. Haglund B. Birthweight distributions by gestational age: comparison of LMP-based and ultrasound-based estimates of gestational age using data from the Swedish Birth Registry. *Paediatr Perinat Epidemiol* 2007;21 Suppl 2:72–8.
13. Henriksen TB, Wilcox AJ, Hedegaard M, Secher NJ. Bias in studies of preterm and postterm delivery due to ultrasound assessment of gestational age. *Epidemiology* 1995;6(5):533–7.
14. Alexander GR, Tompkins ME, Petersen DJ, Hulsey TC, Mor J. Discordance between LMP-based and clinically estimated gestational age: implications for research, programs, and policy. *Public Health Rep* 1995;110(4):395–402.
15. Moore KL, Persaud, TVN. *The Developing Human: Clinically Oriented Embryology*. Philadelphia, PA: Saunders, 2008.
16. Wilcox AJ, Weinberg CR, O'Connor JF, et al. Incidence of early loss of pregnancy. *N Engl J Med* 1988;319(4):189–94.
17. Chamberlain RCG, Howlett B, Claireaux A. *British Births 1970: Volume 1, The First Week of Life*. London: William Heinamann Medical Books Ltd, 1975.

18. Papiernik E, Alexander GR, Paneth N. Racial differences in pregnancy duration and its implications for perinatal care. *Med Hypotheses* 1990;33(3):181–6.
19. NCHS. *Advance Report of Final Natality Statistics, 1980. Monthly Vital Statistics Reports*. Vol. 31, November 30, 1982.
20. Martin JA, Hamilton BE, Sutton PD, Ventura SJ, Menacker F, Kirmeyer S. Births: final data for 2004. *Natl Vital Stat Rep* 2006;55(1):1–101.
21. Rayburn WF, Zhang J. Rising rates of labor induction: present concerns and future strategies. *Obstet Gynecol* 2002;100(1):164–7.
22. Lydon-Rochelle MT, Cardenas V, Nelson JC, Holt VL, Gardella C, Easterling TR. Induction of labor in the absence of standard medical indications: incidence and correlates. *Med Care* 2007;45(6):505–12.
23. Ananth CV, Vintzileos AM. Maternal-fetal conditions necessitating a medical intervention resulting in preterm birth. *Am J Obstet Gynecol* 2006;195(6):1557–63.
24. Minkoff H, Chervenak FA. Elective primary cesarean delivery. *N Engl J Med* 2003;348(10):946–50.
25. Martin JA, Hamilton BE, Sutton PD, et al. Births: final data for 2005. *Natl Vital Stat Rep* 2007;56(6):1–103.
26. Callister LC. Cesarean birth rates: global trends. *MCN Am J Matern Child Nurs* 2008;33(2):129.
27. Villar J, Valladares E, Wojdyla D, et al. Caesarean delivery rates and pregnancy outcomes: the 2005 WHO global survey on maternal and perinatal health in Latin America. *Lancet* 2006;367(9525):1819–29.
28. Churchill F. *The Diseases of Females*. 4th ed. Philadelphia, PA: Lea and Blanchard, 1860.
29. Farr W. *Vital Statistics: A Memorial Volume of Selections from the Reports and Writings of William Farr* Metuchen, NJ: Scarecrow Press, 1975.
30. Budin P. Les enfants debiles. *Presse Med* 1902;10:1155.
31. Anctil AO, Joshi GB, Lucas WE, Little WA, Callagan DA. Prematurity: a more precise approach to identification. *Obstet Gynecol* 1964;24:716–21.
32. Ylppö A. Das Wachstum der Fruehgeborenen von der Geburt bis zum Schulalter. *Eur J Pediatr* 1919;24:111–78.
33. McKeown T, Gibson JR. Observations on all births (23,970) in Birmingham, 1947. IV: "Preterm Birth" *Br Med J* 1951;ii:513–7.
34. Reed DM, Stanley FJ. *The Epidemiology of Prematurity*. Baltimore, MD: Urban and Schwarzenberg, 1977.
35. Silverman WA, Lecey JF, Beard A, et al. Committee on fetus and newborn: nomenclature for duration of gestation, birth weight and intra-uterine growth. *Pediatrics* 1967;39:935–9.
36. Goldenberg RL, Culhane JF, Iams JD, Romero R. Epidemiology and causes of preterm birth. *Lancet* 2008;371(9606):75–84.
37. Bjork C, Mortensen LH, Morgen CS, et al. Socio-economic inequality in preterm birth: a comparative study of the Nordic countries from 1981 to 2000. *Paediatr Perinat Epidemiol*, in press.
38. Leung TN, Roach VJ, Lau TK. Incidence of preterm delivery in Hong Kong Chinese. *Aust N Z J Obstet Gynaecol* 1998;38(2):138–41.
39. Martin JA, Kung HC, Mathews TJ, et al. Annual summary of vital statistics: 2006. *Pediatrics* 2008;121(4):788–801.
40. Savitz DA, Murname, P. Review of epidemiologic research on behaviors and preterm birth. *Epidemiology*. In press.

41. Wood NS, Marlow N, Costeloe K, Gibson AT, Wilkinson AR. Neurologic and developmental disability after extremely preterm birth. EPICure Study Group. *N Engl J Med* 2000;343(6):378–84.
42. Hutcheon JA, Platt RW. The missing data problem in birth weight percentiles and thresholds for "small-for-gestational-age." *Am J Epidemiol* 2008;167(7):786–92.
43. Lie RT. Intersecting perinatal mortality curves by gestational age—Are appearances deceiving? *Am J Epidemiol* 2000;152(12):1117–9.
44. Romero R, Espinoza J, Goncalves LF, Kusanovic JP, Friel L, Hassan S. The role of inflammation and infection in preterm birth. *Semin Reprod Med* 2007;25(1):21–39.
45. Romero R, Garite TJ. Twenty percent of very preterm neonates (23–32 weeks of gestation) are born with bacteremia caused by genital Mycoplasmas. *Am J Obstet Gynecol* 2008;198(1):1–3.
46. Swadpanich U, Lumbiganon P, Prasertcharoensook W, Laopaiboon M. Antenatal lower genital tract infection screening and treatment programs for preventing preterm delivery. *Cochrane Database Syst Rev* 2008(2):CD006178.
47. McDonald HM, Brocklehurst P, Gordon A. Antibiotics for treating bacterial vaginosis in pregnancy. *Cochrane Database Syst Rev* 2007(1):CD000262.
48. Basso O, Rasmussen S, Weinberg CR, Wilcox AJ, Irgens LM, Skjaerven R. Trends in fetal and infant survival following preeclampsia. *JAMA* 2006;296(11):1357–62.
49. Schieve LA, Cohen B, Nannini A, et al. A population-based study of maternal and perinatal outcomes associated with assisted reproductive technology in Massachusetts. *Matern Child Health J* 2007;11(6):517–25.
50. Basso O, Baird DD. Infertility and preterm delivery, birthweight, and Caesarean section: a study within the Danish National Birth Cohort. *Hum Reprod* 2003;18(11):2478–84.
51. Wright VC, Chang J, Jeng G, Chen M, Macaluso M. Assisted reproductive technology surveillance—United States, 2004. *MMWR Surveill Summ* 2007;56(6):1–22.
52. Morgen CS, Bjørk C, Andersen PK, Mortensen LH, Nybo Andersen AM. Socioeconomic position and the risk of preterm birth—a study within the Danish National Birth Cohort. *Int J Epidemiol* 2008;37(5):1109–20.
53. Hauger MS, Gibbons L, Vik T, Belizan JM. Prepregnancy weight status and the risk of adverse pregnancy outcome. *Acta Obstet Gynecol Scand* 2008;87(9):953–9.
54. Walkinshaw SA. Pregnancy in women with pre-existing diabetes: management issues. *Semin Fetal Neonatal Med* 2005;10(4):307–15.
55. Haider BA, Bhutta ZA. Multiple-micronutrient supplementation for women during pregnancy. *Cochrane Database Syst Rev* 2006(4):CD004905.
56. Wigle DT, Arbuckle TE, Turner MC, et al. Epidemiologic evidence of relationships between reproductive and child health outcomes and environmental chemical contaminants. *J Toxicol Environ Health B Crit Rev* 2008;11(5–6):373–517.
57. Goldberg JM, Falcone T. Effect of diethylstilbestrol on reproductive function. *Fertil Steril* 1999;72(1):1–7.
58. Wilcox AJ, Skjaerven R, Lie RT. Familial patterns of preterm delivery: maternal and fetal contributions. *Am J Epidemiol* 2008;167(4):474–9.
59. Ananth CV, Savitz DA. Vaginal bleeding and adverse reproductive outcomes: a meta-analysis. *Paediatr Perinat Epidemiol* 1994;8(1):62–78.
60. Honest H, Bachmann LM, Gupta JK, Kleijnen J, Khan KS. Accuracy of cervicovaginal fetal fibronectin test in predicting risk of spontaneous preterm birth: systematic review. *BMJ* 2002;325(7359):301.

61. Iams JD, Romero R, Culhane JF, Goldenberg RL. Primary, secondary, and tertiary interventions to reduce the morbidity and mortality of preterm birth. *Lancet* 2008;371(9607):164–75.
62. Thornton JG. Progesterone and preterm labor—still no definite answers. *N Engl J Med* 2007;357(5):499–501.
63. Sun Y, Vestergaard M, Pedersen CB, Christensen J, Basso O, Olsen J. Gestational age, birth weight, intrauterine growth, and the risk of epilepsy. *Am J Epidemiol* 2008;167(3):262–70.
64. Moster D, Lie RT, Markestad T. Long-term medical and social consequences of preterm birth. *N Engl J Med* 2008;359(3):262–73.
65. WHO. Recommended definitions, terminology and format for statistical tables related to the perinatal period and use of a new certificate for cause of perinatal deaths: modifications recommended by FIGO as amended Octobrer 14, 1976. *Acta Obstet Gynecol Scand* 1977;56:247–53.
66. Shea KM, Wilcox AJ, Little RE. Postterm delivery: a challenge for epidemiologic research. *Epidemiology* 1998;9(2):199–204.
67. Gülmezoglu AM, Crowther CA, Middleton P. Induction of labour for improving birth outcomes for women at or beyond term. *Cochrane Database Syst Rev* 2007;18(4):CD004945.
68. Steer PJ, Little MP, Kold-Jensen T, Chapple J, Elliott P. Maternal blood pressure in pregnancy, birth weight, and perinatal mortality in first births: prospective study. *BMJ* 2004;329(7478):1312.
69. Chen A, Basso O. Does low maternal blood pressure during pregnancy increase the risk of perinatal death? *Epidemiology* 2007;18(5):619–22.
70. Platt RW, Joseph KS, Ananth CV, Grondines J, Abrahamowicz M, Kramer MS. A proportional hazards model with time-dependent covariates and time-varying effects for analysis of fetal and infant death. *Am J Epidemiol* 2004;160(3):199–206.
71. Wilcox AJ, Weinberg CR. Invited commentary: analysis of gestational-age-specific mortality--on what biologic foundations? *Am J Epidemiol* 2004;160(3):213–4; discussion 215–6.
72. Yudkin PL, Wood L, Redman CW. Risk of unexplained stillbirth at different gestational ages. *Lancet* 1987;1(8543):1192–4.
73. Caughey AB. Measuring perinatal complications: methodologic issues related to gestational age. *BMC Pregnancy Childbirth* 2007;7:18.
74. Cole SR, Hernan MA. Fallibility in estimating direct estimates. *Internat J Epidemiol* 2002;31:163–5.

15

Birth Weight and Fetal Growth

Birth weight is a popular research topic because of the accessibility of data and the strong association of birth weight with perinatal mortality. Birth weight has become a convenient surrogate for infant health as well as a proposed pathway for interventions to improve infant health. There are questions, however, about the role of birth weight as a health surrogate and whether the link between birth weight and mortality is causal.

On the face of it, birth weight is a simple variable, easily and precisely measured. Birth weight is also among the most plentiful of perinatal data. In most developed nations, birth weight is recorded by law as a part of birth certificate data. Birth weight data for millions of births are freely available online (for example, see www.cdc.gov/nchs/births.htm). Most important, low birth weight is strongly and consistently associated with high infant mortality. All these factors have led birth weight to be highly valued as an epidemiologic variable—both as a predictor of perinatal risk and as an outcome in itself.

Despite the central role of birth weight in perinatal studies, there are unresolved questions about its interpretation and its utility. After years of intensive study, there still is not a clear understanding of the underlying relationship between birth weight and mortality. Is low birth weight a cause of infant mortality, or is it simply a marker for other factors that affect infant mortality? Does enhancing fetal growth reduce perinatal risk? Does restricting fetal growth increase perinatal risk? Before we address these questions, it is useful to consider the basic descriptive epidemiology of birth weight.

The Frequency Distribution of Birth Weight

Figure 15-1 shows a typical distribution of birth weights for 400,000 Norwegian live births.[1] This distribution has not been smoothed—the bars show the raw

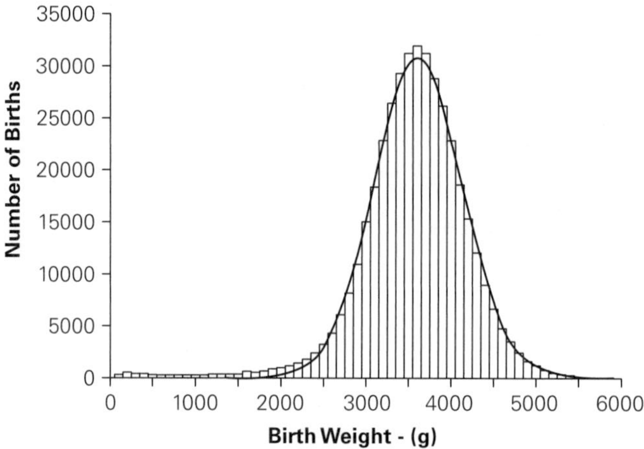

Figure 15-1. An empirical distribution of birth weights, with Gaussian curve (solid line) (400,000 live singleton births, Norway, 1992–98) (Reprinted from Wilcox[1])

data. With large sample sizes, the birth-weight distribution closely approximates a Gaussian distribution (shown in the figure as a solid line). The overall Gaussian distribution of birth weights is characteristic of birth weight in every known population. The one important deviation from the Gaussian distribution is in the lower tail, where there is an excess of low-weight, high-risk babies.

Based on these observations, the birth weight distribution can be divided into two parts. One is the Gaussian distribution, known as the predominant distribution. This distribution typically contains 95% to 98% of births.[1] The other is the excess portion in the lower tail, lying outside the main Gaussian distribution. This is the residual distribution. Although residual births are few, they contribute a major portion of infant deaths.

The excess small babies in the residual distribution presumably would have been part of the Gaussian distribution had not something interfered with their growth. This interference could in principle be either preterm delivery or restriction of fetal growth. In fact, virtually all babies in the residual distribution are preterm. (Many preterm births are also growth restricted, as discussed in Chapter 14.) The contribution of preterm delivery to the residual distribution can be demonstrated by separating the birth-weight distribution into term and preterm births (based on gestational age less than 37 weeks). Figure 15-2 shows these two birth weight distributions.

Among term births, the distribution of birth weights is almost exactly Gaussian. Removing preterm births from the birth weight distribution removes the heavier tail to the left (the residual part of the distribution). The fact that the residual

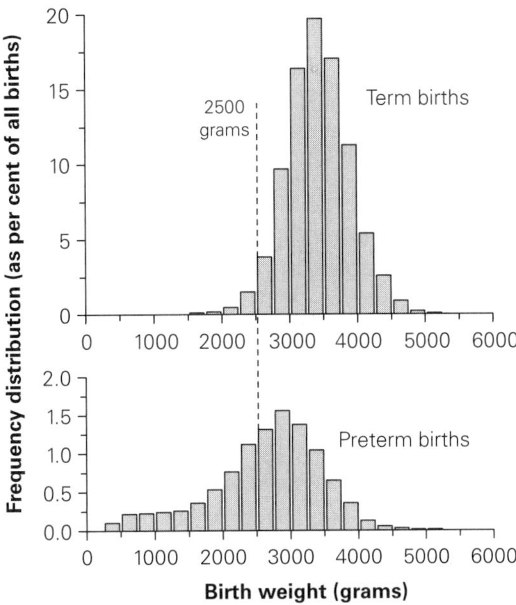

Figure 15-2. The birth weight distributions of preterm and term births (gestational age based on last menstrual period) (11.5 million live singleton births, United States, 2000–2002) (*Source:* U.S. National Center for Health Statistics)

distribution is made up almost entirely of preterm births is not to say that all preterm births are in the residual distribution. As seen in Figure 15-2, there are many preterm births distributed across heavier birth weights. Most of these heavy preterm births are late preterm—35 or 36 weeks of gestation.[2] A few may be term births with errors in gestational age. Even though there are preterm births in the main distribution, they have little impact on the mean or standard deviation of the predominant distribution.

It follows that the predominant distribution (estimated from the complete distribution of births) provides an estimate of the distribution of term birth weights.[3] The residual distribution in turn provides a crude estimate of the proportion of small preterm births. (An online program for estimating the predominant and residual distributions is available at http://eb.niehs.nih.gov/bwt/index.htm.)

These structural characteristics of the birth-weight distribution are important because of their constancy across all known populations. Furthermore, the Gaussian distribution of term births and the residual distribution of small preterm births are independent of each other. That is, populations can differ in the distribution of their term births without differing in their residual distribution, and vice versa. As an empirical observation, all major birth-weight differences between populations can be fully described by these limited options. Populations can have different means and standard deviations of their predominant distribution, and they can have different proportions of births in the residual distribution.

Factors Associated with Birth Weight

There are so many factors associated with birth weight, it might be easier to list the ones *not* associated. Mean birth weight varies by most of the variables that are of interest to reproductive epidemiologists, including ethnicity, social class, parity, plurality, maternal height and weight, parents' birth weights, maternal smoking, and sex of the baby.[4,5] A typical birth weight difference is in the range of 100 to 150 g, with larger differences seen among ethnic groups. There is limited evidence that birth weight is reduced with exposure to certain environmental exposures including lead, DDT/DDE, environmental tobacco smoke, outdoor air pollution, disinfection by-products in drinking water, and nitrate in drinking water.[6]

It is striking that although many factors affect birth weight, one of the most plausible factors—nutrition during pregnancy—has little impact. Even under the starvation conditions of the Dutch famine during World War II, mean birth weight fell by only 300 g.[7] Similarly, there is little evidence for changes in birth weight over time. As women's adult height and weight has increased, birth weights have remained relatively stable. In Norway, mean birth weight since 1860 has fluctuated within a range of 200 g.[8]

Birth-Weight-Specific Mortality

Figure 15-3 shows neonatal mortality at each birth weight. Like the distribution of birth weight, weight-specific mortality has a characteristic shape that varies little among populations. Mortality is highest among the smallest babies, falls rapidly as birth weights increase, reaches a nadir, and then rises slightly among the heaviest babies. (Mortality on the Y axis is shown on a logarithmic scale in order to accommodate the 1,000-fold range of mortality.) Like the distribution of birth weight, this pattern of weight-specific mortality appears to be universal.[9]

Figure 15-4 combines the distribution of birth weights with weight-specific mortality, revealing one additional feature of birth weight: the lowest mortality occurs at a weight above the mean weight. As with other aspects of birth weight and mortality, this is found in every known population.[10]

Figure 15-5 shows birth-weight distributions and weight-specific neonatal mortality for the United States in 1950 and 2000.[11] Birth weights are similar, with slightly heavier weights in 2000. Meanwhile, neonatal mortality declined more than 75% during this half-century, from 20.0 to 4.6 per 1,000. In absolute terms, the improvements were greatest among the smallest babies (under 1,000 g), for whom neonatal mortality fell from 872 to 262 deaths per 1,000 live births. However, the

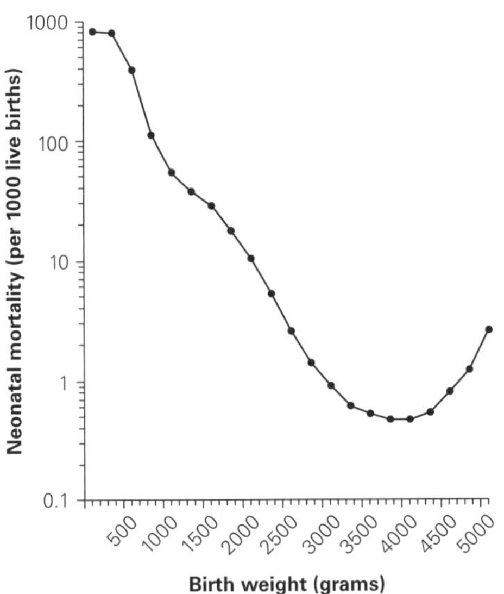

Figure 15-3. Neonatal mortality rates by birth weight (11.5 million live singleton births, United States, 2000–2002) (*Source:* U.S. National Center for Health Statistics)

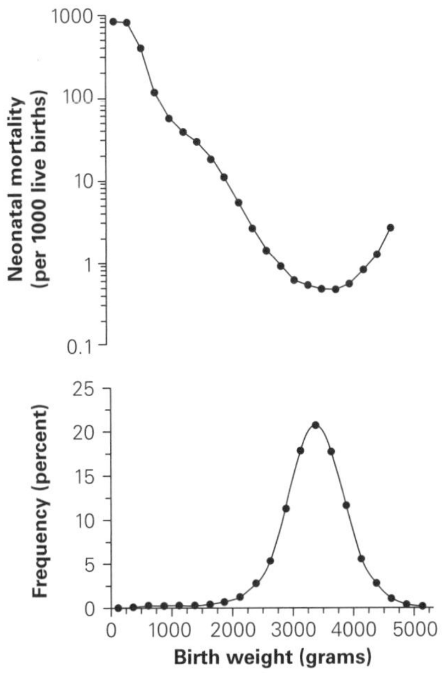

Figure 15-4. Birth-weight distribution and weight-specific neonatal mortality rates (11.5 million singleton live births, United States, 2000–2002) (*Source*: U.S. National Center for Health Statistics)

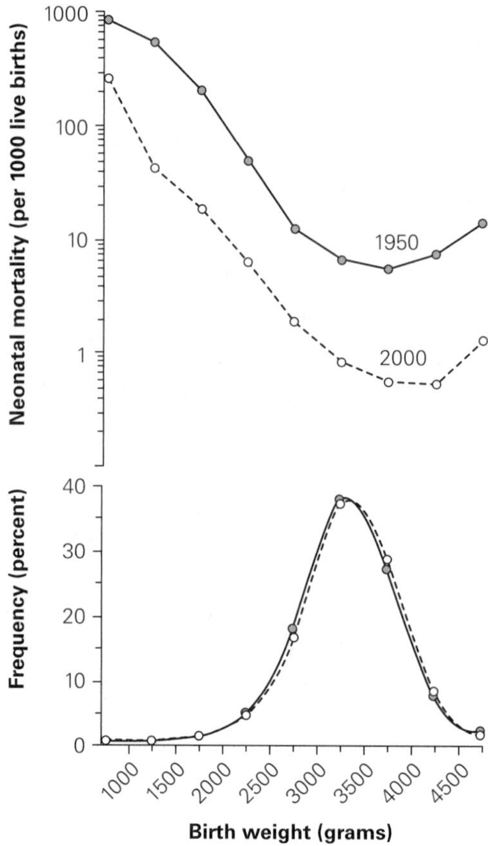

Figure 15-5. Changes in birth weight and weight-specific mortality over time (United States, 1950 and 2000) (US National Center for Health Statistics)

shape of the weight-specific mortality curve (on this log scale) has varied little over time; mainly, the mortality curve has shifted downward. In other words, the *ratio* of mortality decline over time has been similar across the various birth weight groups (with a constant distance on the log scale corresponding to a constant ratio). Babies less than 1,000 g had the largest absolute decline but the least improvement in relative terms: mortality for the smallest babies declined 70%, whereas for all other birth weight groups the declines ranged from 85% to 93%.

Low Birth Weight

Historically, the most common approach to birth weight has been to dichotomize weight at 2,500 g (5.5 lb). This dichotomy identifies a high-risk group of infants, with infant mortality 25 times higher than the mortality of heavier babies.[12] A PubMed search by "low birth weight" yields 30,000 papers, with new papers appearing at the rate of about 100 a month. The majority of low-birth-weight (LBW) studies describe LBW as either an adverse pregnancy outcome in itself or as a risk factor for other adverse outcomes. Unfortunately, any use of LBW presents major problems, as discussed below.

The Association of Birth Weight and Weight-Specific Mortality

The extremely strong gradient of mortality with low birth weight invites a causal interpretation. Over the course of the past century this interpretation has gone through two stages and may be about to go through a third. The first interpretation was that the high mortality of small babies was caused by premature delivery. A second interpretation became necessary when it was recognized that many small babies are not preterm but are still at high risk. The explanation for the observed risk among small term babies was "intrauterine growth retardation." The third possible interpretation is that the association of birth weight with mortality results primarily from confounding by unknown factors.

"Prematurity"

LBW babies were regarded as "premature" for much of the twentieth century. (As discussed in the previous chapter, LBW literally became the definition of prematurity.) Once population-based data on gestational age and birth weight were available, it became clear that as many as half of LBW babies are actually born at term.[13] Thus, population differences in LBW could reflect differences in preterm birth or differences in fetal size—LBW by itself does not distinguish the two. Because preterm delivery and fetal growth are largely distinct biological phenomena, the lack of specificity with LBW is a problem.

The recognition that LBW babies are not all preterm opened up an even more unsettling problem. LBW babies who are not preterm by gestational age nonetheless have very high mortality—even higher, at given birth weights, than preterm births. If their mortality is not caused by preterm delivery, what could be the explanation? A new disease had to be defined.

Intrauterine Growth Retardation

The concept of intrauterine growth retardation (IUGR) was created to explain the high mortality of term LBW babies. Although IUGR sounds like a medical condition, there are no particular clinical signs or symptoms that characterize IUGR. The first definition of intrauterine growth retardation was simply "LBW babies born at term."[14] The IUGR definition was modified to be "small-for-gestational

Fetal Growth Curves

An odd episode in the history of perinatal epidemiology was the interpretation of mean birth weight at each gestational age as an "intrauterine growth curve." The first intrauterine growth curve was constructed by Lulu Lubchenco in 1963 from cross-sectional data of birth weight distributions at specific gestational ages (see figure below).[15] This became known as the "lulugram" and was widely cited. Furthermore, the slopes of these curves were often interpreted biologically (even though Lubchenco herself cautioned against this). For example, the flattening of the slope near term has been regarded as evidence of the placenta reaching its natural limits ("placental insufficiency").[16] To interpret these curves as "growth trajectories" implicitly (and incorrectly) assumes that a baby born at 28 or 33 weeks is a random sample of all babies at that gestational age that continue in utero. Longitudinal interpretations of cross-sectional data are risky under the best of circumstances and misleading in the context of birth weight and gestational age. "Fetal growth curves" constructed from birth data have little to do with the growth pattern of fetuses.

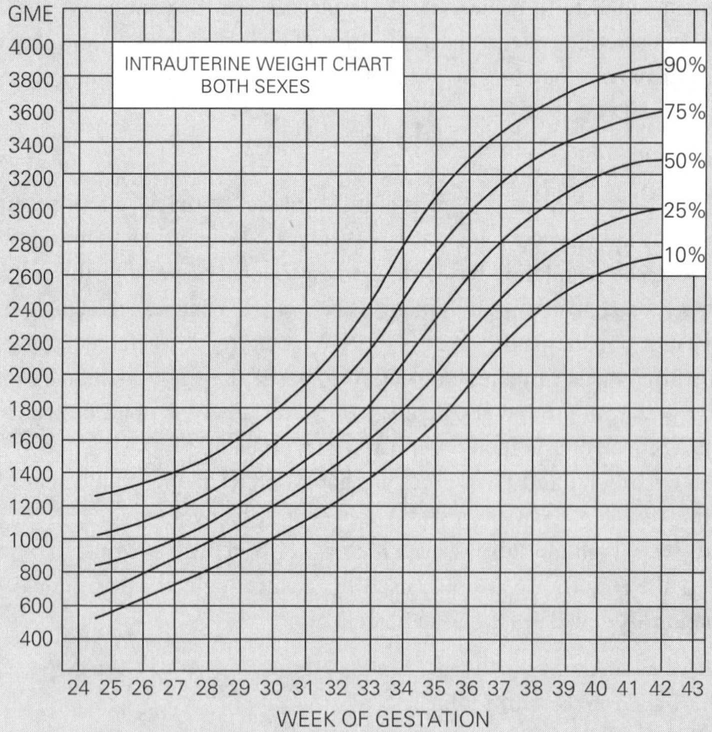

"Lulugram": distribution of birth weights by gestational ages (Reprinted with permission from Lubchenco et al[15] © 1963 by the American Academy of Pediatrics)

age" (or SGA), which is the smallest 10% of babies at each gestational age. The specific standards for SGA are either derived from the data set being analyzed or based on a published referent. This may seem to be a more refined definition than "term LBW," but it is not much different—SGA captures almost all term babies less than 2,500 g plus a few others.

SGA is a marker of high-risk babies independent of gestational age. In this regard, SGA is more useful than LBW. However, SGA has its own limitations. Like LBW, SGA still mixes preterm and term births, although not as badly. (The proportion of SGA births that are preterm is, by definition, the same as the proportion preterm in the general population.)

At first, the extension of the concept of intrauterine growth restriction to preterm births was regarded as an advance, but it has become a problem. By definition, the prevalence of SGA among preterm babies is 10%, just as it is in term births. However, we now know that babies who are born preterm are smaller than the fetuses who continue in utero.[17] Thus, a proper measure of growth restriction should identify more growth-restricted babies among preterm births than among term births. To do so would require SGA criteria based on all fetuses at a given gestational age, which is technically difficult given our limited ability to estimate intrauterine fetal weight. To avoid this problem, SGA is sometimes restricted to term births.

The problem with SGA applied to preterm births points to a larger issue. The fact that SGA (and thus IUGR) is defined as a percentile becomes a tautology. SGA is the smallest 10% of babies, and therefore, the prevalence of SGA is 10%. By definition, such a condition cannot be prevented or alleviated. This circularity creates some embarrassing gaffes—more than one grant proposal has claimed that intrauterine growth restriction is an important outcome because it affects 10% of all births.

Yet another conceptual problem with SGA is that it defines all small babies as growth restricted, and no others. This is wrong in two ways. Not all small babies are growth restricted. Some are small simply because of natural variability in fetal growth.[18] Conversely, there is no reason why a large baby could not be restricted in fetal growth.[19] Factors that restrict fetal growth (such as living at high altitudes) affect the entire birth-weight distribution (Fig. 15-6). Epidemiologic factors that cause growth restriction seem to affect fetuses of all weights more or less equally.

There is one sense in which SGA can be a useful measure (at least on a population level). SGA will detect an exposure that restricts fetal growth (and thereby shifts the distribution of birth weights). The shift of birth weights will cause a higher proportion of babies to fall below a predefined tenth-percentile standard of weight. However, it would be an obvious error to interpret this excess in SGA as "fetal growth restriction" only among SGA babies. SGA can detect shifts of the birth-weight distribution, but it cannot identify specific babies whose growth has been restricted.

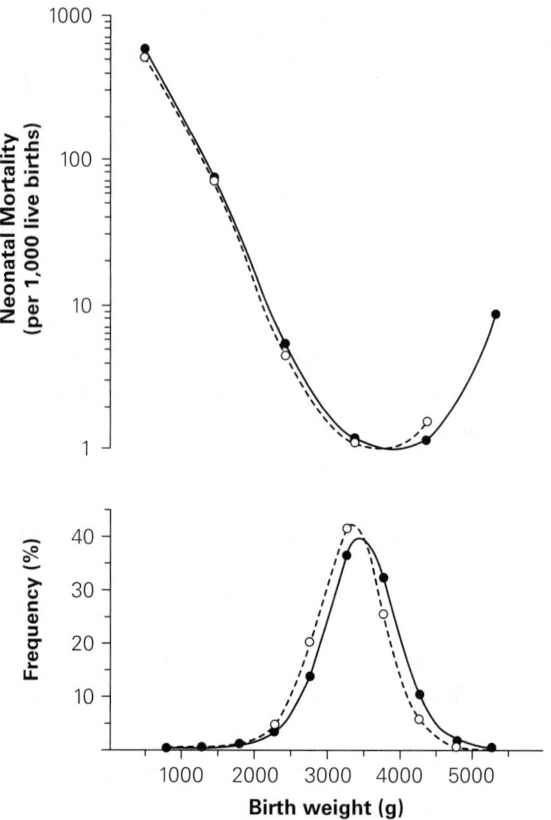

Figure 15-6. Fetal growth restriction in the infants of mothers who live in a high-altitude state (Colorado, dashed line) compared with the whole United States (1984, solid line) (Reprinted from Wilcox[19])

Unmeasured Confounding

Another option for explaining the association between birth weight and mortality is that the association is a result of unmeasured confounding. Epidemiologists routinely invoke the possibility of unknown confounders, but rarely in discussing birth weight and mortality. Perhaps this is because the weight-and-mortality association is so strong. (By definition, the association between the confounder and the outcome has to be even stronger than the confounded association it produces, and such a confounder for birth weight and infant mortality is hard to imagine.) The possibility of confounding, however, is particularly important for birth weight because confounding could explain one of the conundrums of reproductive epidemiology—the low-birth-weight paradox.

THE LOW-BIRTH-WEIGHT PARADOX. It has been acknowledged for many years that small babies from a high-risk population can have lower mortality than small babies from a lower-risk population. Maternal smoking is a classic example. The babies of mothers who smoke have higher infant mortality. However, among LBW babies, mortality is lower if the mother smokes.[20] (This has prompted half-serious suggestions that women who are going to have small babies could improve their baby's chances by smoking.) A similar advantage among small babies of high-risk groups is found in many comparisons, including parity, plurality, and race.[21] Attempts to explain this by differences in gestational age or other known risk factors have proven futile.[22]

In 1966, Brian MacMahon offered a succinct explanation for the paradox. He pointed out that the lower mortality among small babies in the high-risk group would be paradoxical *"only if low weight were causally associated with mortality. But it is not. The marked relationship between weight and mortality is the result of factors... that affect them both."*[23] If the association between low birth weight is not causal but rather produced by unmeasured confounding, then it is to be expected that distortions of risk will occur within a particular group of babies defined by birth weight (such as the LBW babies of smoking mothers).

An example of this distortion is seen in Figure 15-6. The shift of birth weight with high altitude might be expected to produce higher mortality because more babies are subjected to the higher risks at lower weights. In fact, total mortality is the same in the two populations. How could that be possible if one population has smaller babies? It is because weight-specific mortality rates are not the same in the two populations. It is as if the specific mortality rates at high altitude have shifted with the birth weight distribution, leading to no net change in mortality. The LBW paradox is apparent in this figure: at any given weight below 3,000 g, babies born at high altitude have slightly better survival than other babies.

An analysis of weight-specific mortality in this comparison produces a confusing picture: mortality is lower for smaller babies, higher for larger babies, and not different overall. Using the same argument as MacMahon, Meyer and Comstock concluded in 1972 that it is a mistake to analyze birth-weight-specific mortality at all.[21] These cautions by Comstock and MacMahon— two of the most prominent epidemiologists of their day—fell on deaf ears. Researchers continued to ponder the low-birth-weight paradox and to try to glean meaning from weight-specific mortality rates.

MacMahon's argument has recently been enriched through the application of directed acyclic graphs.[24] In a simple example (Figure 15-7), a factor (altitude) affects birth weight but not mortality. If another factor is present that affects both birth weight and mortality, birth weight becomes a "collider,"[25] and stratifying on birth weight (say, by 2,500 g) biases the relationship between altitude and mortality within those weight strata. The same is true if the variable being analyzed (such as smoking) has its own direct effects on mortality (Fig. 15-8).

In these graphs there is no causal arrow between birth weight and mortality. Simulations have shown that the observed patterns of birth weight and mortality

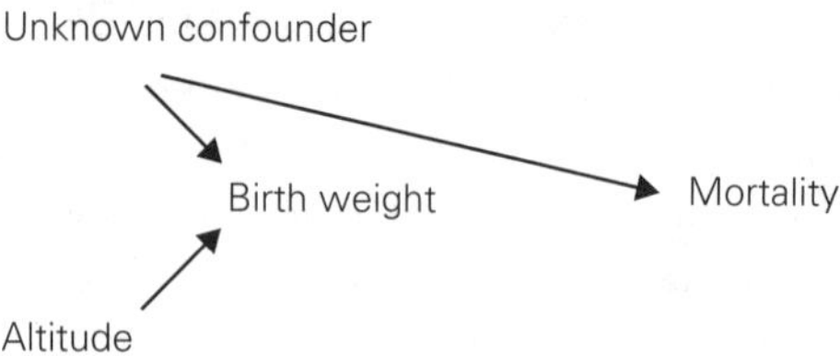

Figure 15-7. Directed acyclic graph for the analysis of the association of altitude with birth weight and neonatal mortality; an unmeasured confounder that affects both birth weight and neonatal mortality will make birth weight a collider and thus disrupt the association between altitude and mortality within strata of birth weight

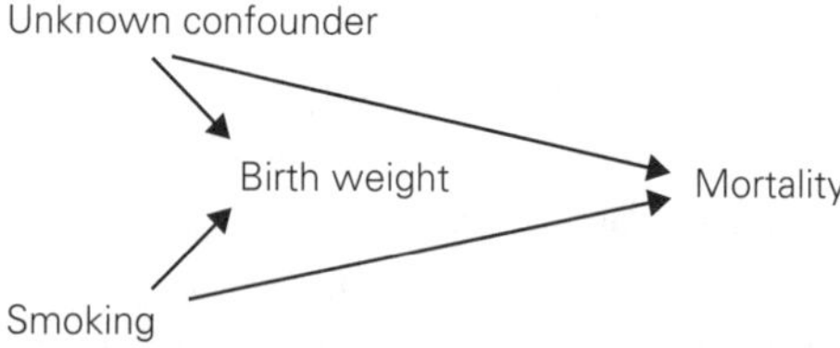

Figure 15-8. Directed acyclic graph for the analysis of the association of smoking with birth weight and neonatal mortality; again, an unmeasured confounder makes birth weight a collider and disrupts the association of smoking with mortality within strata of birth weight

can be produced with no causal effect of birth weight on mortality.[26] Furthermore, the observed patterns of weight-specific mortality cannot be reproduced unless a causal effect of birth weight is either absent or small in comparison to the unmeasured confounder.[26] It is not yet possible to conclude that birth weight has no direct effect on mortality. However, if birth weight does have a causal effect, it is likely to be much weaker than the observed association.

The identity of the inferred unmeasured confounder (or confounders) of birth weight and mortality remains a mystery. It is of course possible that no such factor exists. Still, there is no other option at present that comes close to explaining the observed patterns of weight-specific mortality. MacMahon's insight may be the correct one, even if we are far from understanding its biological underpinnings.

High Birth Weight and Mortality

The slightly higher mortality among babies with the heaviest weights (see Fig. 15-3) is generally given less attention than the risk among small babies. This may be because the excess mortality contributed by heavier babies is relatively inconsequential. Maternal obesity and diabetes are often mentioned as contributors to this risk, although this pattern is also prominent in developing countries where obesity or diabetes are rare.[9] Birth injuries are another frequent explanation, but this does not fit the data either. Higher mortality with heavy birth weight is found for all the major causes of death.[27] Like the rest of the mortality curve, this pattern persists in all populations and over time. It is possible that additional unknown confounding is present, in which unmeasured factors contribute to both large birth weight and higher mortality.

The Association of Birth Weight and Later Morbidity

In addition to its strong associations with perinatal risk, birth weight is associated with morbidity and mortality later in life. The reverse-J shape of birth-weight-specific mortality persists (albeit in a steadily weakened form) throughout childhood[28] and even into adulthood. Cardiovascular disease in adults follows the reverse-J-shaped pattern of risk, as do other causes excluding cancer (Fig. 15-9).[29] Cancer mortality, in contrast, steadily increases with birth weight.

Birth weight is also associated with morbidity, especially morbidity related to neurologic function. In children a reverse-J pattern with birth weight is found for mental handicap (Fig. 15-10).[30] There are similar patterns for IQ,[31] hearing and vision,[32] and the risk of schizophrenia.[33]

The association of birth weight with cardiovascular disease (seen in Fig. 15-9) has been energetically pursued by David Barker and others in an evolving hypothesis about fetal nutrition and long-term effects on cardiovascular health.[34] Barker's theories have stimulated an extensive scientific literature spotlighting the links between fetal life and adult life. These links undoubtedly deserve attention. However, the present focus on nutrition and cardiovascular-related diseases has perhaps distracted from the strong patterns between low birth weight and neurologic diseases, between low birth weight and other causes of death, and between high birth weights and cancer risk—relationships that are not addressed in the current theories of fetal adaptive response.

Birth Length

A birth characteristic strongly related to mortality (independent of birth weight) is length of the baby. Even though this association was featured on the cover of the 1984 textbook, *Perinatal Epidemiology*, the topic has had little attention from epidemiologists. Length independent of birth weight is fundamentally a measure of leanness. Both extremes (i.e., leanness and fatness) are associated with increased mortality.[35] None of the usual measures used to combine weight and length (BMI, ponderal index, Rohrer's index) are statistically optimal, in the sense that none of them fully expresses leanness independent of birth weight.

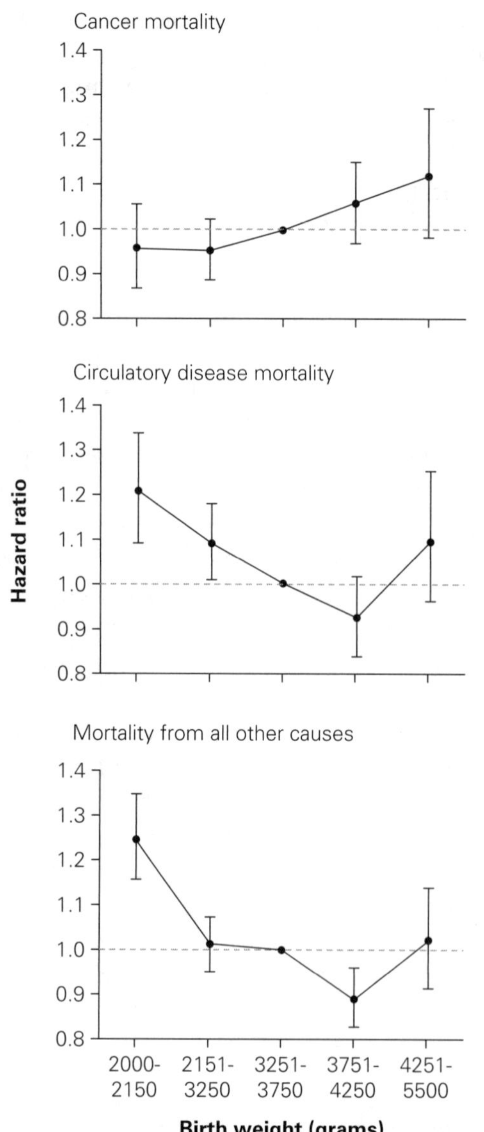

Figure 15-9. Birth weight as a predictor of adult mortality (in major categories of death) (Adapted from Baker et al[29])

The Analysis of Birth Weight

For all the misunderstandings surrounding birth weight and its interpretation, this variable can be useful in reproductive epidemiology, although perhaps in more limited ways than has generally been thought.

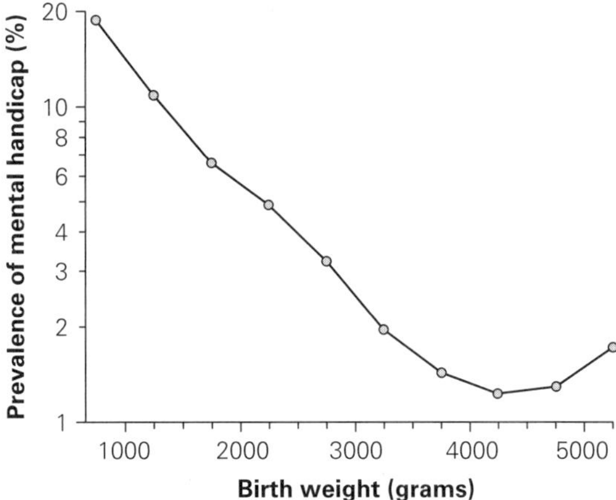

Figure 15-10. Birth weight as a predictor of mental handicap among school children (ages 12–15, Florida, 1996–97)[30]

Fetal Growth Restriction

On a clinical level, a slowing of fetal growth during pregnancy is a sign that the fetus is encountering difficulties. This is not true on the population level, at least not for the type of fetal growth restriction we are able to detect through the study of birth weight (i.e., a wholesale shift of the birth-weight distribution).

Even so, a shift in birth weight to lower weights is not necessarily benign. The shift may be a sign of exposure to a hazard that also increases risk. Maternal smoking is a good example. Smoking reduces birth weights, and it increases infant mortality (although apparently not because of smaller birth weights).[20] Thus, even though a shift in the birth weight distribution is not evidence in itself of fetal distress, it may mark the influence of an exposure that harms the fetus in other ways.

The most direct measure of population-level fetal growth restriction is to examine the whole distribution of birth weight (rather than LBW or SGA). Summary measures such as mean birth weight are also appropriate. It may be useful to control for gestational age, which can be done as simply as excluding preterm births. SGA also controls for gestational age, although SGA presumably has less power to detect a shift in birth weight than an analysis of the complete weight distribution.

When differences in SGA are found between populations, these differences are sometimes mistakenly interpreted as an effect on small babies only. Fetal growth restriction could in theory produce an accumulation of very small babies in the lower tail of the birth-weight distribution without otherwise affecting the distribution of birth weights, but there is no known example of this.

A more subtle problem in the interpretation of SGA is related to preterm SGA babies. An "improvement" in fetal growth in the preterm gestational ages could be caused by a factor that increases the risk of preterm delivery among normally growing fetuses. Such an effect would not be good for fetuses but would nonetheless look like improved "growth" among preterm babies. Any assessment of birth weight among preterm births should take careful account of preterm delivery itself as an outcome.

Adjusting for Birth Weight

One of the recurring errors of reproductive epidemiology has been analyses that stratify or otherwise "control" for absolute birth weight in assessing associations between risk factors and infant mortality. As demonstrated in the previous discussion of the LBW paradox, there is strong evidence that birth weight is a collider—a variable affected by unmeasured confounders linked to infant mortality. To adjust, standardize, or stratify by birth weight in any manner as part of the analysis of a factor that affects birth weight runs the risk of introducing bias.

Birth Weight as a Surrogate for Preterm Birth

Although low birth weight is a poor surrogate for preterm birth, birth weight can be used to provide an indirect window on preterm delivery. The extreme category of "very low birth weight" or VLBW (defined as babies less than 1,500 g) comprises about 1% to 2% of all births and is made up almost entirely of preterm babies. VLBW is specific as a measure of preterm but not sensitive—it captures only a small portion of all preterm births. The residual distribution of the birth weight distribution is another surrogate for preterm. The residual captures a larger proportion of preterm deliveries but requires large sample sizes (thousands if not tens of thousands of births) to obtain stable estimates of the residual distribution. Also, there are no established methods to estimate the precision of such estimates. Whenever possible, preterm births should be studied directly using available data on gestational age.

Assessment of Birth-Weight-Specific Mortality

Population differences in weight-specific mortality are uninterpretable if there are also population differences in birth-weight distributions. In the presentation of weight-specific mortality in 1950 and 2000 (Fig. 15-5), the comparisons of weight-specific mortality rates are valid because the two birth-weight distributions are nearly identical.

It is possible to adjust sets of weight-specific mortality rates to a standard birth-weight distribution by the use of *z*-scores for birth weight.[1] This removes the distortion caused by adjustment by a collider and allows two sets of weight-specific mortality rates to be compared. However, such analysis seldom provides more information than could be obtained from simple comparison of overall mortality in the two populations.

Birth Weight and Public Health Policy

Birth weight has occupied a central position in public health policy for decades. The World Health Organization describes birth weight as having "undisputed value as a public health indicator."[36] Strategies to increase birth weight are regarded as necessary to reduce infant mortality and even childhood mortality.[37]

Despite the prominence of birth weight in public policy, there are many reasons why one might question the public health value of birth weight. First, population differences in birth weight are unreliable predictors of mortality. Some of the countries with the lowest infant mortality rates are Asian, where mean birth weights are relatively small. Second, interventions to improve birth weights have been largely ineffective.[38] Third, where such interventions may be most effective (among undernourished women in developing countries), there is a concern that increased fetal growth may raise the risk of obstructed labor.[39] When obstetric rescue is not available, obstruction during labor is a life-threatening condition for both mother and baby. Finally, historical trends provide no support for the idea that improved infant survival requires the prevention of LBW. The great secular declines in infant mortality have occurred with little or no change in birth weight (Fig. 15-5). If past improvement in infant mortality has not depended on changes in birth weight, there is little reason to suppose that future improvement depends on it.

References

1. Wilcox AJ. On the importance—and the unimportance—of birthweight. *Int J Epidemiol* 2001;30(6):1233–41.
2. Wilcox AJ, Skjaerven R. Birth weight and perinatal mortality: the effect of gestational age. *Am J Public Health* 1992;82(3):378–82.
3. Wilcox AJ, Russell IT. Birthweight and perinatal mortality: I. On the frequency distribution of birthweight. *Int J Epidemiol* 1983;12(3):314–8.
4. Lie RT, Wilcox AJ, Skjaerven R. Maternal and paternal influences on length of pregnancy. *Obstet Gynecol* 2006;107(4):880–5.
5. Kramer MS, Olivier M, McLean FH, Dougherty GE, Willis DM, Usher RH. Determinants of fetal rowth and body proportionality. *Pediatrics* 1990;86(1):18–26.
6. Wigle DT, Arbuckle TE, Turner MC, et al. Epidemiologic evidence of relationships between reproductive and child health outcomes and environmental chemical contaminants. *J Toxicol Environ Health B Crit Rev* 2008;11(5–6):373–517.
7. Stein Z, Susser M, Saenger G, Marolla F. *Famine and Human Development: The Dutch Hunger Winter of 1944–45*. New York: Oxford University Press, 1975.

8. Rosenberg M. Birth weights in three Norwegian cities, 1860–1984. Secular trends and influencing factors. *Ann Hum Biol* 1988;15(4):275–88.
9. Habib N, Wilcox A, Dalveit A, et al. Birth weight, preterm birth and perinatal mortality: a comparison of Black babies in Tanzania and the US, personal communication.
10. Graafmans WC, Richardus JH, Borsboom GJ, et al. Birth weight and perinatal mortality: a comparison of "optimal" birth weight in seven Western European countries. *Epidemiology* 2002;13(5):569–74.
11. Mathews TJ, Menacker F, MacDorman MF. Infant mortality statistics from the 2000 period linked birth/infant death data set. *Natl Vital Stat Rep* 2002;50(12):1–28.
12. Mathews TJ, MacDorman MF. Infant Mortality Statistics from the 2005 Period Linked Birth/Infant Death Data Set. In: *Natl Center for Health Statistics* 2008;57:1–32.
13. McKeown T, Gibson JR. Observations on all births (23,970) in Birmingham, 1947. IV: "Preterm Birth." *Br Med J* 1951;ii:513–17.
14. Yerushalmy J. The classification of newborn infants by birth weight and gestational age. *J Pediatr* 1967;71(2):164–72.
15. Lubchenco LO, Hansman C, Dressler M, Boyd E. Intrauterine growth as estimated from liveborn birth-weight data at 24 to 42 weeks of gestation. *Pediatrics* 1963;32:793–800.
16. Gruenwald P. Growth of the human fetus. I. Normal growth and its variation. *Am J Obstet Gynecol* 1966;94(8):1112–9.
17. Hutcheon JA, Platt RW. The missing data problem in birth weight percentiles and thresholds for "small-for-gestational-age". *Am J Epidemiol* 2008;167(7):786–92.
18. Chard T, Yoong A, Macintosh M. The myth of fetal growth retardation at term. *Br J Obstet Gynaecol* 1993;100(12):1076–81.
19. Wilcox AJ. Intrauterine growth retardation: beyond birthweight criteria. *Early Hum Dev* 1983;8(3–4):189–93.
20. Wilcox AJ. Birth weight and perinatal mortality: the effect of maternal smoking. *Am J Epidemiol* 1993;137(10):1098–104.
21. Meyer MB, Comstock GW. Maternal cigarette smoking and perinatal mortality. *Am J Epidemiol* 1972;96(1):1–10.
22. Collins JW Jr, David RJ. Differential survival rates among low-birth-weight black and white infants in a tertiary care hospital. *Epidemiology* 1990;1(1):16–20.
23. Macmahon B, Alpert M, Salber EJ. Infant weight and parental smoking habits. *Am J Epidemiol* 1965;82(3):247–61.
24. Hernandez-Diaz S, Schisterman EF, Hernan MA. The birth weight "paradox" uncovered? *Am J Epidemiol* 2006;164(11):1115–20.
25. Greenland S. Quantifying biases in causal models: classical confounding vs collider-stratification bias. *Epidemiology* 2003;14(3):300–6.
26. Basso O, Wilcox AJ, Weinberg CR. Birth weight and mortality: causality or confounding? *Am J Epidemiol* 2006;164(4):303–11.
27. Wilcox AJ, Russell IT. Birthweight and perinatal mortality: II. On weight-specific mortality. *Int J Epidemiol* 1983;12(3):319–25.
28. Samuelsen SO, Magnus P, Bakketeig LS. Birth weight and mortality in childhood in Norway. *Am J Epidemiol* 1998;148(10):983–91.
29. Baker JL, Olsen LW, Sorensen TI. Weight at birth and all-cause mortality in adulthood. *Epidemiology* 2008;19(2):197–203.
30. Avchen RN, Scott KG, Mason CA. Birth weight and school-age disabilities: a population-based study. *Am J Epidemiol* 2001;154(10):895–901.

31. Sorensen HT, Sabroe S, Olsen J, Rothman KJ, Gillman MW, Fischer P. Birth weight and cognitive function in young adult life: historical cohort study. *BMJ* 1997;315(7105):401–3.
32. Olsen J, Sorensen HT, Steffensen FH, et al. The association of indicators of fetal growth with visual acuity and hearing among conscripts. *Epidemiology* 2001; 12(2):235–8.
33. Gunnell D, Rasmussen F, Fouskakis D, Tynelius P, Harrison G. Patterns of fetal and childhood growth and the development of psychosis in young males: a cohort study. *Am J Epidemiol* 2003;158(4):291–300.
34. Barker DJ. Human growth and cardiovascular disease. *Nestle Nutr Workshop Ser Pediatr Program* 2008;61:21–38.
35. Melve KK, Gjessing HK, Skjaerven R, Oyen N. Infants' length at birth: an independent effect on perinatal mortality. *Acta Obstet Gynecol Scand* 2000;79(6):459–64.
36. WHO. Promoting optinmal fetal development: Report of a technical consultation. *WHO Technical Consultation Towards the Development of a Strategy for Promoting Optimal Fetal Development.* Geneva: WHO, 2003.
37. Shrimpton R. Preventing low birthweight and reduction of child mortality. *Trans R Soc Trop Med Hyg* 2003;97(1):39–42.
38. Haider B, Bhutta ZA. Multiple-micronutrient supplementation for women during pregnancy. *Cochrane Database Syst Rev* 2006;4:CD004905.
39. Rush D. Nutrition and maternal mortality in the developing world. *Am J Clin Nutr* 2000;72(1 Suppl):212S-40S.

16

Birth Defects

A common worry among expectant parents is that their baby will have a birth defect—and that mother may inadvertently have contributed to that risk. There are well-known examples of medications that cause birth defects and concerns about environmental toxicants that might damage the fetus. Even so, most birth defects have no known cause, and the prevalence of most birth defects remains steady.

In 1941, an Australian ophthalmologist named Norman Gregg noticed an unusual number of infants born with cloudy lenses—congenital cataracts. In his words, the cataracts had "remarkable similarity" across his patients, even though the infants came from diverse backgrounds. To Gregg, this temporal clustering of birth defects had the appearance of an epidemic.[1]

In Gregg's time, the prevailing scientific view was that birth defects were inherited. The term "congenital" was virtually synonymous with "hereditary." Indeed, to suggest even the possibility that environmental factors might cause malformations was considered by some to be unscientific.[2] Nonetheless, the outbreak of cataracts in newborns seemed to Gregg to be evidence that a nongenetic teratogen had emerged. In a paper published in 1941, he suggested that the cause of these cataracts was "of infective nature rather than a purely developmental defect."[1] Gregg took note of a severe epidemic of rubella that had swept Australia in 1940. Most of the mothers of the affected babies reported having had rubella early in their pregnancy. Gregg's observations were at first met with skepticism, but the rapid accumulation of data soon became persuasive. Recognition of the teratogenic properties of rubella opened the door to a radically new scientific idea—that external exposures of minor consequence to the mother could have serious consequences for her baby.

In 1961 another epidemic of birth defects challenged the medical establishment even more profoundly. Beginning in the late 1950s, an unusual number of children were born without the long bones of their arms and legs. This defect, in which the hands or feet are attached to the torso like seal flippers, is known as phocomelia (from the Greek for "seal limbs"). In 1961, two clinicians independently recognized an association between this defect and a popular sedative known as thalidomide.[3,4] Thalidomide had been introduced by a German pharmaceutical firm in 1958, and the drug quickly became widely used as a treatment for the morning-sickness of early pregnancy. Thalidomide was marketed in 46 countries under at least 37 names. (Thalidomide was never approved by the U.S. Food and Drug Administration, which had concerns about safety of the drug.) Once the link with phocomelia emerged, the drug was withdrawn from the market, and the epidemic came to a halt. By this time, at least 8,000 children had been affected.[5]

The thalidomide disaster had an immediate impact on public policy. The fact that a seemingly mild medication recommended by doctors could cause such a dramatic, crippling, and untreatable birth defect led to new laws regarding the process of drug approval. Population-based birth defects registries were established to detect new outbreaks of birth defects as early as possible. There was rapid expansion of teratology, the medical specialty studying the causes of birth defects.

These two examples show the evolution of our understanding about the damage that exposures during pregnancy can inflict on the fetus. Both examples demonstrate biological mechanisms of fetal pathogenesis that had not previously been considered a danger to humans. Although these examples are disturbing, such occurrences have been infrequent. In the four decades that birth defects registries have been monitoring time trends in birth defects, we have not yet discovered another teratogen equal to thalidomide.

McBride and the Temptations of Fame

As one of the "alert clinicians" who observed that thalidomide might be the cause of the phocomelia epidemic, William McBride found himself thrust into the limelight, reaping a sheaf of professional honors including Commander of the British Empire.

In the 1970s, McBride became convinced that Bendectin (another drug used to relieve the nausea of early pregnancy) also caused birth defects. Courtroom testimony by McBride and others led Bendectin to be withdrawn from the market. This time, however, the data did not support his position. Careful review of the evidence has established that Bendectin has no measurable teratogenic effects.[6]

Still later, McBride produced laboratory results suggesting that scopolamine (yet another drug used to treat nausea) causes malformations in rabbits. His data had been falsified. McBride was found guilty of scientific fraud by an Australian tribunal in 1993, and his medical license was revoked.[7]

The Epidemiology of Birth Defects

Birth defects have been subject to intensive study over the past five decades in the hopes of uncovering preventable causes. The summary below mentions factors that are likely to be associated with birth defects. It is important to put these results into perspective: the vast majority of defects occur without known cause. Parents who have a child with a birth defect often carry guilt over past actions of theirs that might have produced the defect. With few exceptions, there is little way to know the cause of a particular defect.

Some specialists distinguish between "congenital malformations" (a category that includes only structural defects) and "birth defects" (which can be construed more broadly to include functional problems such as phenylketonuria). Epidemiologists tend to use the two terms interchangeably.

Occurrence

Major malformations can be found in roughly 3% of live births.[8] Prevalence is strongly affected by the vagaries of case ascertainment. For example, the prevalence of congenital malformations depends on how long babies are followed after birth. Cardiac defects are a classic example of a major defect that may not become apparent until after the newborn has been discharged from the hospital. Thus, registries based only on newborn records are less complete than those that include later ascertainment. Prevalence also depends on how carefully babies are examined and on the examiner's criteria for distinguishing a birth defect from a natural variant of normal. Minor defects are probably at least as common as the major defects but are less completely reported.

Birth defects, like the cancers, are a collection of diverse diseases. Unlike cancers, the specific major types of birth defects are all relatively rare, with the most common occurring among only a few per 1,000 births (Table 16-1). Each type of malformation tends to have its own distribution in the population and its own set of risk factors. Epidemiologic studies typically focus on major categories (such as neural tube defects or cleft lip). However as with cancer, there is no standard number of categories and no easy answer to the question of how narrowly such categories should be defined. Birth defects epidemiologists must balance the gains in statistical power that come from aggregating similar conditions against the advantages of having more homogeneous cases in narrowly defined subtypes (a dilemma shared by all epidemiologists). The clinically based ICD codes may not be as useful as more epidemiologically based guidelines.[9]

The occurrence of birth defects (both as a whole and in the major subtypes) has been fairly stable in the time since the establishment of the major birth defects registries in the 1960s and 1970s. When changes have occurred, they have most often been attributable to changes in ascertainment, as with the improved diagnosis of heart defects by ultrasound.[10] Subtle and minor defects may fluctuate in their detection according to the standards of the examiners; malformations of the male genitalia are an example.[11]

Table 16-1. Birth prevalence of major defects[a]

Categories of major birth defects	Prevalence per 1,000 births
Total affected births	35
Musculoskeletal	11
Cardiovascular	9
Gastrointestinal tract (including cleft lip and palate)	6
Reproductive	6
Male	10
Female	1
Ear, face, neck	4
Central nervous system	3
Skin	3
Eye	2
Urinary tract	2
Respiratory tract	2
Aneuploidy (autosomal)	2
Miscellany	1

[a] Data from Metropolitan Atlanta Congenital Defects Program, 1968–95. Each major defect is counted separately, even if there are accompanying defects in the same baby.[12]

Birth defects are commonly cited as among the main causes of infant mortality in developed countries. Malformations are the leading cause of infant mortality in the United States, accounting for 20% of deaths.[13] Babies with birth defects are more likely to be born preterm, which may contribute to their increased risk of mortality.[14] In developing countries, birth defects are probably no less common, but they are a minor contributor to mortality compared with infection.[15]

Etiology

HERITABLE CAUSES. Even though birth defects are no longer ascribed solely to heritable causes, genes play an important role. About 10% of defects are attributable to chromosomal anomalies.[16] Among the defects occurring to chromosomally normal babies, familial recurrence is high. Recurrence in the siblings of babies with various types of birth defects ranges from 5- to 50-fold (see Table 7-2).[17] Similar recurrence risks are found among the offspring of affected parents.[18,19] Although these high recurrence rates suggest the presence of heritable factors, the patterns of birth defects recurrence are not those of single genes transmitted in simple Mendelian fashion. There are probably multiple genes acting together for most birth defects, perhaps in concert with environmental conditions (see discussion of the multifactorial/threshold model in Chapter 5). The investigation of genes that contribute to specific birth defects is an active area of genetic epidemiologic research.

SEX DIFFERENCES. Birth defects are about 40% more common in boys than in girls.[12] Half of this excess represents the high risk of malformations in the male reproductive tract. This difference may reflect easier detection of malformations of the male reproductive organs or more error-prone development for male genitalia. Boys also have an excess of defects in most other major categories including gastrointestinal tract and cardiovascular defects. Girls have a higher risk of neural tube defects and cleft palate (but lower risk of cleft lip).[12] The mechanisms for these sex differences are unknown.

ETHNIC AND REGIONAL DIFFERENCES. The quality of data on birth defects varies widely among countries, which complicates national comparisons of risk. Within countries, there are some variations among ethnic groups. For example, Americans of African descent have about the same overall risk of malformations as Americans of European descent, but with about half the risk of cleft lip and palate and about 10 times the risk of polydactyly (extra fingers or toes).[20] Ethnic differences may reflect differences in exposures or in the distribution of susceptibility genes. Ethnic differences may also reflect differences in customs regarding marriage among relatives. In Norway, a 40% excess of birth defects among the offspring of Pakistani immigrants was attributable to marriages between first cousins.[21] Infants of parents who are first cousins had about twice the occurrence of birth defects.

MATERNAL CONDITIONS AND CHARACTERISTICS. Uncontrolled maternal diabetes substantially increases the risk of birth defects. Mothers with Type 1 or Type 2 diabetes before pregnancy have at least a threefold increased risk of major malformations in their offspring.[22] The defects associated with diabetes are diverse and are especially likely to be multiple defects. The mechanisms by which diabetes produces birth defects are related to blood levels of glucose. With good control of blood glucose, risk is reduced.[23] Mothers who develop gestational diabetes during their pregnancy are at much less risk, and what risk there is may be attributable to undetected diabetes before conception.[22] Obesity has been weakly associated with neural tube defects and perhaps heart defects.[24] Although such studies attempt to control for diabetes, the association with obesity may nonetheless reflect unmeasured irregularities in glucose regulation among overweight women.

Increased risk of birth defects is seen among older mothers, in part because of the increased risk of aneuploidy with age. However, even among babies with no apparent aneuploidy, the risk of some malformations rises with maternal age.[25] There is less evidence for an effect of father's age on risk of birth defects, at least for the major categories.[26]

A slight increase in malformations is sometimes seen among young mothers. Gastroschisis (a defect of the abdominal wall) is unusual among malformations in that it is more common in younger than older mothers.[27] This strongly suggests an environmental cause, a possibility made more urgent by the fact that this rare defect is increasing over time.[28]

MEDICATIONS. Prescription and over-the-counter drugs have the express purpose of affecting physiologic function. Some of the best examples of human teratogens are medications. In addition to thalidomide and diethylstilbestrol, isotretinoin (trade name Accutane©) is an established cause of multiple malformations. A derivative of vitamin A, isotretinoin provides highly effective treatment for severe acne. Those seeking treatment for acne are often young women, and they are prescribed the drug only if they agree to use effective methods of birth control during their treatment. Although this stipulation has been generally successful, it has not completely prevented Accutane-associated birth defects.[29]

A general problem in assessing the side effects of medications is whether the association is with the drug or with the disease that the drug is treating (confounding by indication). This problem is seen in the associations of anticonvulsant drugs with major defects. Drugs used to treat epilepsy have long been suspected of being teratogenic. This interpretation was called into question by data suggesting that women with epilepsy might also have a genetic susceptibility to birth defects.[30] The weight of evidence now implicates the drugs, not the disease, although the role of specific anticonvulsant drugs remains difficult to untangle.[31]

Testing drugs for teratogenicity is an imperfect system at best (see below). It is impossible to guarantee that a new drug will not have teratogenic effects. Postmarketing surveillance is the logical alternative, but there is no systematic process at present to accomplish this.[32]

NUTRITION. Two of the most important public health advances of recent decades have been the discoveries that low maternal levels of folate contribute to the risk of neural tube defects and that maternal intake of folic acid at the earliest stages of pregnancy substantially reduces that risk.[33] (Women, in fact, must start folic acid supplements before they conceive in order to be sure that the fetus is protected at the crucial early stages of development.) Folic acid may also reduce the risk of facial clefts.[34] It is possible that supplemental vitamins protect against other birth defects,[35] although associations with specific vitamins have been slow to emerge.

At least one vitamin has been suggested as a teratogen. Vitamin A is closely related to the teratogen isotretinoin, and one study found an association of vitamin A at high doses with defects.[36] Subsequent data have not clearly supported a risk with vitamin A.[37] At lower doses, vitamin A may be protective for facial clefts.[38]

ALCOHOL. Very high levels of alcohol consumption by mothers during pregnancy are associated with a condition known as fetal alcohol syndrome. The syndrome consists of subtle but characteristic facial anomalies, growth restriction, and abnormalities of neurodevelopment.[39] Estimates of prevalence are hampered by lack of consistent case definition, but range from 0.5 to 2 per 1,000 births.[40] Lower consumption of alcohol may also contribute to specific defects, although these associations are not well established.

STRESS. There is a long history of laboratory experiments showing that stressing the pregnant mouse (for example by physical restraint) can induce birth defects.[41,42] Studies of stress in humans have been less conclusive, although there is a small body of evidence suggesting that a pregnant woman's experience of highly stressful events may harm the fetus.[43,44]

ENVIRONMENTAL CAUSES. One of the most dramatic examples of an environmental teratogen took place in Japan. The fish in Minamata Bay were contaminated by methylmercury, which had been discharged into the bay by a local factory. These fish accumulated levels of methylmercury so high as to cause severe neurologic damage to the offspring of pregnant women who ate the fish.[45] Radiation is also a known teratogen, causing microcephaly and mental retardation among fetuses exposed to the Hiroshima atomic blast.[46] Both of these examples are characterized by very high exposures.

The Most Famous Photograph You Will Never See

W. Eugene Smith was a photojournalist famous for his brutally honest photographs in World War II. He and his wife moved to Japan in the early 1970s, during which time Smith created a stunning photoessay that documented the human tragedy of Minamata disease. In 1972 Smith was attacked and beaten by employees of the polluting company in an effort to discourage him from this project. Smith lost vision in one eye and never fully regained his health. He died in 1978 at the age of 60.

His photographs are credited with bringing the world's attention to the Minamata tragedy. The most moving photograph was of a mother cradling her naked, severely damaged teenage daughter in her lap while bathing her. Published with consent of the family, this photograph became the symbol of the Minamata disaster.

In 1997, 20 years after the daughter's death, the photograph was withdrawn from circulation at the request of the family.

The possible effects of lower-level exposures to environmental contaminants are much less clear. Maternal smoking is consistently associated with increased risk of facial clefts,[47] but there is no clear evidence that other forms of air pollution produce birth defects. More generally, there are no convincing associations between ambient environmental contaminants and birth defects, despite hundreds of studies on this topic. Among the factors with limited evidence of teratogenicity are disinfection by-products in drinking water and residential proximity to toxic waste dumps.[48]

Sequelae of Birth Defects

Many birth defects are treatable and compatible with normal function. Even so, there are detectable reductions in the proportion who survive and, among the survivors, a reduction in the chances of having children of their own.[18,19] Survivors have an increased risk of cancer, particularly persons born with neural tube defects or multiple defects.[49] The mechanisms of this cancer risk are unknown.

The Role of Timing

The timing of fetal exposure to a teratogen is of paramount importance. Fetal development is rigidly sequenced with specific organ systems being formed at particular stages of pregnancy. The vulnerability of the fetus to teratogenic insult varies by the stage of development at which exposure occurs. Figure 16-1 provides a broad overview of the stages at which organ systems are vulnerable to structural damage. The upper limbs are susceptible to major anomalies during the fourth and fifth weeks of fetal life (obstetric weeks 5 and 6), whereas the oral palate is vulnerable during the seventh and eighth fetal weeks. For most organ systems, the vulnerable period lasts only 2–3 weeks. The brain is a notable exception, with a period of developmental vulnerability that extends to delivery and beyond.

The fact that organ vulnerability occurs at certain stages is useful in making causal inferences about possible teratogens. An exposure in the seventh or eighth month of pregnancy obviously cannot be blamed for a limb defect that develops in the second month of pregnancy. Conversely, an exposure that is associated with a birth defect only when the exposure occurs at a specific stage of fetal development has added plausibility as a true cause.

Biological Noise

Variability and genetic error are intrinsic elements of biology, and there is no reason to suppose that this does not include embryologic development. The assembly of a human embryo is bafflingly complex, carried out along pathways that have developed (and are still developing) through the processes of evolution. A certain amount of randomness (and thus random error) in fetal development is inevitable.[50] A demonstration of this is the less-than-100% concordance of birth defects in monozygotic twins. Even though monozygotic twins share virtually identical genotypes and fetal environments, they do not necessarily have the same birth defects. Only 60% of monozygotic twins with facial cleft are concordant for the defect.[51]

To go a step further, it is possible that the "noise" (or random error) of embryologic processes plays a positive role in human biology. Genetic theorists have proposed that noise is not only constructive, it is necessary to maximize population fitness by helping to purge mutations.[52] The importance of these ideas from an epidemiologic perspective is to dispel any illusion that birth defects could be completely prevented, even in theory. It is far more realistic to aim for the discovery of the preventable causes (such as folic acid insufficiency) than to suppose that the discovery of all causes would one day eliminate all birth defects.

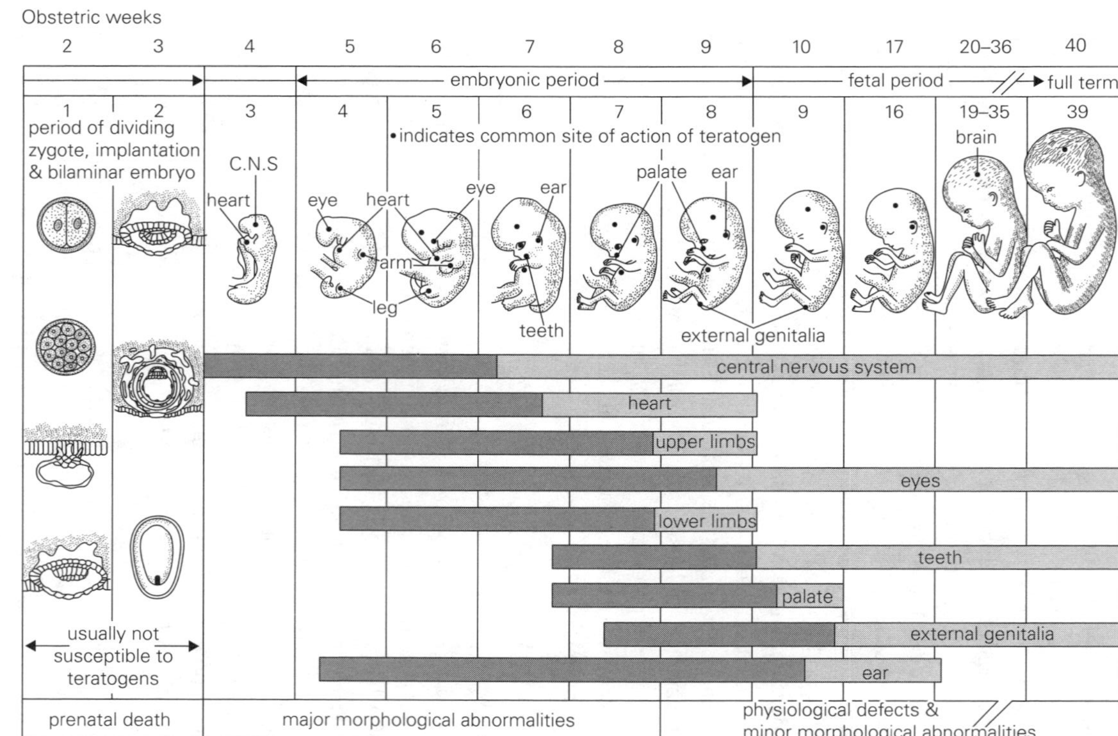

Figure 16-1. Stages of embryologic development and fetal vulnerability. Dark shading on bars indicates the most sensitive time-periods. (Adapted from Moore and Persaud © Elsevier 2008[53])

Methodologic Challenges

The Limits of Teratology

The field of teratology focuses on the biochemical and histologic mechanisms by which the developing fetus can be damaged. This work has provided many of the basic principles of birth defects epidemiology, for example, the importance of dose, timing, and genetic susceptibility to the outcome.[54] Still, teratology has limitations. One is the variation of teratogenic effects across species. What is teratogenic in a given laboratory species is not necessarily teratogenic in humans (aspirin, for example).[55] Similarly, what is teratogenic in humans may not be teratogenic in other species. An example is thalidomide, which is not a strong teratogen in mice or rats (the most commonly tested animals) but is in rabbits.[56] Although animal testing provides a useful screen for substances that might cause birth defects, the absence of harm in test animals is not proof of an absence of harm in humans. Most human teratogens have been identified first in humans and then confirmed in laboratory species.

A second limitation is that an understanding of molecular structure or pharmacologic function does not necessarily predict the safety of new chemical products. Toxicology often extrapolates the effects of well-tested chemicals with known structure and activity to untested chemicals in the same general class of structure and activity. Unfortunately, this extrapolation does not work for teratogens. Two chemicals can be very similar (for example thalidomide and glutethimide, both sedatives), with one causing birth defects and the other not.[57]

The Missing Denominator

A conspicuous problem of birth defects epidemiology is the inability to describe disease incidence (defined as the proportion of a defined population that develops the disease in a given time). Incidence requires a denominator, and the true denominator for fetal defects—that is, the number of fetuses at risk for defects—is unobtainable. We can describe only the prevalence of defects at the time they become observable (prevalence being the proportion of a given population who have the disease). Historically, the period of observation for birth defects has started at birth, although today structural birth defects can be identified at midpregnancy using ultrasound.

The prevalence we can observe (at midpregnancy or later) is not a good estimate of incidence. A large proportion of fetuses are lost early in pregnancy through either miscarriage or induced abortion. To the degree that malformed fetuses are overrepresented among these losses, prevalence measures at birth or beyond will be biased. Furthermore, it is impossible to know the extent of this bias because it is practically impossible to identify all malformations among the losses.

This fact of fetal life has implications for epidemiologists. When we speak of the occurrence of birth defects, we should be careful to recognize (and state) this as prevalence, not incidence. A change in prevalence does not necessarily reflect a change in incidence. Prevalence can change because of a change in the proportion of affected fetuses lost in early pregnancy.

This is not a minor point. When folic acid supplements were found to reduce the birth prevalence of neural tube defects, some researchers suggested that folic acid has this effect by increasing the miscarriage of affected infants.[58] The possibility that folic acid might act as an abortifacient for defective fetuses was regarded as unacceptable by those who oppose abortion. This created tension over folic acid supplementation as a public policy until the hypothesis could be definitively dismissed.[59]

Birth Defects as Rare Diseases

Because birth defects are rare, the case-control design is a common epidemiologic approach. A case-control study has the potential advantage of short recall intervals (if mothers can be recruited shortly after delivery), but there is still the possibility of biased recall related to pregnancy outcome. Mothers who have given birth to an affected baby may scour their memories more thoroughly in search of a possible cause—or may deny certain exposures out of guilt. (This has been a rationale for using other birth defects as controls.[60]) Although such methodologic concerns can never be entirely dismissed, there is evidence that women are relatively unbiased (at least with regard to the case or control status of their infant) in their recall of exposures during pregnancy.[61] Within a given study, the specificity of effect for one exposure among several similar exposures can also help to rule out recall bias.

"Isolated" versus "Multiple" versus "Syndromic"

A baby can have more than one birth defect. The prevalence of accompanying defects varies for different types of defects; for example, babies with cleft palate (and no cleft lip) are twice as likely to have another defect as babies with cleft lip. Furthermore, the completeness of registration for accompanying defects can vary widely. Minor defects are often unrecorded.

Sometimes multiple defects are referred to as "syndromic," and isolated defects are called "nonsyndromic." Alternatively, cases with multiple defects may be divided into those with recognized or suspected syndromes, those with structurally related defects, and others.[62] Although all these strategies for grouping and dividing can be argued on biological grounds, an argument can also be made for studying all cases of a given defect regardless of accompanying defects, given that the data are available.[63] In this way, evidence of heterogeneity among the isolated and nonisolated cases can be tested empirically rather than assumed.

Problems of Ascertainment

The accurate ascertainment of cases is a problem in birth defects research as in most other areas of epidemiology. Hospital records and registries seldom (if ever) capture all birth defects among live births. Even conspicuous defects such as cleft lip are not recorded with 100% accuracy. Among Norwegian babies with cleft lips serious enough to need surgery, 17% are not noted in the birth records.[64] Less obvious defects are even less completely ascertained. Birth records miss 43% of cleft palate cases that eventually go to surgery.[64] The prevalence of birth defects is presumably even higher among stillbirths than among live births, but ascertainment is worse.[65] It follows that any factor associated with better ascertainment can mistakenly appear as a cause in an analysis of ascertained cases. (This can be a problem, for example, in assessing teratogenic effects of ART procedures, if ART pregnancies receive closer scrutiny than naturally conceived pregnancies.[66]) Problems of ascertainment would be greatly reduced by standardized clinical examination of all births; however, such standardization is seldom possible.

Another problem of ascertainment arises with prenatal screening and induced abortion. Where babies with major structural defects are electively aborted, the birth prevalence of those defects will be reduced. A decline in anencephaly and spina bifida in the 1970s and 1980s was likely a result of prenatal screening and abortion.[11] Birth defects registries often try to include information about terminations performed for fetal defects, but those data can be difficult to obtain.[67]

Detection of New Epidemics

An abrupt increase in the prevalence of a birth defect would provide strong evidence that a teratogen is at work. The epidemics of congenital cataracts and phocomelia were such examples. It is a curious if welcome fact that no such outbreaks have been identified since the establishment of population birth defects registries in the 1960s and 1970s. This has prompted reflections on the limitations of such registries—for example, their inability to detect teratogens when only a small proportion of mothers are exposed, or when the strength of teratogenic effect is only moderate (in the range of two- to threefold).[68] Predictably, the political will to maintain these registries has weakened in the absence of a dramatic reminder of their usefulness. It would be short-sighted, however, to dismantle these early-warning systems, given the proliferation of new chemicals and drugs and the difficulties of adequately screening new products. It may be wiser to supplement the registries with case-control surveillance, allowing the collection of more detailed exposure data that could help flag new teratogens.[32]

References

1. Gregg N. Congenital cataract following German measles in the mother. *Trans Ophthalmol Soc Aust* 1941;3:35–46.
2. Warkany J. Trends in teratological research. In: Perrin VD, Finegold MJ, ed. *Pathobiology of Development, or Ontogeny Revisited*. Baltimore, MD: Williams & Wilkins, 1973;1–10.
3. McBride WG. Thalidomide and congenital abnormalities. *Lancet* 1961;278(7216):1358.
4. Lenz W. Klinische Misbilduengen nach Medikament: einnahme Waehrend der Gravidataet? *Dtsch Med Wochenschr* 1961;86:2555–65.
5. Annas GJ, Elias S. Thalidomide and the Titanic: reconstructing the technology tragedies of the twentieth century. *Am J Public Health* 1999;89(1):98–101.
6. Brent RL. Bendectin: review of the medical literature of a comprehensively studied human nonteratogen and the most prevalent tortogen-litigen. *Reprod Toxicol* 1995;9(4):337–49.
7. Specialist life—William McBride. *Eur J Obstet Gynecol Reprod Biol* 2001;95:139–40.
8. Kalter H, Warkany J. Congenital malformations: etiologic factors and their role in prevention (Part 1). *N Engl J Med* 1983;308(8):424–31.
9. Rasmussen SA, Olney RS, Holmes LB, Lin AE, Keppler-Noreuil KM, Moore CA. Guidelines for case classification for the National Birth Defects Prevention Study. *Birth Defects Res A Clin Mol Teratol* 2003;67(3):193–201.
10. Edmonds LD, James LM. Temporal trends in the prevalence of congenital malformations at birth based on the birth defects monitoring program, United States, 1979–1987. *MMWR CDC Surveill Summ* 1990;39(4):19–23.
11. Toppari J, Kaleva M, Virtanen HE. Trends in the incidence of cryptorchidism and hypospadias, and methodological limitations of registry-based data. *Hum Reprod* Update 2001;7(3):282–6.
12. Lary JM, Paulozzi LJ. Sex differences in the prevalence of human birth defects: a population-based study. *Teratology* 2001;64(5):237–51.
13. Mathews TJ, MacDorman, MF. Infant Mortality Statistics from the 2005 Period Linked Birth/Infant Death Data Set. In: *Nastional Center for Health Statistics* Vol. 57, 2008;1–32.
14. Shaw GM, Savitz DA, Nelson V, Thorp JM Jr. Role of structural birth defects in preterm delivery. *Paediatr Perinat Epidemiol* 2001;15(2):106–9.
15. Lawn JE, Cousens S, Zupan J. 4 million neonatal deaths: when? where? why? *Lancet* 2005;365(9462):891–900.
16. Nelson K, Holmes LB. Malformations due to presumed spontaneous mutations in newborn infants. *N Engl J Med* 1989;320(1):19–23.
17. Lie RT, Wilcox AJ, Skjaerven R. A population-based study of the risk of recurrence of birth defects. *N Engl J Med* 1994;331(1):1–4.
18. Skjaerven R, Wilcox AJ, Lie RT. A population-based study of survival and childbearing among female subjects with birth defects and the risk of recurrence in their children. *N Engl J Med* 1999;340(14):1057–62.
19. Lie RT, Wilcox AJ, Skjaerven R. Survival and reproduction among males with birth defects and risk of recurrence in their children. *JAMA* 2001;285(6):755–60.
20. Erickson JD. Racial variations in the incidence of congenital malformations. *Ann Hum Genet* 1976;39(3):315–20.

21. Stoltenberg C, Magnus P, Lie RT, Daltveit AK, Irgens LM. Birth defects and parental consanguinity in Norway. *Am J Epidemiol* 1997;145(5):439–48.
22. Correa A, Gilboa SM, Besser LM, et al. Diabetes mellitus and birth defects. *Am J Obstet Gynecol* 2008;199(3):237 e1–9.
23. Loeken MR. Advances in understanding the molecular causes of diabetes-induced birth defects. *J Soc Gynecol Investig* 2006;13(1):2–10.
24. Shaw GM, Carmichael SL. Prepregnant obesity and risks of selected birth defects in offspring. *Epidemiology* 2008;19(4):616–20.
25. Hollier LM, Leveno KJ, Kelly MA, McIntire DD, Cunningham FG. Maternal age and malformations in singleton births. Obstet Gynecol 2000;96(5 Pt 1): 701–6.
26. Kazaura M, Lie RT, Skjaerven R. Paternal age and the risk of birth defects in Norway. *Ann Epidemiol* 2004;14(8):566–70.
27. Rasmussen SA, Frias JL. Non-genetic risk factors for gastroschisis. *Am J Med Genet C Semin Med Genet* 2008;148C(3):199–212.
28. Castilla EE, Mastroiacovo P, Orioli IM. Gastroschisis: international epidemiology and public health perspectives. *Am J Med Genet C Semin Med Genet* 2008; 148C(3):162–79.
29. Mitchell AA, Van Bennekom CM, Louik C. A pregnancy-prevention program in women of childbearing age receiving isotretinoin. *N Engl J Med* 1995;333(2):101–6.
30. Shapiro S, Hartz SC, Siskind V, et al. Anticonvulsants and parental epilepsy in the development of birth defects. *Lancet* 1976;1(7954):272–5.
31. Perucca E. Birth defects after prenatal exposure to antiepileptic drugs. *Lancet Neurol* 2005;4(11):781–6.
32. Mitchell AA. Systematic identification of drugs that cause birth defects—a new opportunity. *N Engl J Med* 2003;349(26):2556–9.
33. Botto LD, Moore CA, Khoury MJ, Erickson JD. Neural-tube defects. *N Engl J Med* 1999;341(20):1509–19.
34. Wilcox AJ, Lie RT, Solvoll K, et al. Folic acid supplements and risk of facial clefts: national population based case-control study. *BMJ* 2007;334(7591):464.
35. Werler MM, Hayes C, Louik C, Shapiro S, Mitchell AA. Multivitamin supplementation and risk of birth defects. *Am J Epidemiol* 1999;150(7):675–82.
36. Rothman KJ, Moore LL, Singer MR, Nguyen US, Mannino S, Milunsky A. Teratogenicity of high vitamin A intake. *N Engl J Med* 1995;333(21):1369–73.
37. Azais-Braesco V, Pascal G. Vitamin A in pregnancy: requirements and safety limits. *Am J Clin Nutr* 2000;71(5 Suppl):1325S-33S.
38. Johansen AM, Lie RT, Wilcox AJ, Andersen LF, Drevon CA. Maternal dietary intake of vitamin A and risk of orofacial clefts: a population-based case-control study in Norway. *Am J Epidemiol* 2008;167(10):1164–70.
39. Stratton K, Howe C, Battaglia F. *Fetal Alcohol Syndrome: Diagnosis, Epidemiology, Prevention, and Treatment.* Washington DC: Institute of Medicine, 1996.
40. May PA, Gossage JP. Estimating the prevalence of fetal alcohol syndrome. A summary. *Alcohol Res Health* 2001;25(3):159–67.
41. Greene RM, Kochhar DM. Some aspects of corticosteroid-induced cleft palate: a review. *Teratology* 1975;11(1):47–55.
42. Lee YE, Byun SK, Shin S, et al. Effect of maternal restraint stress on fetal development of ICR mice. *Exp Anim* 2008;57(1):19–25.
43. Carmichael SL, Shaw GM, Yang W, Abrams B, Lammer EJ. Maternal stressful life events and risks of birth defects. *Epidemiology* 2007;18(3):356–61.

44. Hansen D, Lou HC, Olsen J. Serious life events and congenital malformations: a national study with complete follow-up. *Lancet* 2000;356(9233):875–80.
45. Harada M. Minamata disease: methylmercury poisoning in Japan caused by environmental pollution. *Crit Rev Toxicol* 1995;25(1):1–24.
46. National Research Council. *The Effects on Populations of Exposure to Low Levels of Ionizing Radiation: 1980. Committee on the Biological Effects of Ionizing Radiation (BIER).* Washington DC: National Academy Press, 1980.
47. Little J, Cardy A, Munger RG. Tobacco smoking and oral clefts: a meta-analysis. *Bull WHO* 2004;82(3):213–18.
48. Wigle DT, Arbuckle TE, Turner MC, et al. Epidemiologic evidence of relationships between reproductive and child health outcomes and environmental chemical contaminants. *J Toxicol Environ Health B Crit Rev* 2008;11(5–6):373–517.
49. Bjorge T, Cnattingius S, Lie RT, Tretli S, Engeland A. Cancer risk in children with birth defects and in their families: a population based cohort study of 5.2 million children from Norway and Sweden. *Cancer Epidemiol Biomarkers Prev* 2008;17(3):500–6.
50. Brent RL. The complexities of solving the problem of human malformations. *Clin Perinatol* 1986;13(3):491–503.
51. Christensen K. The 20th century Danish facial cleft population—epidemiological and genetic-epidemiological studies. *Cleft Palate Craniofac J* 1999;36(2):96–104.
52. Krakauer DC, Sasaki A. Noisy clues to the origin of life. *Proc Biol Sci* 2002;269(1508):2423–8.
53. Moore KL, Persaud TVN. *The Developing Human: Clinically Oriented Embryology.* Philadelphia, PA: Saunders, 2003.
54. Wilson JG. *Environment and Birth Defects. Environmental Science Series.* London: Academic Press, 1973.
55. Warkany J. Problems in applying teratologic observations in animals to man. *Pediatrics* 1974;53:820.
56. Webster WS, Brown-Woodman PD, Ritchie HE. A review of the contribution of whole embryo culture to the determination of hazard and risk in teratogenicity testing. *Int J Dev Biol* 1997;41(2):329–35.
57. Mitchell AA. Studies of drug-induced birth defects. In: Strom BL, ed. *Pharmacoepidemiology.* New York: John Wiley & Sons, 2005.
58. Hook EB, Czeizel AE. Can terathanasia explain the protective effect of folic-acid supplementation on birth defects? *Lancet* 1997;350(9076):513–15.
59. Gindler J, Li Z, Berry RJ, et al. Folic acid supplements during pregnancy and risk of miscarriage. *Lancet* 2001;358(9284):796–800.
60. Lieff S, Olshan AF, Werler M, Savitz DA, Mitchell AA. Selection bias and the use of controls with malformations in case-control studies of birth defects. *Epidemiology* 1999;10(3):238–41.
61. Khoury MJ, James LM, Erickson JD. On the use of affected controls to address recall bias in case-control studies of birth defects. *Teratology* 1994;49(4):273–81.
62. Khoury MJ, Moore CA, James LM, Cordero JF. The interaction between dysmorphology and epidemiology: methodologic issues of lumping and splitting. *Teratology* 1992;45(2):133–8.
63. Lie RT. Flawed epidemiology of birth defects? *Lancet* 1995;346(8981):1037.
64. Kubon C, Sivertsen A, Vindenes HA, Abyholm F, Wilcox A, Lie RT. Completeness of registration of oral clefts in a medical birth registry: a population-based study. *Acta Obstet Gynecol Scand* 2007;86(12):1453–7.

65. Greb AE, Pauli RM, Kirby RS. Accuracy of fetal death reports: comparison with data from an independent stillbirth assessment program. *Am J Public Health* 1987;77(9):1202–6.
66. Schieve LA, Rasmussen SA, Reefhuis J. Risk of birth defects among children conceived with assisted reproductive technology: providing an epidemiologic context to the data. *Fertil Steril* 2005;84(5):1320–4; discussion 1327.
67. Cragan JD, Khoury MJ. Effect of prenatal diagnosis on epidemiologic studies of birth defects. *Epidemiology* 2000;11(6):695–9.
68. Holtzman NA, Khoury MJ. Monitoring for congenital malformations. *Annu Rev Public Health* 1986;7:237–66.

17

Sex Ratio

The ratio of boys to girls at birth is easy to calculate and just as easy to misinterpret. Environmental toxicants, war, and many other factors have been reported to affect the sex ratio. The vast majority of these findings are false positives. There are books instructing couples on how to affect the sex ratio of their pregnancies (that is, how to choose the sex of their offspring). These methods are successful half the time.

The first question about a new baby is whether it is a boy or a girl. This information is important more than socially. Infant sex is recorded in all medical records and vital statistics, and these data are easily accessible for analysis on a population level. The boy-to-girl ratio at birth is 51 to 49. Sometimes this is presented in scientific papers as the proportion of boys among all births (that is, 0.51, as in this chapter). Another way of expressing the sex ratio is as the ratio of boys to girls (1.06; also sometimes 106 per 100 girls, or 1,060 per 1,000 girls).

Biological Basis for the Sex Ratio

As with other aspects of reproductive biology, the sex ratio at birth varies across species.[1] Biologists have theorized that the ability of species to adjust their sex ratio may be advantageous to species survival.[2] Among certain reptiles, including crocodiles, turtles, and lizards, the offspring's sex is determined by ambient temperature of the incubating egg.[3] Some shrimp and mollusks are born as males, reproduce as males when young, and then change sex to reproduce as females later on. Some fish change in the other direction. Snails, tapeworms, and earthworms come fully equipped to perform reproductively as both male and female.[4] By comparison, mammals are a bit dull. Sex is determined at conception by the X and Y chromosomes, and (with a few surgical exceptions) sex does not change.

The biological mechanisms that cause the slight excess of boys are unknown. Human sperm have an equal probability of carrying X or Y chromosomes,[5] as predicted by Mendelian inheritance. There is no evidence that Y-bearing sperm survive better in the female reproductive tract or that Y-bearing sperm are more able than X-bearing sperm to fertilize an egg. An excess of female deaths during pregnancy could cause an excess of males at birth, but (based on our limited evidence) just the opposite occurs: male fetuses have higher mortality than female fetuses at all observable stages of pregnancy. Thus, it remains a puzzle as to how the consistent excess of males at birth is produced.

"Middlesex"

The sex of a baby is not necessarily obvious at birth. Ambiguity of the genitalia can result from rare hormonal or genetic conditions and affects roughly 6 per 10,000 babies.[6] Such ambiguity can lead to errors in assigned sex, creating considerable difficulties for the persons involved. *Middlesex* is a Pulitzer-Prize-winning novel on the coming of age of a man incorrectly labeled as a girl at birth, and raised as a girl. Such errors are too few to have measurable effect on the sex ratio.

Biological Factors Hypothesized to Affect the Sex Ratio

No biological mechanisms are known to alter the human sex ratio, but there is a rich literature of speculation.

Radiation

In 1958, geneticists proposed that the mutational effects of radiation exposure of men and women might produce opposite effects on the sex ratio.[7] They suggested that the genetic inertness of the Y chromosome makes the Y less susceptible than the X chromosome to the mutational effects of radiation. If so, radiation to men would selectively produce more mutations in the sperm X chromosome than the Y chromosome. This would damage the resulting female conceptuses more than the male, thus causing the exposed men to father more boys. Conversely, if mothers were exposed, the X chromosomes of their eggs would be damaged, producing a greater disadvantage for the resulting male conceptus (which lack another X chromosome to compensate). This would cause exposed women to produce more girls. The theory is appealing but it has not been empirically validated.

Parental Hormones at Conception

William James has proposed that the sex ratio is increased by high levels of testosterone and estrogen in either parent around the time of conception and decreased by high levels of progesterone.[8] There is a large body of circumstantial evidence that supports the hypothesis,[9] although as yet no experimental proof.

Males as the Weaker Sex

The male organism seems to be the more delicate of the sexes, perhaps because of its dependence on only one X chromosome. If so, male embryos may be the first to die under an assault by environmental toxicants, thus reducing the sex ratio. This argument has been used to suggest that sex ratio might be a useful "sentinel event" for the detection of environmental toxicants.[10] This suggestion remains speculative.

The Myth of the Speedy Y Sperm

There is a widely held idea that sperm carrying the Y chromosome swim faster in the woman's reproductive tract. This is supposedly because the Y chromosome is smaller than the X, and thus the Y sperm are not carrying as heavy a load. This notion was suggested 50 years ago on the basis of primitive laboratory tools[11] and has since been soundly refuted.[12] Even so, the idea persists as the scientific equivalent of an urban myth, perhaps because it seems so plausible.

Factors Associated with Variations in Natural Sex Ratio

The sex ratio is a highly accessible epidemiologic endpoint, recorded universally and with near-perfect accuracy. Its abundance is also its weakness: there is perhaps no other endpoint in all of epidemiology with more opportunities to publish small differences made to seem important and for selective publication of false-positive findings. As a general rule, the factors dependably associated with sex ratio work mostly at the third decimal place without nudging the overall 51:49 sex ratio. Factors associated with dramatic divergence from 51:49 are usually based on small sample sizes with low precision.

Variations over Time

The sex ratio drifts up and down over time for reasons that remain completely unknown. Although these changes are more than can be attributed to chance, they are nonetheless minuscule. Consider the sex ratio in the United States over the past 60 years (Fig. 17-1). Even though the trends are highly statistically significant, the difference between the highest and lowest sex ratio during this 60-year period represents only a 1% difference in male births.

Biological Predisposition of Parents

Many families have only boys or only girls, even with large numbers of children. This raises the question of whether there are characteristics of individual parents

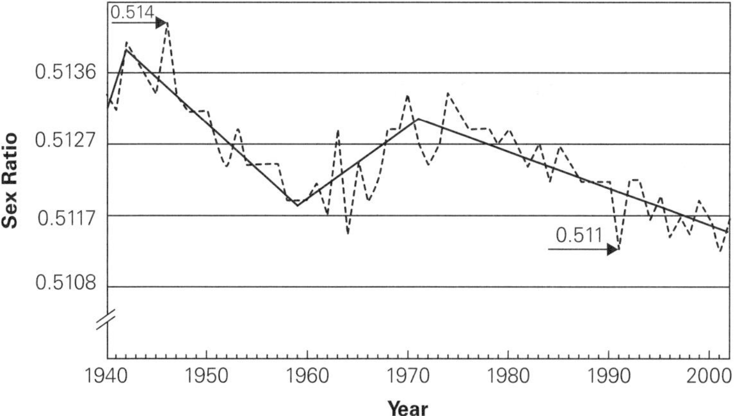

Figure 17-1. U.S. sex ratio over time (1940–2002) (Adapted from Mathews and Hamilton[13])

or couples that predispose them to produce children of one sex or the other. There is no evidence for this. The sex ratio of future children does not differ among families depending on the sex of their previous children.[14]

Racial/Ethnic Differences

There are slight but consistent differences in sex ratio among racial/ethnic groups in the United States. The highest sex ratio is found among U.S. mothers of European descent (0.513), with lower ratios for mothers of African descent (0.507) and Native American descent (0.506).[13,15] An analysis of interracial couples suggests that the father, not the mother, is responsible for these differences.[16]

Parental Age

There is a small decline in the sex ratio with maternal age (from 0.513 among 15- to 19-year-olds to 0.509 among 40- to 44-year-olds).[13] This may be a combination of age effects in both men and women.[14]

Times of War

One of the most intriguing claims about sex ratio is that the proportion of boys at birth increases during and after war, as if nature were doing her part to replenish the supply of men lost in conflict. However, the data are not consistent. Where associations have been seen, they are, once again, exceedingly small. In an analysis restricted to whites in five U.S. states, the sex ratio peaked at 0.517 in 1946 and fell to 0.514 by 1949.[17]

Stress

A possible effect of stress on sex ratio has been suggested. By linking hospital and death records to birth records, Danish researchers found a deficit of boys among the offspring of women who experienced severe stress (hospitalization or death of their partner or another child) near the time of conception.[18] The sex ratio was 49:51 in the exposed, compared with 51:49 in the unexposed. The pathway is presumed to be stress experienced by the mother, although an effect could also be working through stress on her partner. A slight decline in sex ratio (to 50:50) was also observed after the Kobe earthquake.[19]

Environmental Toxicants

In 1976, an explosion at a factory in Seveso, Italy, exposed the surrounding population to high levels of dioxin, one of the most toxic chemicals produced by humans. During the next 7 years, the proportion of boys among 72 births in exposed families was only 36% (95% confidence interval 25% to 47%).[20] Although this dramatic incident suggests that the sex ratio may be sensitive to environmental toxicants, there has not been much evidence subsequently to support the association.[21] As an intermediate measure of sex ratio, slight differences in the ratio of Y- and X-bearing sperm have been reported in association with PCB and DDE contaminants in semen.[22] Exposures to factors known to be human reproductive toxicants (such as cigarette smoking) have produced no consistent or convincing evidence of effects on sex ratio.[23]

The Propensity for False-Positive Findings

In 2005, the *British Medical Journal* published a paper showing an association between decreased fertility and increased sex ratio.[24] Within 4 days other researchers had posted data on the *BMJ* website showing an utter lack of association in another study.[25] Within weeks a second negative study was posted.[26] Although this sequence played out with remarkable briskness, the basic plot line is familiar: a dramatic sex-ratio finding is published (complete with imaginative hypotheses for biological mechanisms, and broadcast across many news media) followed by multiple boring refutations of the association. Epidemiologists are not alone—biologists are also prone to publication bias on sex ratios in mammals,[27] although these findings get less press.

The sex ratio is sure to remain a popular topic of conversation and an attractive endpoint for epidemiologic studies. Whether it will ever be a useful barometer of reproductive health, however, is doubtful. As a rule of thumb, a skeptical attitude toward dramatic new sex-ratio findings is a safe bet. In today's rapid-response environment, it may be only a matter of days until a new finding is overruled.

Selecting the Sex of the Baby

Couples sometimes have a strong preference for the sex of a planned offspring. This has led to countless folk remedies and a number of scientific-sounding recommendations for tipping the scales in favor of one sex or the other. These recommendations always come with success stories—an abundant supply of which is guaranteed by the fact that all methods succeed half the time. Best-selling books notwithstanding,[28] there is no reliable evidence that changes in intercourse timing (or frequency, or position) will budge the 51:49 odds by even a small amount.

Sperm Sex Selection

After numerous attempts, methods are slowly emerging to sort sperm by their sex chromosome. This research is primarily applied in veterinary medicine. The principle is to fluorescently stain sperm based on their relative content of DNA and then to sort the X- and Y-bearing sperm by their differential fluorescence. The procedure is now efficient enough to be used commercially in animal husbandry, mostly for production of cattle.[29] There is optimism for the eventual application of this technology to humans, although the process is not benign for the sperm. The sorted sperm have a shorter life-span in the female reproductive tract, suffer destabilization of their membranes, and are less effective at fertilizing. There is also evidence that the resulting blastocysts are not as viable.[29,30] The stain applied to the sperm and the intense laser light during sorting may cause genetic damage.[31] Clinical trials are being conducted to explore short-term efficacy and safety of the procedure in humans.[32] Implications for longer-term health of human offspring are unknown.

Embryo Sex Selection

Far more effective (and controversial) are the methods of preimplantation genetic diagnosis. This procedure involves removing a single cell from an in-vitro-fertilized egg at an early stage of cell division (see Figure 1-15) and determining the sex by genetic testing. Fertilized eggs of the chosen sex can then be transferred to the woman. This procedure may not be entirely benign to the blastocyst.[33]

Fetal Sex Selection

The most extreme form of sex selection is infanticide.[34] Sex selection can also be performed during pregnancy, using fetal ultrasound to determine the sex of the fetus and then abortion to remove the unwanted fetus. This is illegal in virtually all countries, but it is not uncommon.[35] Presumptive evidence of the use of ultrasound for sex selection can be found in the sex ratios of countries where sons are highly prized. Keeping in mind that few if any preconception factors can cause the sex ratio to deviate from 51:49, the sex ratio is 0.53 in Korea, 0.54 in Singapore and Taiwan, 0.55 in China, and up to 0.63 in provinces of India.[36] U.S. corporations export a large number of ultrasound machines to India, where they are found even in villages that lack clean water or dependable electricity.[37] Beyond the legal issues, fetal sex selection has long-term implications for the affected birth cohorts, creating, for example, a dearth of future partners for men.

References

1. Clutton-Brock TH, Iason GR. Sex ratio variation in mammals. *Q Rev Biol* 1986;61(3):339–74.
2. Trivers RL, Willard DE. Natural selection of parental ability to vary the sex ratio of offspring. *Science* 1973;179(68):90–2.
3. Miller D, Summers J, Silber S. Environmental versus genetic sex determination: a possible factor in dinosaur extinction? *Fertil Steril* 2004;81(4):954–64.
4. Andersson M. Sex ratios and reversals. *Science* 1983;220(4599):853–4.
5. Boklage CE. The epigenetic environment: secondary sex ratio depends on differential survival in embryogenesis. *Hum Reprod* 2005;20(3):583–7.
6. Irgens A, Irgens LM. Secular trends in uncertain-sex births and proportion of male births in Norway, 1967–1998. *Arch Environ Health* 2003;58(9):554–9.
7. Schull WP, Neel JV. Radiation and the sex ratio in man. *Science* 1958;128:343–8.
8. James WH. Evidence that mammalian sex ratios at birth are partially controlled by parental hormone levels at the time of conception. *J Theor Biol* 1996;180:271–86.
9. James WH. Further evidence that mammalian sex ratios at birth are partially controlled by parental hormone levels around the time of conception. *Hum Reprod* 2004;19(6):1250–6.
10. Davis DL, Gottlieb MB, Stampnitzky JR. Reduced ratio of male to female births in several industrial countries: a sentinel health indicator? *JAMA* 1998;279(13):1018–23.
11. Shettles LB. Nuclear morphology of human spermatozoa. *Nature* 1960;186:648–9.
12. Grant VJ. Entrenched misinformation about X and Y sperm. *BMJ* 2006; 332(7546):916.
13. Mathews TJ, Hamilton BE. Trend analysis of the sex ratio at birth in the United States. *Natl Vital Stat Rep* 2005;53(20):1–17.
14. Jacobsen R, Moller H, Mouritsen A. Natural variation in the human sex ratio. *Hum Reprod* 1999;14(12):3120–5.
15. Martin JA, Hamilton BE, Sutton PD, et al. Births: final data for 2005. *Natl Vital Stat Rep* 2007;56(6):1–103.
16. Khoury MJ, Erickson JD, James LM. Paternal effects on the human sex ratio at birth: evidence from interracial crosses. *Am J Hum Genet* 1984;36(5):1103–11.
17. MacMahon B, Pugh TF. Sex ratio of white births in the United States during the Second World War. *Am J Hum Genet* 1954;6(2):284–92.
18. Hansen D, Moller H, Olsen J. Severe periconceptional life events and the sex ratio in offspring: follow up study based on five national registers. *BMJ* 1999;319(7209):548–9.
19. Fukuda M, Fukuda K, Shimizu T, Moller H. Decline in sex ratio at birth after Kobe earthquake. *Hum Reprod* 1998;13(8):2321–2.

20. Mocarelli P, Gerthoux PM, Ferrari E, et al. Paternal concentrations of dioxin and sex ratio of offspring. *Lancet* 2000;355(9218):1858–63.
21. Rogan WJ, Ragan NB. Some evidence of effects of environmental chemicals on the endocrine system in children. *Int J Hyg Environ Health* 2007;210(5):659–67.
22. Tiido T, Rignell-Hydbom A, Jonsson BA, et al. Impact of PCB and *p,p*'-DDE contaminants on human sperm Y:X chromosome ratio: studies in three European populations and the Inuit population in Greenland. *Environ Health Perspect* 2006;114(5):718–24.
23. Mills JL, England L, Granath F, Cnattingius S. Cigarette smoking and the male-female sex ratio. *Fertil Steril* 2003;79(5):1243–5.
24. Smits LJ, de Bie RA, Essed GG, van den Brandt PA. Time to pregnancy and sex of offspring: cohort study. *BMJ* 2005;331(7530):1437–8.
25. Olsen J, Zhou W, Zhu JL. Time to pregnancy and sex of offspring. *BMJ* rapid response published online December 21, 2005.
26. Slama R, Bouyer J, Ducot B, Spira A, Blonde B. Are subfertile couples more likely to have boys? A comprehensive nationwide study. *BMJ* rapid response published online January 6, 2006.
27. Festa-Bianchet M. Offspring sex ratio studies of mammals: does publication depend upon the quality of the research or the direction of the results? *Ecoscience* 1996;3(1):42–4.
28. Shettles LB. *How to Choose the Sex of your Baby: A Complete Update on the Method Best Supported by the Scientific Evidence.* New York: Harper-Collins Publishers, 1985.
29. Maxwell W, Evans G, Hollinshead F, et al. Integration of sperm sexing technology into the ART toolbox. *Anim Reprod Sci* 2003;82–83:79–95.
30. Palma GA, Olivier NS, Neumuller C, Sinowatz F. Effects of sex-sorted spermatozoa on the efficiency of in vitro fertilization and ultrastructure of in vitro produced bovine blastocysts. *Anat Histol Embryol* 2008;37(1):67–73.
31. Garner DL, Seidel GE Jr. History of commercializing sexed semen for cattle. *Theriogenology* 2008;69(7):886–95.
32. Schulman JD, Karabinus DS. Scientific aspects of preconception gender selection. *Reprod Biomed Online* 2005;10 Suppl 1:111–15.
33. Mastenbroek S, Twisk M, van Echten-Arends J, et al. In vitro fertilization with preimplantation genetic screening. *N Engl J Med* 2007;357(1):9–17.
34. Egozcue J. Control of human sex ratios: sex selection: why not? *Hvm Reprod* 1993;8(11):1777.
35. Wu Z, Viisainen K, Hemminki E. Determinants of high sex ratio among newborns: a cohort study from rural Anhui province, China. *Reprod Health Matters* 2006;14(27):172–80.
36. Ding QJ, Hesketh T. Family size, fertility preferences, and sex ratio in China in the era of the one child family policy: results from national family planning and reproductive health survey. *BMJ* 2006;333(7564):371–3.
37. Wonacott P. India's skewed sex ratio puts GE sales in spotlight. *Wall Street Journal.* New York, April 18, 2007.

18

Maternal Mortality and Morbidity

The biological mechanisms that enable a woman to conceive and bear children also make her vulnerable to a unique set of health problems. Many of these problems occur in connection with pregnancy, but not all. These pathologic conditions have no counterpart in men and have been relatively understudied.

By most measures, women are healthier than men and live longer. Nonetheless, the capacity to bear children comes with specific liabilities that, in other eras, put women of reproductive age at severe disadvantage. Even today, women suffer from serious morbidity related to their reproductive system.

Maternal Mortality

Pregnancy is a time of risk for women as well as for their offspring. Over most of human history, this risk has been substantial. In recent times, maternal mortality has fallen to extremely low levels in developed countries, although it remains relatively high in some developing countries. In poor countries, a mother's death can have the further consequence of imperiling the survival of her newborn and other children.[1]

Definitions

The pattern of maternal mortality is similar to that of infant mortality in that the risk is highest in the first 24 hours after delivery and then steadily declines (Fig. 18-1).[2] The World Health Organization defines a maternal death as death while pregnant or within 42 days of termination of pregnancy, from any cause related to the pregnancy but not from accidental or incidental causes.[3] One difficulty with this definition is in deciding whether a woman's death is "related" to

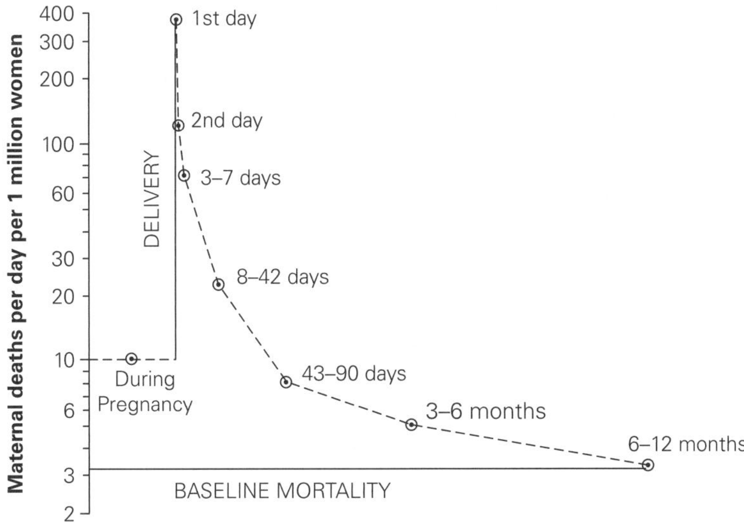

Figure 18-1. Maternal mortality in relation to delivery (160,000 live births, Bangladesh, 1983–2001)[4]

pregnancy. An alternative definition is to include deaths to women from *any* cause if the death occurs within 42 days of delivery (Tenth International Classification of Diseases). Maternal mortality can be expressed as maternal deaths per woman of reproductive age in a year, or more specifically as the ratio of maternal deaths to live births.

Data from Bangladesh provide information on the underlying pattern of maternal risk around delivery. A woman's risk of death is increased about threefold during pregnancy and then jumps to more than 100-fold higher on the day of delivery (Fig. 18-1). (These data are presented on a log scale to accommodate the extreme changes in risk.) Although maternal risk falls rapidly thereafter, it does not return to prepregnancy levels until about 6 months after delivery. This extended period of maternal risk is captured in the category of "late maternal mortality," comprising deaths of women from direct or indirect obstetric causes between 42 days and 1 year.[3]

Occurrence

As with infant mortality (Chapter 12), estimates of maternal mortality vary 100-fold across nations.[2] The maternal mortality ratio in developed countries is around 20 per 100,000 live births, with a few countries below 10 per 100,000 (0.01%).[5] In contrast, the ratio in developing countries is around 400 per 100,000 births (0.4%) and reaches up to 1% of pregnancies in sub-Saharan Africa.[6]

There are a half-million women who die of pregnancy complications each year; 99% of these deaths occur in developing countries.[7] This high maternal risk per pregnancy in the developing countries is compounded by the fact that women in these countries also have more pregnancies. Thus, the lifetime risk of dying from the complications of pregnancy is 1 out of 16 women in Sierra Leone and Afghanistan, compared with 1 out of 30,000 women in Sweden.[2]

Problems of Estimation

Most statistics on maternal mortality are underestimates,[8] especially in developing countries. Making the link between a woman's death and her recent pregnancy is not simple even when vital statistics systems are functioning. Demographers have developed indirect approaches to estimate maternal mortality in poor countries, for example, by conducting detailed interviews of women about their sisters.[9] To further complicate the estimation process, the connection of a death with the occurrence of pregnancy may be concealed (if the death resulted from an illegal abortion) or missed altogether (for example, if a ruptured tubal pregnancy is not recognized as the cause of death). Many countries have no data from any source.[3]

Secular Trends

In the United States and Europe before the twentieth century, 1% to 2% of pregnancies resulted in maternal death. Maternal death was a virtual death sentence for the infant as well.[10] In the United States, maternal mortality plummeted between 1920 and 1950 and has declined slowly since (Fig. 18-2).

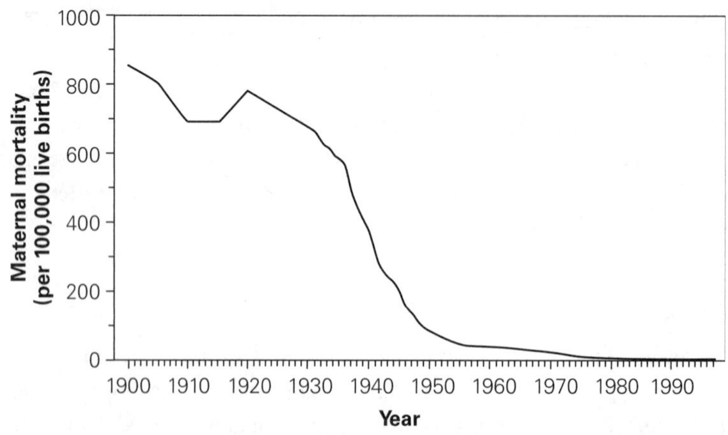

Figure 18-2. Decline in maternal mortality over time (per 100,000 live births, United States, 1900–97) (Reprinted from MMWR[11])

General Risk Factors

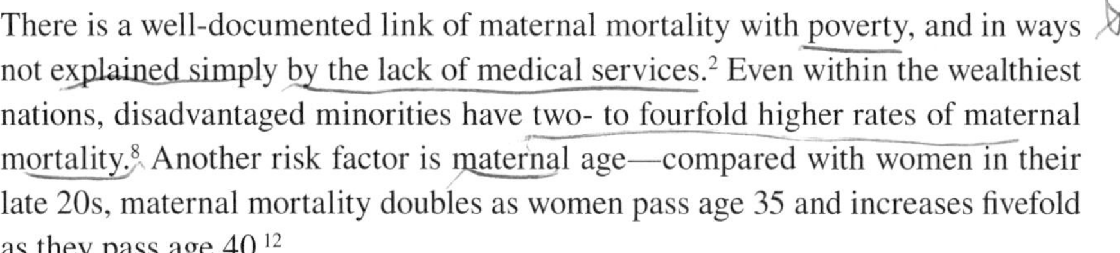

There is a well-documented link of maternal mortality with poverty, and in ways not explained simply by the lack of medical services.[2] Even within the wealthiest nations, disadvantaged minorities have two- to fourfold higher rates of maternal mortality.[8] Another risk factor is maternal age—compared with women in their late 20s, maternal mortality doubles as women pass age 35 and increases fivefold as they pass age 40.[12]

Specific Causes of Maternal Mortality

The most common causes of maternal death are hemorrhage, hypertensive disorders (preeclampsia and eclampsia), infection, and obstructed labor.[2] The relative contributions of these causes vary across regions. For example, hypertensive disorders are a larger contributor in Latin America, whereas hemorrhage is more important in Africa.[13] Lethal infection is especially common in countries where abortion is illegal. Obstructed labor is a problem wherever women deliver without access to skilled obstetric care.[13] About two-thirds of pregnant women in sub-Saharan Africa and South Asia deliver without benefit of a trained birth attendant.[14] In the developed countries, maternal deaths are more likely to be from preexisting conditions in the mother.[15] Violence against women—often by the woman's partner—is a component of maternal mortality in all countries. Women may be at increased risk of partner violence during pregnancy as well as in the months following delivery.[16]

Vaginal Fistulae

For every woman who dies of labor complications, there are others who sustain serious injuries. One type of injury is the vaginal fistula, in which prolonged pressure of the baby's head on the vaginal wall damages the wall. One result of such injury is that an opening develops between the woman's bladder or rectum and her vagina. Such fistulas result in urinary or fecal incontinence and require surgical repair. In traditional societies, incontinence makes women social outcasts and can be grounds for divorce and abandonment. There are few data on the extent of this condition; estimates range from 2 to 4 million women, almost entirely in the developing countries, where skilled management of labor is least available.[17]

Preeclampsia

Preeclampsia is a multisystem disorder of pregnancy that seems to occur only in humans.[18] Its cause remains unknown. Its progression to the full-blown form of eclampsia can cause maternal death. The syndrome is characterized by dysfunction of the blood vessels that produces hypertension and sometimes clotting disorders. A key sign is protein in urine. The peculiarities of preeclampsia, along with its prevalence and risk, have made this disease an intensely researched and hotly debated topic. For this reason, preeclampsia is the subject of its own chapter (Chapter 19).

The remaining causes of maternal mortality may seem more ordinary, although there is surprisingly little known about their prevalence or etiologies.

Postpartum Hemorrhage

Postpartum hemorrhage is the most commonly reported cause of maternal mortality, causing about 30% of maternal deaths worldwide.[19] In the United States, hemorrhage accounts for about 20% of maternally related deaths.[20]

The average woman loses 300 to 500 cc of blood in the first 24 hours after delivery without serious consequence.[21] If the uterus has trouble contracting after delivery (sometimes because pieces of placenta have been retained), or if the uterus has been damaged during delivery, then blood loss can be more serious. WHO defines postpartum hemorrhage as the loss of more than 500 cc of blood in the 24 hours after a vaginal delivery.[21] There is little agreement on the prevalence of postpartum hemorrhage. One U.S. study reports 4%,[22] an obstetrics textbook says 2% to 11%,[23] and a recent review 40%.[21] Few studies have considered what risk factors might be associated.[24]

Hyperemesis

Perhaps three-quarters of pregnant women have nausea with pregnancy, and about half of women experience vomiting.[25] A very few—about 0.5%—have intractable vomiting known as hyperemesis gravidarum, usually defined as a loss of at least 5% of prepregnancy body weight. This is a serious source of pregnancy morbidity and (before intravenous fluids were available) mortality. Death rates among women with hyperemesis were 3% to 10% before the era of modern medicine.[25,26] Hyperemesis may be related to the production of hCG, although this is still in dispute.[25] The condition is twice as common with multiple fetuses and in pregnancies that later develop preeclampsia.[27]

Placental Abruption

In normal pregnancy, the placenta separates from the uterus after the baby has been delivered. In 6–10 pregnancies out of 1,000, the placenta begins to separate before delivery, producing pain and vaginal bleeding. Premature separation is an obstetric emergency. The mother's risk with good obstetric care is relatively small, but there is substantial risk of losing the baby. In the United States, perinatal mortality is 15-fold higher with abruption.[28] Although abruption can occur without warning, it is likely that the underlying cause has been present since early in pregnancy (as is true for many pathologies of the placenta). Consistent with this, babies from pregnancies with placental abruption are on average several hundred grams smaller than other babies born at the same gestational age.[28] Maternal smoking is associated with a doubling of risk.[29] Other risk factors include preeclampsia and hypertension.[30]

Placenta Previa

The placenta usually attaches to the upper portion of the uterus, well away from the cervix. Attachment of the placenta to the lower part of the uterus is known as placenta previa and occurs in 3 to 5 per 1,000 pregnancies.[31] In the worst case, the placenta covers the opening of the cervix, such that the baby cannot be delivered vaginally without dislodging the placenta. In the United States, neonatal mortality is increased fourfold in the presence of placenta previa.[32] Maternal age is one of the strongest risk factors for placenta previa, with an eightfold increased risk among mothers 35 years and older. Relative risk with maternal smoking is around 1.6.[33]

Other Bleeding during Pregnancy

Bleeding before 20 weeks of pregnancy is not in itself a threat to the mother, although it is associated with moderately increased risks of preterm delivery, fetal growth restriction, and perinatal death.[34] Ten percent to 20% of pregnant women report at least 1 day with signs of bleeding, especially during the first 2 months.[34,35] Other than impending miscarriage, hydatidaform mole or the rare pathologies of placentation discussed above, the reasons for bleeding in early pregnancy are unclear. It may be a general sign of less-than-optimum placental attachment. The blood itself may contribute to fetal troubles by irritating thc fctal membranes. There is no evidence that early vaginal bleeding occurs with implantation, as is sometimes suggested.[36]

Preventing Maternal Mortality

The high rates of maternal mortality in developing countries are a public health challenge. Because many of the ostensible causes are preventable, the prevention of maternal mortality is sometimes discussed as "simple and relatively inexpensive."[37] This has not proven to be the case. As with infant mortality, specific interventions to prevent maternal mortality have produced little in demonstrable improvements.[38] This may be because the interventions were too narrow or because the evaluations were not large enough to demonstrate an effect.

Female Reproductive-Organ Morbidity

In addition to the life-threatening conditions connected with pregnancy, women are vulnerable to an array of nonmalignant ailments specific to their reproductive organs. These ailments can cause substantial morbidity in the absence of pregnancy and, in fact, often interfere with pregnancy.

Fibroids

Uterine fibroids (or leiomyomas) are benign tumors of the muscular wall of the uterus, with tumors sometimes reaching the size of a closed fist. Fibroids are associated with pain, increased menstrual bleeding, and infertility. In the United States, fibroids are the leading cause of hysterectomy.[39] The prevalence of fibroids increases with age, affecting 70% to 80% of women by the time they approach menopause.[40] There is racial and ethnic disparity in the prevalence of fibroids. African-Americans have earlier onset,[41] and the tumors are larger when first diagnosed.[42] In black women, fibroids do not show the decline in growth rate with age that is seen in whites.[43] Although hormonally dependent, the etiology and pathogenesis of fibroids remain obscure, and there have been few etiologic studies.[44] Early age of menarche and nulliparity have been consistently associated with increased risk.[45] Fibroids may reduce fecundability and increase pregnancy loss and preterm birth, although these associations are less clear.[46]

Hysterectomy

Surgical removal of the uterus is a common surgical procedure, with about one-third of U.S. women having hysterectomy by age 60.[47] Most indications for hysterectomy are for noncancerous conditions such as fibroids, endometriosis, excessive menstrual bleeding, and uterine prolapse. About half of U.S. hysterectomies include the removal of the ovaries ("surgical menopause").[48] Even if one or both ovaries are left intact, hysterectomy accelerates natural menopause by about 4 years, perhaps because of the residual trauma of the hysterectomy.[49] Hysterectomy must be taken into account in any epidemiologic study of female reproductive function. A high prevalence of hysterectomy in the population can affect estimates of age-specific fertility rates, age at menopause, risk of diseases of the uterus, and other uterine-related functions.

Endometriosis

Endometriosis is the presence of endometrial tissue outside the uterus (usually attached to the surfaces of the pelvic cavity). It is not clear whether this tissue escapes from the uterus (perhaps in retrograde menstrual flow through the oviducts) or grows from embryologic cells scattered early in development. In either case, the misplaced tissue responds like normal uterine endometrium to menstrual hormones, producing cyclic bleeding. Blood is an irritant, and the bleeding is painful. Endometriosis has also been associated with infertility. Although endometriosis is not rare, the difficulties of diagnosis have made population-based estimates nearly impossible.[50] Its prevalence remains unknown.

Polycystic Ovary Syndrome

The most common endocrine problem among women is polycystic ovary syndrome. This syndrome is characterized by irregular menses and ovulatory disturbance (often with infertility), overproduction of androgens (producing hairiness and acne), and obesity. Numerous enlarged ovarian follicles (or "cysts") may be visible on the surface of the ovary. Clinicians have been unable to agree on a definition of the disease,[51] which contributes to the difficulties of epidemiologic study. When defined by the clinical features of anovulation and hyperandrogenism, the syndrome is present in an estimated 5% of women of reproductive age.[52] Many women with this syndrome have insulin resistance and are at risk of Type 2 diabetes and gestational diabetes. Women with polycystic ovarian syndrome are also at increased risk for poor pregnancy outcomes, including preterm birth and perinatal death.[53] The causes of this syndrome remain obscure.

References

1. Zaba B, Whitworth J, Marston M, et al. HIV and mortality of mothers and children: evidence from cohort studies in Uganda, Tanzania, and Malawi. *Epidemiology* 2005;16(3):275–80.
2. Ronsmans C, Graham WJ. Maternal mortality: who, when, where, and why. *Lancet* 2006;368(9542):1189–200.
3. WHO. *Maternal Mortality in 2005: Estimates developed by WHO, UNESCO, UNFPA and the World Bank*. Geneva: WHO, 2007.
4. Hurt LS, Alam N, Dieltiens G, Aktar N, Ronsmans C. Duration and magnitude of mortality after pregnancy in rural Bangladesh. *Int J Epidemiol* 2008;37(2):397–404.
5. WHO. *Maternal Mortality in 2000: Estimates Developed by WHO, UNICEF and UNFPA*. Geneva: WHO, 2004.
6. Mukuria A, Aboulafia C, Themme A. *The Context of Women's Health: Results from the Demographic and Health Surveys, 1994–2001. DHS Comparative Reports No. 11*. Calverton, MD: USAID, 2005.
7. WHO. Maternal mortality ratio falling too slowly to meet goal. London/Geneva: WHO, 2007; http://www.who.int/mediacentre/news/releases/2007/pr56/en/print.html, last accessed October 27, 2009.
8. Atrash HK, Alexander S, Berg CJ. Maternal mortality in developed countries: not just a concern of the past. *Obstet Gynecol* 1995;86(4 Pt 2):700–5.
9. Stanton C, Abderrahim N, Hill K. DHS maternal mortality indicators: an assessment of data quality and implications for data use. *Demographic and Health Surveys Analytical Reports*. Calverton, MD, 1997.
10. Hogberg U, Brostrom G. The demography of maternal mortality—seven Swedish parishes in the 19th century. *Int J Gynaecol Obstet* 1985;23(6):489–97.
11. MMWR. Achievements in Public Health, 1900–1999: Healthier Mothers and Babies. *MMWR Weekly* 1999;48(38):849–58.
12. Callaghan WM, Berg CJ. Pregnancy-related mortality among women aged 35 years and older, United States, 1991–1997. *Obstet Gynecol* 2003;102(5 Pt 1):1015–21.

13. Khan KS, Wojdyla D, Say L, Gulmezoglu AM, Van Look PF. WHO analysis of causes of maternal death: a systematic review. *Lancet* 2006;367(9516):1066–74.
14. Kruk ME, Prescott MR, Galea S. Equity of skilled birth attendant utilization in developing countries: financing and policy determinants. *Am J Public Health* 2008;98(1):142–7.
15. Rochat RW, Koonin LM, Atrash HK, Jewett JF. Maternal mortality in the United States: report from the Maternal Mortality Collaborative. *Obstet Gynecol* 1988;72(1):91–7.
16. Shadigian E, Bauer ST. Pregnancy-associated death: a qualitative systematic review of homicide and suicide. *Obstet Gynecol Surv* 2005;60(3):183–90.
17. Wall LL. Obstetric vesicovaginal fistula as an international public-health problem. Lancet 2006;368(9542):1201–9.
18. Sibai B, Dekker G, Kupferminc M. Pre-eclampsia. Lancet 2005;365(9461):785–99.
19. Kwast BE. Postpartum haemorrhage: its contribution to maternal mortality. Midwifery 1991;7(2):64–70.
20. Berg CJ, Chang J, Callaghan WM, Whitehead SJ. Pregnancy-related mortality in the United States, 1991–1997. *Obstet Gynecol* 2003;101(2):289–96.
21. Jansen AJ, van Rhenen DJ, Steegers EA, Duvekot JJ. Postpartum hemorrhage and transfusion of blood and blood components. *Obstet Gynecol Surv* 2005;60(10):663–71.
22. Combs CA, Murphy EL, Laros RK Jr. Factors associated with postpartum hemorrhage with vaginal birth. *Obstet Gynecol* 1991;77(1):69–76.
23. Norwitz E, Arulkumaran S, Symonds IM, Fowlie A. *Oxford American Handbook of Obstetrics and Gynecology*. New York: Oxford University Press, 2004.
24. Waterstone M, Bewley S, Wolfe C. Incidence and predictors of severe obstetric morbidity: case-control study. *BMJ* 2001;322(7294):1089–93; discussion 1093–4.
25. Goodwin TM. Hyperemesis gravidarum. *Obstet Gynecol Clin North Am* 2008; 35(3):401–17, viii.
26. Verberg MF, Gillott DJ, Al-Fardan N, Grudzinskas JG. Hyperemesis gravidarum, a literature review. *Hum Reprod* Update 2005;11(5):527–39.
27. Basso O, Olsen J. Sex ratio and twinning in women with hyperemesis or pre-eclampsia. *Epidemiology* 2001;12(6):747–9.
28. Ananth CV, Wilcox AJ. Placental abruption and perinatal mortality in the United States. *Am J Epidemiol* 2001;153(4):332–7.
29. Ananth CV, Savitz DA, Luther ER. Maternal cigarette smoking as a risk factor for placental abruption, placenta previa, and uterine bleeding in pregnancy. *Am J Epidemiol* 1996;144(9):881–9.
30. Oyelese Y, Ananth CV. Placental abruption. *Obstet Gynecol* 2006;108(4):1005–16.
31. Iyasu S, Saftlas AK, Rowley DL, Koonin LM, Lawson HW, Atrash HK. The epidemiology of placenta previa in the United States, 1979 through 1987. *Am J Obstet Gynecol* 1993;168(5):1424–9.
32. Ananth CV, Smulian JC, Vintzileos AM. The effect of placenta previa on neonatal mortality: a population-based study in the United States, 1989 through 1997. *Am J Obstet Gynecol* 2003;188(5):1299–304.
33. Faiz AS, Ananth CV. Etiology and risk factors for placenta previa: an overview and meta-analysis of observational studies. *J Matern Fetal Neonatal Med* 2003;13(3):175–90.
34. Ananth CV, Savitz DA. Vaginal bleeding and adverse reproductive outcomes: a meta-analysis. *Paediatr Perinat Epidemiol* 1994;8(1):62–78.

35. Yang J, Savitz DA, Dole N, et al. Predictors of vaginal bleeding during the first two trimesters of pregnancy. *Paediatr Perinat Epidemiol* 2005;19(4):276–83.
36. Harville EW, Wilcox AJ, Baird DD, Weinberg CR. Vaginal bleeding in very early pregnancy. *Hum Reprod* 2003;18(9):1944–7.
37. Kantrowitz B. "What kills one woman every minute of every day?" *Newsweek* July 9, 2007;56–7.
38. Ronsmans C. In: Semba RD, Bloem MW, ed. *Nutrition and Health in Developing Countries*. Totowa, NJ: Humana Press; 2001:31–56.
39. Stewart EA. Uterine fibroids. *Lancet* 2001;357(9252):293–8.
40. Baird DD, Dunson DB, Hill MC, Cousins D, Schectman JM. High cumulative incidence of uterine leiomyoma in black and white women: ultrasound evidence. *Am J Obstet Gynecol* 2003;188(1):100–7.
41. Laughlin SK, Baird DD, Savitz DA, Herring AH, Hartmann KE. Prevalence of uterine leiomyomas in the first trimester of pregnancy: an ultrasound-screening study. *Obstet Gynecol* 2009;113(3):630–5.
42. Kjerulff KH, Langenberg P, Seidman JD, Stolley PD, Guzinski GM. Uterine leiomyomas. Racial differences in severity, symptoms and age at diagnosis. *J Reprod Med* 1996;41(7):483–90.
43. Peddada SD, Laughlin SK, Miner K, et al. Growth of uterine leiomyomata among premenopausal black and white women. *Proc Natl Acad Sci USA* 2008; 105(50):19887–92.
44. Flake GP, Andersen J, Dixon D. Etiology and pathogenesis of uterine leiomyomas: a review. *Environ Health Perspect* 2003;111(8):1037–54.
45. Baird DD. Invited commentary: uterine leiomyomata—we know so little but could learn so much. *Am J Epidemiol* 2004;159(2):124–6.
46. Coronado GD, Marshall LM, Schwartz SM. Complications in pregnancy, labor, and delivery with uterine leiomyomas: a population-based study. *Obstet Gynecol* 2000;95(5):764–9.
47. Pokras R, Hufnagel VG. Hysterectomies in the United States. Vital Health Stat 13 1987(92):1–32.
48. Whiteman MK, Hillis SD, Jamieson DJ, Morrow B, Podgornik MN, Brett KM, Marchbanks PA. Inpatient hysterectomy surveillance in the United States, 2000-2004. Am J Obstet Gynecol 2008;198(1):34 e1–7.
49. Farquhar CM, Sadler L, Harvey SA, Stewart AW. The association of hysterectomy and menopause: a prospective cohort study. Br J Obstet Gynaecol 2005;112(7):956–62.
50. Missmer SA, Cramer DW. The epidemiology of endometriosis. *Obstet Gynecol Clin North Am* 2003;30(1):1–19, vii.
51. Azziz R, Carmina E, Dewailly D, et al. The Androgen Excess and PCOS Society criteria for the polycystic ovary syndrome: the complete task force report. *Fertil Steril* 2009;91(2):456–88.
52. Solomon CG. The epidemiology of polycystic ovary syndrome. Prevalence and associated disease risks. *Endocrinol Metab Clin North Am* 1999;28(2):247–63.
53. Boomsma CM, Eijkemans MJ, Hughes EG, Visser GH, Fauser BC, Macklon NS. A meta-analysis of pregnancy outcomes in women with polycystic ovary syndrome. *Hum Reprod Update* 2006;12(6):673–83.

19

Preeclampsia

Preeclampsia is a serious obstetric complication that can escalate to maternal convulsions and death. It is also a peculiar entity in many ways. It requires two people—the mother and the fetus—and it is their interaction that produces the syndrome. The cure is to separate the two.

Preeclampsia is an enigmatic syndrome that is both common (occurring in up to 5% of primiparous women) and dangerous (being a major contributor to maternal and infant death).[1] The history of research into the causes of preeclampsia is littered with failed hypotheses, and even today investigators disagree about its origins.

For all these reasons, preeclampsia occupies a special place among the diseases of pregnancy. There is a courtyard set among the corridors of Chicago's famed Lying-In Hospital for Women that contains limestone tablets carved with names of the giants of obstetrics. One tablet has been left blank—reserved for the person who discovers the cause of preeclampsia (Fig. 19-1).

Clinical Features of Preeclampsia

Preeclampsia is defined by its signs. It can occur to any pregnant woman, but especially to women in their first pregnancy. The main criteria for the diagnosis of preeclampsia are hypertension and protein in urine that emerge in the second half of pregnancy.[2] These signs are not necessarily accompanied by symptoms, which is why pregnant women must have their blood pressure and urine checked regularly after 20 weeks of pregnancy.

If preeclampsia is detected, the woman requires close surveillance. The purpose of surveillance is to identify as early as possible the small proportion of women in whom the condition progresses. This can happen with alarming speed.

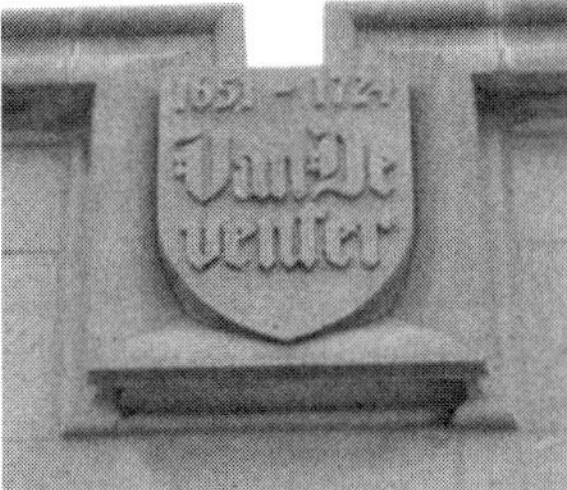

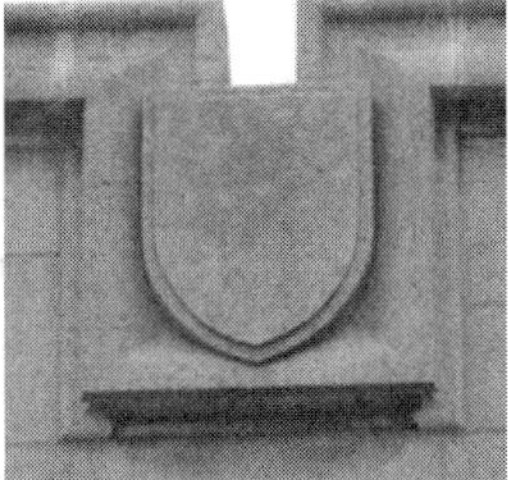

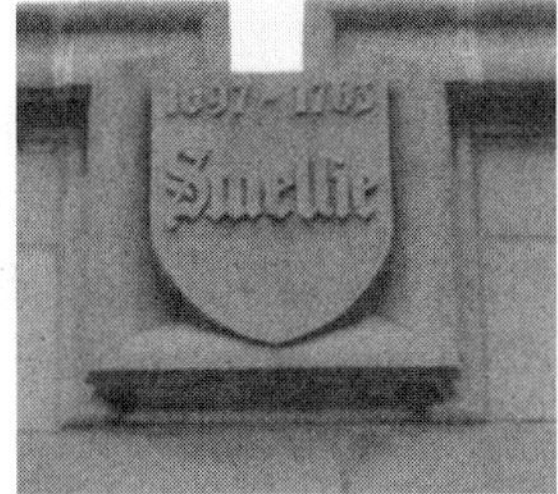

Figure 19-1. Tablets at the University of Chicago Lying-In Hospital commemorating major historical figures in obstetrics. The blank tablet is reserved for the discoverer of the cause of preeclampsia (Photographs courtesy of Diane Anderson, University of Chicago)

(*Preeclampsia* is Greek for "before the lightning strikes.") Eclampsia can produce seizures, cerebral hemorrhage, and maternal and infant death. Another severe variant is the HELLP syndrome, a disorder of blood-clotting mechanisms expressed as Hemolytic anemia, Elevated Liver enzymes and Low Platelet count.[3]

The most effective treatment for preeclampsia is delivery of the fetus. Women with severe preeclampsia are often induced or delivered by cesarean section once they reach 34 weeks of gestation.[1] Preeclampsia can also emerge shortly after delivery (although this is uncommon), in which case the diagnosis can easily be missed.

Two Types of Preeclampsia?

Although any attempt to categorize preeclampsia is inexact (and controversial), the condition is sometimes discussed as having two broad types. One is more severe, less common, and occurs earlier in pregnancy. The fetus is often smaller than expected for its gestational age.[4] The milder form of preeclampsia occurs later in pregnancy, with normal fetal growth. Recurrence is more likely following the severe than the mild form.[5]

Pathogenesis

Most experts agree that the placenta is key to the origins of preeclampsia, with pathologic processes present even as early as implantation.[6] However, it is unclear whether the problem begins with abnormal placentation or stems from a mother's exaggerated inflammatory response to the invading trophoblast cells.[1]

The theoretical biologist David Haig has suggested that preeclampsia might be an extreme expression of a more general struggle between mother and fetus. In this framework, a fetus improves its own nutrition by producing substances that increase resistance in the mother's blood vessels. This benefits the fetus by causing higher maternal blood pressure and better vascular perfusion of the placenta.[7] The observation that preeclampsia is more common with twin pregnancies[8] is consistent with this hypothesis.

Another widely discussed mechanism for preeclampsia is as an immunologic process. Repeated exposure of the mother to the semen of her partner has been proposed to improve her immunologic tolerance of paternal antigens carried by her fetus.[9] This immunologic hypothesis was originally prompted by epidemiologic data showing that the risk of preeclampsia is higher if the pregnancy is fathered by a new partner, compared with the mother's risk in additional pregnancies by the same partner.[10] Further epidemiologic work has raised questions about this observation (more below).

Changes in placental biomarkers (including placental growth factor and factors associated with the growth of blood vessels) are associated with preeclampsia.[11–14] These biomarkers may shed light on the pathophysiology of preeclampsia. Although the power of these markers to predict later preeclampsia is limited, the development of better predictors is likely. These may offer useful tools to epidemiologists exploring the causes of preeclampsia.

Incidence

Incidence of preeclampsia is highest among first pregnancies (3% to 5%) and falls to less than 2% in later pregnancies.[15] The higher risk in first pregnancies is well known but not understood. The occurrence of preeclampsia seems to have increased over time,[16] although such changes are difficult to interpret because of changes in clinical definition and improvements in ascertainment and recording. As with most pregnancy outcomes, there is a high recurrence risk, with a sevenfold higher risk (incidence of about 14%) among women with preeclampsia in the previous pregnancy.[17]

Familial Risk

The highest risk of familial recurrence (2.2-fold) is seen in mothers who were themselves born into a preeclamptic pregnancy. Genes may contribute to this risk in two ways. Such women potentially inherit their mother's genetic predisposition, and they also could pass to their fetus the genetic traits that triggered preeclampsia when the mother was a fetus. In contrast, fathers who were born into preeclamptic pregnancies can pass to their offspring only those genetic traits that operate in the fetus. The recurrence risk through fathers is lower but not absent (1.5-fold).[18] These data support the presence of two different pathways by which genetic factors can contribute to preeclampsia: one through the mother and the other through the fetus.

Pregnancy Interval

The risk of preeclampsia is reduced after the first pregnancy. However, as time passes, preeclampsia risk rises (Fig. 19-2).[15] If the first pregnancy reduces the mother's subsequent risk of preeclampsia, it seems to do so only transiently.

This increased risk with longer time since pregnancy may explain the risk seen with a change in male partner (discussed above). The basis for the immune hypothesis of preeclampsia has been that a change in partners increases risk.[10] However, those studies did not take into account the time between pregnancies. Women who dissolve their partnership after a delivery and find a new partner take longer to have their next pregnancy than women who stay with the same partner.[15] When pregnancy interval is taken into account, there is no increased risk among women who change partners (Fig. 19-3).[15]

Smoking

Mothers who smoke are only about half as likely as other women to have preeclampsia.[19] The biological explanation for this finding is not known. Also, although

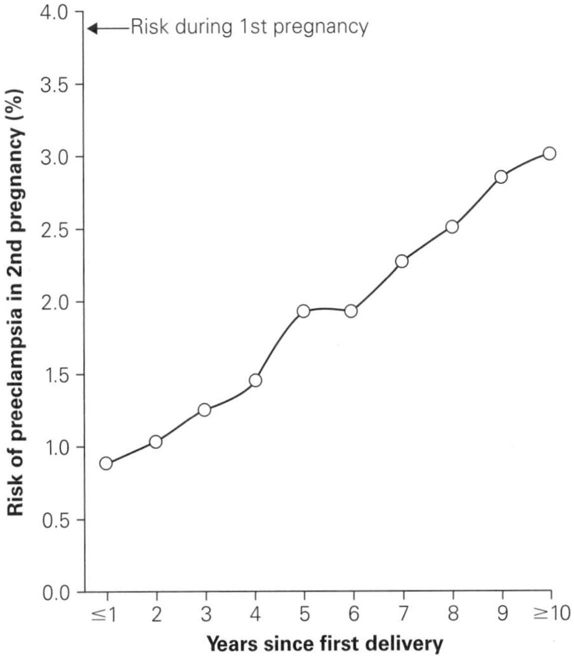

Figure 19-2. Risk of preeclampsia in the second pregnancy, given the time elapsed since the mother's first delivery (Norway, 1967–98) (Reprinted from Skjaerven et al[15])

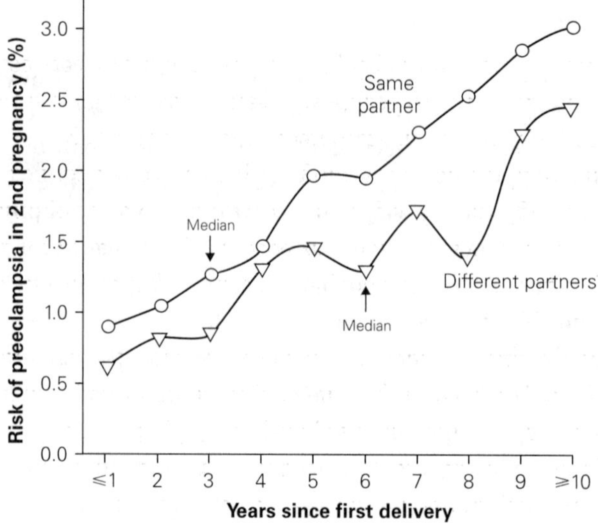

Figure 19-3. Risk of preeclampsia in the second pregnancy by time elapsed since first delivery, and stratified by whether the second pregnancy is by the same partner or a different partner (Norway, 1967–98) (Reprinted from Skjaerven et al[15])

the incidence of preeclampsia is lower among women who smoke, the severity of the preeclampsia (if it occurs) may be worse.[20]

Maternal Characteristics

Mothers are at substantially higher risk of preeclampsia if they are obese, or have diabetes or preexisting hypertension.[21] Because the prevalence of maternal obesity (and its sequelae of hypertension and diabetes) is increasing over time, the occurrence of preeclampsia is also expected to rise.[22] Women with preeclampsia have been observed to have a higher risk of cardiovascular disease.[23] This association may be explained by the fact that the risk factors for preeclampsia are also strong risk factors for cardiovascular disease.[24]

Risks for Offspring

The risk of neonatal mortality is doubled among babies born from preeclamptic pregnancies.[25] This increased mortality is largely a result of the early delivery of the fetus. Stillbirth risk can also be high among preeclamptic pregnancies, although the preemptive delivery of preeclamptic pregnancies (done primarily to protect the mother) seems to have reduced the excess risk of stillbirth with preeclampsia.[25]

References

1. Sibai B, Dekker G, Kupferminc M. Pre-eclampsia. *Lancet* 2005;365(9461):785–99.
2. Report of the National High Blood Pressure Education Program Working Group on High Blood Pressure in Pregnancy. *Am J Obstet Gynecol* 2000;183(1):S1-S22.
3. Rath W, Faridi A, Dudenhausen JW. HELLP syndrome. *J Perinat Med* 2000; 28(4):249–60.
4. Vatten LJ, Skjaerven R. Is pre-eclampsia more than one disease? *Br J Obstet Gynaecol* 2004;111(4):298–302.
5. Moore LE. Recurrent risk of adverse pregnancy outcome. *Obstet Gynecol Clin North Am* 2008;35(3):459–71, ix.
6. Huppertz B. Placental origins of preeclampsia: challenging the current hypothesis. *Hypertension* 2008;51(4):970–5.
7. Haig D. Genetic conflicts in human pregnancy. *Q Rev Biol* 1993;68(4):495–532.
8. Krotz S, Fajardo J, Ghandi S, Patel A, Keith LG. Hypertensive disease in twin pregnancies: a review. *Twin Res* 2002;5(1):8–14.
9. Dekker GA, Sibai BM. Etiology and pathogenesis of preeclampsia: current concepts. *Am J Obstet Gynecol* 1998;179(5):1359–75.
10. Robillard PY, Hulsey TC, Alexander GR, Keenan A, de Caunes F, Papiernik E. Paternity patterns and risk of preeclampsia in the last pregnancy in multiparae. *J Reprod Immunol* 1993;24(1):1–12.
11. Levine RJ, Lam C, Qian C, et al. Soluble endoglin and other circulating antiangiogenic factors in preeclampsia. *N Engl J Med* 2006;355(10):992–1005.
12. Levine RJ, Maynard SE, Qian C, et al. Circulating angiogenic factors and the risk of preeclampsia. *N Engl J Med* 2004;350(7):672–83.
13. Levine RJ, Thadhani R, Qian C, et al. Urinary placental growth factor and risk of preeclampsia. *JAMA* 2005;293(1):77–85.
14. Romero R, Nien JK, Espinoza J, et al. A longitudinal study of angiogenic (placental growth factor) and anti-angiogenic (soluble endoglin and soluble vascular endothelial growth factor receptor-1) factors in normal pregnancy and patients destined to develop preeclampsia and deliver a small for gestational age neonate. *J Matern Fetal Neonatal Med* 2008;21(1):9–23.
15. Skjaerven R, Wilcox AJ, Lie RT. The interval between pregnancies and the risk of preeclampsia. *N Engl J Med* 2002;346(1):33–8.
16. Wallis AB, Saftlas AF, Hsia J, Atrash HK. Secular trends in the rates of preeclampsia, eclampsia, and gestational hypertension, United States, 1987–2004. *Am J Hypertens* 2008;21(5):521–6.
17. Trogstad L, Skrondal A, Stoltenberg C, Magnus P, Nesheim BI, Eskild A. Recurrence risk of preeclampsia in twin and singleton pregnancies. *Am J Med Genet A* 2004;126A(1):41–5.
18. Skjaerven R, Vatten LJ, Wilcox AJ, Ronning T, Irgens LM, Lie RT. Recurrence of pre-eclampsia across generations: exploring fetal and maternal genetic components in a population based cohort. *BMJ* 2005;331(7521):877.
19. England L, Zhang J. Smoking and risk of preeclampsia: a systematic review. *Front Biosci* 2007;12:2471–83.

20. Pipkin FB. Smoking in moderate/severe preeclampsia worsens pregnancy outcome, but smoking cessation limits the damage. *Hypertension* 2008;51(4):1042–6.
21. Eskenazi B, Fenster L, Sidney S. A multivariate analysis of risk factors for preeclampsia. *JAMA* 1991;266(2):237–41.
22. Villamor E, Cnattingius S. Interpregnancy weight change and risk of adverse pregnancy outcomes: a population-based study. *Lancet* 2006;368(9542):1164–70.
23. Irgens HU, Reisaeter L, Irgens LM, Lie RT. Long-term mortality of mothers and fathers after pre-eclampsia: population based cohort study. *BMJ* 2001;323(7323):1213–17.
24. Bellamy L, Casas JP, Hingorani AD, Williams DJ. Pre-eclampsia and risk of cardiovascular disease and cancer in later life: systematic review and meta-analysis. *BMJ* 2007;335(7627):974.
25. Basso O, Rasmussen S, Weinberg CR, Wilcox AJ, Irgens LM, Skjaerven R. Trends in fetal and infant survival following preeclampsia. *JAMA* 2006;296(11):1357–62.

20

Fetal Exposures and Adult Disease

Many diseases have been proposed to have their origins in fetal life. Much research has been conducted on the possibility that fetal and infant nutrition has long-term effects on health. Toxic exposures to the mother during pregnancy can also have long-term effects on the fetus. The extent of this threat is not easily assessed, and relatively little research on this topic has been carried out.

Imagine a toxic exposure that damages women's ability to reproduce. This exposure doubles the woman's risk of infertility and, for women who get pregnant, triples their risk of preterm delivery and quadruples neonatal deaths. Now imagine that 2 million women have been exposed to this toxicant.

You might think that the discovery of this toxic exposure would be straightforward. All the ingredients for a solid epidemiologic result would seem to be present: the exposed population is large, the endpoints are measurable, and the risks are substantial. A study of even moderate size would have power to link the exposure to the risk—that is, if the investigators knew where to look for the exposure. The remarkable thing is that this exposure really happened, and we came perilously close to missing it completely. The reason is that exposure occurred where no one expected it—during the fetal lives of the affected women.

The exposure is diethylstilbestrol, or DES, a synthetic estrogen that had been prescribed to these women's mothers a generation earlier—while pregnant with them.[1]

The Story of DES

Diethylstilbestrol provides a parable with many lessons. The story begins in 1938, when the drug was first synthesized by British university researchers. DES is a synthetic estrogen with high oral potency, and thus an estrogen that could be taken as a pill. Furthermore, DES is simple and cheap to make. Because it was discovered in a government-supported laboratory, there are no patent restrictions.

The only thing the drug lacked was a purpose. This was no obstacle—many medical uses were soon proposed. By 1941, DES was approved by the US Food & Drug Administration (FDA) for the treatment of vaginal gonorrhea, menopausal symptoms, and suppression of postpartum lactation.[2] (In those simpler times, drug approval required little evidence of either safety or effectiveness.) DES was soon being manufactured by dozens of companies and then hundreds.

Treatment of High-Risk Pregnancies

In the 1940s, the DES story moved to Boston. George and Olive Smith, a distinguished husband-and-wife research team at Harvard, proposed that the administration of DES in pregnancy might help avert miscarriage. A popular theory at the time was that miscarriage was caused by hormonal problems. The Smiths conducted uncontrolled clinical studies among high-risk women and became convinced that DES was effective in improving pregnancy outcomes.[3] (Recall that women with a history of miscarriages have a good chance of a successful pregnancy at their next attempt regardless of treatment [Chapter 11].) In 1947, the FDA approved the drug for use in pregnancy, and soon DES was being promoted not just for women with a history of pregnancy problems but for all healthy women (Fig. 20-1). Women were prescribed daily DES treatment starting at the first prenatal visit and given steadily increasing doses until delivery.

The DES Clinical Trial

There were skeptics. One was William Dieckmann, an obstetrician at the University of Chicago. He regarded the Smiths' clinical studies as flawed, and he set out in 1950 to conduct a proper randomized, placebo-controlled clinical trial of DES. (This study was one of the pioneering clinical trials, conducted just 2 years after the first randomized clinical trial by Bradford Hill and his colleagues on the treatment of tuberculosis with streptomycin.[4])

With admirable briskness, Dieckmann completed his trial in 1952 and published the results in 1953.[5] In carefully worded conclusions, he and his coauthors stated that DES "did not reduce the incidence of [miscarriage], prematurity...or perinatal mortality." One might expect that these conclusive findings would settle any question of DES effectiveness. In fact, the study met a storm of resistance. The Smiths, as well as Eli Lilly (a major manufacturer of DES), scrutinized the data and criticized the trial on various counts (see, for example, the discussion published with Dieckmann's original report[5]). Drug companies continued to market DES, even in the absence of evidence for its efficacy. The advertisement in Fig. 20-1 was published 3 years after Dieckmann's negative clinical trial—and in the same journal that had published Dieckmann's paper.

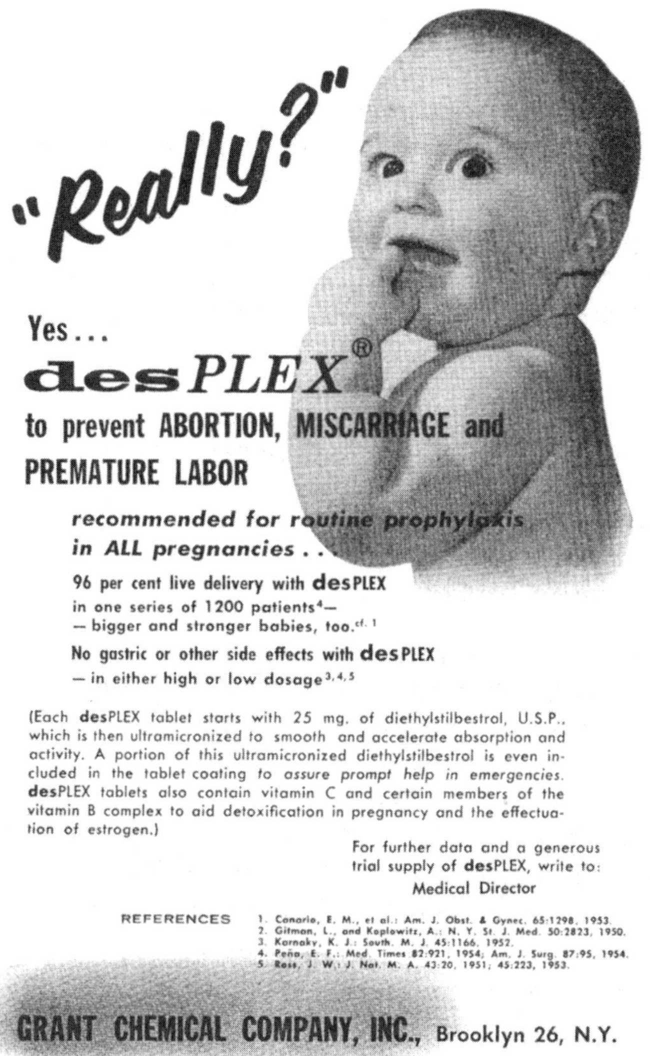

Figure 20-1. "Bigger and Stronger Babies": an advertisement for DES that appeared in the *American Journal of Obstetrics and Gynecology*, June 1956

Vaginal Adenocarcinoma

DES might still be prescribed to pregnant women today were it not for an almost accidental discovery. In 1966, a 15-year-old girl with cancer of the vagina was seen by gynecologists at Massachusetts General Hospital. This rare cancer is ordinarily found only in elderly women. Over the next 3 years, five more young women with this cancer were seen at the hospital—more than had ever been reported in the world literature. Something was clearly amiss. The young women and their mothers were asked about every imaginable exposure, but no common thread emerged. It was one of the mothers who finally raised the possibility that the cause might be DES, which she had taken while pregnant.[6] When questioned, other mothers also reported that they had taken DES.

In 1971, Arthur Herbst and his colleagues published a case-control study with eight patients with clear-cell carcinoma of the vagina and 32 controls.[7] All but one of the cases and none of the controls had been exposed to DES in utero. Very shortly thereafter, the FDA withdrew approval for the use of DES in pregnant women.

Wider Consequences

In the wake of Herbst's paper, DES daughters (as well as sons) became the subject of intense clinical concern and research. The risk of vaginal cancer among the DES daughters, although markedly increased, is low in absolute terms. About 500 women out of the roughly 2 million exposed DES daughters have been diagnosed with vaginal or cervical adenocarcinoma—less than 3 per 10,000 exposed.[8]

Although the adenocarcinoma is rare, other risks are not. The exposed daughters have substantially increased risks of infertility, miscarriage, and preterm delivery.[1,9] As a conservative estimate, DES contributed 300,000 preterm babies and 10,000 neonatal deaths. Were it not for the emergence of the unusually rare cancer among DES-exposed women, it is possible that their increased risk of these other problems would never have been recognized, much less attributed to DES.

Animal studies are now discovering DES effects into the third generation (once regarded as biologically implausible, and perhaps related to epigenetic effects).[10] The DES story is unlikely to be closed any time soon.

Dieckmann Revisited

In the eventful narrative of DES, there is a plot twist as odd as any you are likely to find in clinical research. In 1978, two epidemiologists noticed that the original Dieckmann report was only partly correct in concluding that DES had no benefits. What the published tables plainly show (but the original authors did not discuss) is that the pregnancies randomized to DES treatment were worse off. Late miscarriages were twice as common among the treated group (95% confidence interval 1.1 to 3.5). Neonatal death was increased fourfold (confidence interval 1.3 to 12). Why were these results not mentioned by the original authors? Were the harmful effects simply too contrary to the prevailing clinical opinion to be credible?

Perhaps the more pertinent question is, why did it take a quarter-century after publication of the clinical trial for anyone to notice and comment on these results? (If nothing else, be forewarned about drawing conclusions from abstracts alone.) How many women might have been spared later exposure to DES if the full message of the 1953 clinical trial had been recognized sooner? Even in 1978 this reanalysis was not welcome news. The authors published their findings as a letter[11] after several well-known clinical journals rejected the full manuscript.

The Dieckmann Legacy

Dieckmann's clinical trial provided not only the definitive evidence regarding DES's lack of efficacy but an important resource for documenting its long-term effects. After Herbst's paper on vaginal cancer was published in 1971, the women in the Dieckmann cohort were contacted so that their daughters and sons (unexposed as well as the exposed) could be examined. Herbst later moved from Harvard to Dieckmann's old position as chair of the obstetrics department at the University of Chicago, and he continued to follow these daughters and sons. As a study group, the offspring of the Dieckmann trial have one sterling virtue: their exposure was randomized. Although this study population is limited in size (about 1,000 of the original 1,600 offspring are still being actively followed), they have provided some of the best evidence on the harmful effects of DES.[1,9,12]

Adverse Effects of Prenatal Exposures

DES provides a robust example of a prenatal exposure with major health consequences to the exposed fetus. However, the drug was administered at high doses through many months of pregnancy. How plausible is it that other prenatal exposures might damage adult health? The answer remains unclear. Most research on fetal toxicants has been conducted in animals, with a focus on cancer, although effects on neurologic diseases[13] and behavior[14] have also been proposed.

Animal Studies

The DES experience stimulated intense interest in transplacental carcinogenesis. Laboratory researchers have shown in animal models that fetal exposure to carcinogens can produce cancers of the lung, ovary, central nervous system, kidney, liver, and breast as well as lymphoma and leukemia.[15]

In humans, we still know very little about carcinogens that might work through fetal exposures. Carcinogens in adults have a typical latency of 20 to 30 years from exposure to diagnosis of disease. On this basis, we might expect transplacental effects of carcinogens to be detectable within a few decades of birth (as was the case with DES and vaginal carcinoma). However, fetal exposures to carcinogens may work differently. It appears that breast cancer risk among DES-exposed daughters is doubled as these women reach their late 40s and 50s.[16] This result presents the unsettling possibility that prenatal exposures might amplify the substantial risks of cancer that occur later in life.

Maternal Smoking and Male Fertility

Another outcome that may be related to prenatal exposures is fertility. Fertility effects have been proposed as part of the "testicular dysgenesis syndrome," a collection of effects on the male reproductive system attributed to environmental pollutants (see Chapter 9).[17] A mother's smoking has also been suggested as a factor that decreases the fertility of her sons as well as her daughters.[18] Although evidence is limited, the sons of mothers who smoked during pregnancy have been reported to have poorer semen quality.[19]

The Search for Toxic Effects on the Fetus

Given that prenatal toxicants can affect disease in adult humans, what can we say about the extent of this danger? Very little. The general categories of diseases that are most likely to be affected (based on limited human and laboratory information) are cancer, neurologic diseases, and reproduction. There is some small measure of comfort to be taken from the fact that cancer rates for most sites are steady or falling. It is unclear whether fertility is changing over time (see Chapter 9).

When encountering an unexpected increase in disease incidence, epidemiologists of any specialty should be aware of the possibility of prenatal exposures. Such exposures would include drugs and other medical therapies during pregnancy. Medications are provided at doses intended to have physiologic impact, and exposures can easily occur at vulnerable stages of fetal development. Low-dose environmental exposures may also have more indirect effects, for example, through disruption of the developing immune system.[20] Prenatal exposures are extremely difficult to determine in retrospect, but worse than measuring these exposures poorly would be to neglect altogether the possibility of toxic damage to the fetus.

Fetal Nutrition and Adult Disease

Another possible mechanism linking prenatal experience to adult disease is fetal nutrition. The fetal nutrition hypothesis sprang from the robust associations of low birth weights with increased risk of cardiovascular disease in adulthood (see Chapter 15). Based on these observations, David Barker and others have developed the hypothesis that birth weight is a marker of nutrition during pregnancy and that fetal deficiencies in nutrition put the adult at risk of cardiovascular disease.[21] In a prolific and imaginative series of papers, Barker and his colleagues have conjectured that inadequate fetal nutrition "programs" the fetus—making permanent changes in fetal tissue function and structure—in ways that create a later susceptibility to cardiovascular disease and related ailments.

There is a host of animal research supporting the general principles that nutrition can affect fetal growth and that the manipulation of nutrition can permanently change the structure and function of fetal organs in ways that influence adult health. At first, this area of research emphasized mothers' nutrition during pregnancy. However, in humans the ordinary variations in mother's nutritional intake appear to affect birth weight only slightly,[22] leading to adjustments in the hypothesis. The observation that twins are smaller at birth but suffer no increased risk of cardiovascular disease has also required further refinements of the nutrition hypothesis.[23]

Accordingly, the hypothesis has evolved to focus on fetal rather than maternal nutrition.[24] Factors that interfere with the nutritional "supply line" to the fetus (uterine blood flow to the placenta, placental function itself, and umbilical blood flow to the fetus) are hypothesized to limit fetal nutrition in crucial ways that affect its growth. One difficulty with this refinement is that whereas maternal nutrition is observable, fetal nutrition is not. (Fetal growth is sometimes regarded as a surrogate for fetal nutrition, but this simply assumes the hypothesis is true rather than providing a test of it.) In support of the "supply-line" theory, there are well-established placental problems (e.g., infarcts and maternal hypertension with reduced uterine blood flow) associated with smaller fetuses.[24] Given that the placenta is a fetal organ, there is also the possibility of reverse causation: conditions of the fetus that retard its growth may also produce placental pathology. Despite the strengths of the nutrition hypothesis, there does not yet seem to be enough evidence to justify interventions "to correct micronutrient and macronutrient imbalances" during pregnancy, as some have suggested.[25]

Fetal Nutrition and Epigenetics

A fascinating extension of the fetal origins hypothesis has been provided by molecular advances in epigenetics. A fetus with a given genome may have "developmental plasticity," that is, the ability to develop in various ways depending on the signals received from the mother (including nutrition) that activate or suppress the expression of certain genes.[26] These maternal signals might represent aspects of the external environment that the fetus will face later and thus allow the fetus to prepare for its postuterine life by adjusting aspects of its growth and development. These epigenetic adjustments may also predispose the adult to cardiovascular diseases, perhaps in interaction with the external environment. It remains to be seen whether developmental plasticity can be manipulated for the benefit of later health, or whether the epigenetic mechanisms involved might apply to other diseases associated with birth weight.

Alternative Hypotheses

Alternative explanations for the associations of birth size and adult disease have been proposed. For example, unmeasured genes that predispose to both heart disease and small size at birth could produce the observed associations.[27] Such genes could work directly through the fetus or more indirectly through the mother. Evidence for genetic effects is found in the fact that a father's or mother's risk of heart disease is related to the size of their infants.[28]

Another limitation of the fetal nutrition hypothesis (discussed in Chapter 15) is its relatively narrow focus on cardiovascular disease. Birth weight is associated just as strongly with a host of neurologic endpoints and with mortality from other causes.[29] Furthermore, the relation of birth weights and cancer mortality is markedly different, with bigger babies having the higher risk.[29] This association is especially well established for breast cancer.[30] The breadth of associations between birth weight and a range of health outcomes leaves open the possibility of other, more unifying hypotheses to link birth weight to adult health.

Other Perinatal Factors Associated with Adult Health

Seasonal Effects

A range of health effects has been associated with season of birth. Season-of-birth effects presumably act during relatively short windows of vulnerability during which the short-term changes associated with season can make a difference. It is most plausible that these short windows of vulnerability occur during embryonic and fetal development. Data from Europe show that adults who were born in the second half of the calendar year live longer (by about half a year) than those born in the first half of the year. This pattern is reversed in Australia.[31] In these data, the causes of death associated with season of birth include cardiovascular disease, respiratory diseases, and infectious diseases. These mortality patterns may reflect long-term effects of seasonal fluctuations in fetal nutrition or infectious diseases, either during pregnancy or early in postnatal life.

Schizophrenia is another disease related to season of birth. Once again, the highest risk (in the Northern Hemisphere) is among people born during the first half of the year.[32]

Interpreting Cohort Effects

A cohort effect is a change in the risk of disease seen specifically among a cohort of people born at a certain time. One possibility for a cohort effect is an exposure that affects the cohort during fetal life. There are data to suggest a cohort effect in the obesity epidemic beginning with people born in the late 1960s.[33] This pattern of obesity may be related to age-specific changes in behaviors of that cohort of children, but it could also be the result of prenatal exposures that began in the late 1960s.

One of the best examples of prenatal exposure creating a cohort effect comes from the influenza pandemic of 1918. This outbreak erupted in the United States with ferocious intensity in October of 1918, killing around 500,000 people and then dissipating by February of 1919. Using census data and an ecologic approach, economists have shown that men and women who were in utero at the peak of the epidemic were less likely to graduate from high school and had higher disability rates and lower salaries over their lifetimes than people born just before or after.[34] The risk of diabetes and stroke may also have been increased among this cohort of survivors.[35]

Prenatal Exposures and Health

There is a remarkable array of links between the prenatal period and health outcomes in the adult, with little insight into their basis. A full understanding of human health requires integration of events starting with conception. The poet William Wordsworth wrote that "the child is the father of the man."[36] In the study of human health, we might venture a step further and say that it is the fetus who is the "father of the man." To the extent that a person's experience as a fetus can influence health decades into the future, an understanding of reproductive epidemiology and its tools may prove useful beyond the usual topics of fertility and pregnancy.

References

1. Kaufman RH, Adam E, Hatch EE, et al. Continued follow-up of pregnancy outcomes in diethylstilbestrol-exposed offspring. *Obstet Gynecol* 2000;96(4):483–9.
2. Meyers R. *D.E.S., The Bitter Pill.* New York: Seaview/Putnam, 1983.
3. Gillam R, Bernstein BJ. Doing harm: the DES tragedy and modern American medicine. *Public Hist* 1987;9(1):57–82.
4. Hill AB. Suspended judgment. Memories of the British streptomycin trial in tuberculosis. The first randomized clinical trial. *Control Clin Trials* 1990;11(2):77–9.
5. Dieckmann WJ, Davis ME, Rynkiewicz LM, Pottinger RE. Does the administration of diethylstilbestrol during pregnancy have therapeutic value? *Am J Obstet Gynecol* 1953;66(2):1062–81.
6. Herbst AL. Diethylstilbestrol and adenocarcinoma of the vagina. *Am J Obstet Gynecol* 1999;181(6):1576–8; discussion 1579.
7. Herbst AL, Ulfelder H, Poskanzer DC. Adenocarcinoma of the vagina. Association of maternal stilbestrol therapy with tumor appearance in young women. *N Engl J Med* 1971;284(15):878–81.
8. *Registry for Research on Hormonal Transplacental Carcinogenesis.* Chicago, IL: University of Chicago. Available at http://www.cdc.gov/DES/consumers/research/understanding_cohort.html, last accessed October 27, 2009.
9. Giusti RM, Iwamoto K, Hatch EE. Diethylstilbestrol revisited: a review of the long-term health effects. *Ann Intern Med* 1995;122(10):778–88.
10. Newbold RR, Padilla-Banks E, Jefferson WN. Adverse effects of the model environmental estrogen diethylstilbestrol are transmitted to subsequent generations. *Endocrinology* 2006;147(6 Suppl):S11–7.

11. Brackbill Y, Berendes HW. Dangers of diethylstilboestrol: review of a 1953 paper. *Lancet* 1978;2(8088):520.
12. Herbst AL, Kurman RJ, Scully RE, Poskanzer DC. Clear-cell adenocarcinoma of the genital tract in young females. Registry report. *N Engl J Med* 1972;287(25):1259–64.
13. Miller DB, O'Callaghan JP. Do early-life insults contribute to the late-life development of Parkinson and Alzheimer diseases? *Metabolism* 2008;57 Suppl 2:S44–9.
14. Ecker DJ, Stein P, Xu Z, et al. Long-term effects of culture of preimplantation mouse embryos on behavior. *Proc Natl Acad Sci USA* 2004;101(6):1595–600.
15. Anderson LM, Diwan BA, Fear NT, Roman E. Critical windows of exposure for children's health: cancer in human epidemiological studies and neoplasms in experimental animal models. *Environ Health Perspect* 2000;108 Suppl 3:573–94.
16. Palmer JR, Wise LA, Hatch EE, et al. Prenatal diethylstilbestrol exposure and risk of breast cancer. *Cancer Epidemiol Biomarkers Prev* 2006;15(8):1509–14.
17. Sharpe RM, Skakkebaek NE. Testicular dysgenesis syndrome: mechanistic insights and potential new downstream effects. *Fertil Steril* 2008;89(2 Suppl):e33–8.
18. Jensen TK, Henriksen TB, Hjollund NH, et al. Adult and prenatal exposures to tobacco smoke as risk indicators of fertility among 430 Danish couples. *Am J Epidemiol* 1998;148(10):992–7.
19. Ramlau-Hansen CH, Thulstrup AM, Storgaard L, Toft G, Olsen J, Bonde JP. Is prenatal exposure to tobacco smoking a cause of poor semen quality? A follow-up study. *Am J Epidemiol* 2007;165(12):1372–9.
20. Hertz-Picciotto I, Park HY, Dostal M, Kocan A, Trnovec T, Sram R. Prenatal exposures to persistent and non-persistent organic compounds and effects on immune system development. *Basic Clin Pharmacol Toxicol* 2008;102(2):146–54.
21. Barker DJ. Human growth and cardiovascular disease. *Nestle Nutr Workshop Ser Pediatr Program* 2008;61:21–38.
22. Kramer MS. Balanced protein/energy supplementation in pregnancy. *Cochrane Database Syst Rev* 2000;2:CD000032.
23. Christensen K, McGue M. Academic achievement in twins. *BMJ* 2008;337:a651.
24. Harding JE. The nutritional basis of the fetal origins of adult disease. *Int J Epidemiol* 2001;30:15–23.
25. Gluckman PD, Hanson MA, Cooper C, Thornburg KL. Effect of in utero and early-life conditions on adult health and disease. *N Engl J Med* 2008;359(1):61–73.
26. Bateson P, Barker D, Clutton-Brock T, et al. Developmental plasticity and human health. *Nature* 2004;430(6998):419–21.
27. Hattersley AT, Tooke JE. The fetal insulin hypothesis: an alternative explanation of the association of low birthweight with diabetes and vascular disease. *Lancet* 1999;353(9166):1789–92.
28. Smith GD, Sterne J, Tynelius P, Lawlor DA, Rasmussen F. Birth weight of offspring and subsequent cardiovascular mortality of the parents. *Epidemiology* 2005;16(4):563–9.
29. Baker JL, Olsen LW, Sorensen TI. Weight at birth and all-cause mortality in adulthood. *Epidemiology* 2008;19(2):197–203.
30. dos Santos Silva I, De Stavola B, McCormack V. Birth size and breast cancer risk: re-analysis of individual participant data from 32 studies. *PLoS Med* 2008;5(9):e193.
31. Doblhammer G, Vaupel JW. Lifespan depends on month of birth. *Proc Natl Acad Sci USA* 2001;98(5):2934–9.

32. Davies G, Welham J, Chant D, Torrey EF, McGrath J. A systematic review and meta-analysis of Northern Hemisphere season of birth studies in schizophrenia. *Schizophr Bull* 2003;29(3):587–93.
33. Olsen LW, Baker JL, Holst C, Sorensen TI. Birth cohort effect on the obesity epidemic in Denmark. *Epidemiology* 2006;17(3):292–5.
34. Almond D. Is the 1918 influenza pandemic over? Long-term effects of in utero influenza exposure in the post-1940 US population. *J Political Econ* 2006;114(4):672–712.
35. Almond D, Mazumder B. The 1918 influenza pandemic and subsequent health outcomes: an analysis of SIPP data. *Am Econ Rev* 2005;95(2):258–62.
36. Wordsworth W. *The Complete Poetical Works*. London: Macmillan and co., 1888.

21

Unanswered Questions in Reproductive Epidemiology

Reproductive epidemiology has made at least two major contributions to public health in recent decades—the prevention of neural tube defects by folic acid and the prevention of sudden infant death syndrome (SIDS) by placing babies to sleep on their backs. What other discoveries might lie over the horizon?

Textbooks by necessity focus on what we know. But to discuss only what we know (or what we think we know) can give a misleading perspective. What we know covers only a small patch of what there is to know. Even perfect knowledge of what is known is imperfect without this realization.

The job of the researcher is to extend that small patch. Choosing the right question is in some ways the most important challenge a researcher faces. This is especially true for epidemiologists, whose research projects can easily take a decade from concept to data collection to analysis to publication. The selection of a good question depends on intuition, a sound grasp of the field, rational assessment of the opportunities, and plain good luck.

This chapter discusses some research questions in the area of reproductive epidemiology. The questions are grouped into broad categories of basic clinical biology, clinical practice, and public health. Some have already been heavily studied, whereas others have not attracted much attention. Needless to say, not every good research idea is on this list. Just because your idea is not here does not mean it is not a good one. (If you would like to suggest new ideas to share with your colleagues, please go to www.oup.com/us/fertility.) And of course, the ideas discussed here come with no warranties. Some will no doubt turn out to be duds or dead ends. We will know better in 20 or 40 years.

Clinical Biology

How Can Women Identify Their Fertile Days?

A simple and reliable prospective marker of the first fertile day of the cycle would be extremely useful for women trying to conceive (and also for those trying not to). Women apparently conceive only if they have intercourse on the five days before ovulation or on the day of ovulation itself (see Chapter 2).[1] The complication is that the timing of these six fertile days is unpredictable from cycle to cycle.[2] There are now reasonably reliable ways to identify ovulation (with over-the-counter kits that measure LH surge), but by then most fertile days have already passed. Methods have been proposed to identify fertile days by cervical mucus,[3] although effectiveness has not yet been proven. If the 6-day fertile interval could be prospectively determined, women who want to become pregnant could focus their efforts, and women who do not would know when birth control is necessary.

Do Couples Who Adopt a Baby Have Improved Fertility?

A persistent anecdote related to adoption is the couple who tries for years to conceive, finally gives up and adopts a baby, and shortly thereafter becomes pregnant.[4] Of course, many infertile couples are eventually able to conceive, and a careful analysis would have to rule out the role of chance. If an association were found, the phenomenon might offer insights into the biological mechanisms of fertility in the mother (and perhaps the father). There are virtually no epidemiologic data on this question.

Do Environmental Factors Contribute to Aneuploidy?

Humans are highly susceptible to chromosomal aberrations compared with other species.[5] Might humans have a susceptibility to environmental factors that cause such aberrations? Preliminary studies in this area have been stymied by the difficulties of studying aneuploidy in humans. Although the condition is common, it usually ends in early pregnancy loss without the possibility of diagnosis. A further difficulty is that there are several biological pathways by which aneuploidy can occur, and a given environmental toxicant might contribute only a small portion of all aneuploidy, making its detection even more difficult.

Even more daunting, most aneuploidy events have their origins in the oocyte—specifically in the first meiotic division of the oocyte, which takes place when the woman is a fetus. A woman's exposures during her time as a fetus are not easy to reconstruct. The threat is not merely hypothetical. In mouse models, the common chemical bisphenol A has been found to cause aneuploidy in oocytes when the female has been exposed in utero.[6]

What Causes Preeclampsia?

As discussed in Chapter 19, preeclampsia is a particularly enigmatic disorder (perhaps several disorders). Whoever discovers the basis for preeclampsia will be guaranteed a place in history. Researchers are discovering earlier and earlier precursors of preeclampsia, but we seem no closer to understanding the reasons why preeclampsia emerges in some pregnancies and not others.

What Initiates Natural Labor?

Both mother and fetus seem to play a part in the cascade of events leading to onset of labor,[7] but their specific roles are yet to be worked out. Some progress has been made in identifying markers for impending preterm delivery (e.g., salivary estriol, serum corticotropin-releasing hormone [CRH], and vaginal fetal fibronectin). Still, these markers have limited predictive value, and the key initiating events remain obscure. A better grasp of the events that initiate labor might allow selective delay of preterm labor and more effective induction of labor when indicated.

What Explains the High Mortality of Small Babies Born at Term?

Term babies with the smallest birth weights have high mortality (see Chapter 15). Unknown confounders contribute at least part (and perhaps a large part) of this mortality.[8,9] The question remains what those confounders might be. They would have to include rare conditions that sharply increase mortality and drastically reduce fetal growth.[9] Possibilities include chromosomal mosaicism of the placenta and errors in gene imprinting. Were such entities found to explain the birth weight–mortality association, this would seriously revise our understanding of birth-weight-related risk.

Are Birth Defects Inevitable?

Most epidemiologists approach their work assuming that a better understanding of etiology will yield opportunities for prevention. Removing the pump handle from a contaminated well is one of epidemiology's most compelling paradigms. For chronic diseases, postponement is often a more realistic goal than prevention. For birth defects, prevention may be even more elusive. The biological systems by which an embryo assembles itself are inevitably imperfect. Even so, a better understanding of the built-in limitations ("noise") of embryogenesis may improve our capacity to recognize the external (and preventable) aspects that derail development.

Can Twins Help Demonstrate the "Plasticity" of Fetal Development?

Barker and others have proposed that commonplace variations in physiologic conditions during pregnancy can shape the long-term development of the fetus (see Chapter 20). To the extent that developmental plasticity in pregnancy affects long-term health, one might predict more concordance of crucial health and disease endpoints between dizygotic twins than between full siblings—especially between siblings who are born longer apart. Birth registries with long-term follow-up provide an opportunity for such exploration. Endpoints would have to avoid conditions that are known to be more common in dizygotic twins than in singletons (for example, cerebral palsy). The possibility of unrecorded differences in paternity (extremely unlikely for dizygous twins but possible for siblings) would also have to be taken into account.

Are Infections a Preventable Cause of Preterm Delivery?

Large population differences in risk of preterm point to the presence of preventable causes. Infections are increasingly implicated in early preterm delivery and would seem to be a good candidate for prevention. Antibiotic treatment has so far provided limited improvement in pregnancy outcome. Earlier interventions to prevent infection may be another approach. We have only a limited understanding of factors that predispose women to infection in pregnancy.

What Are the Origins of Cerebral Palsy?

Cerebral palsy is a nonprogressive motor disease that becomes apparent some time after birth.[10] About 2 per 1,000 babies are affected, a prevalence that has been relatively steady over time.[11] Cerebral palsy was once attributed to brain damage during difficult labor but is now thought to stem at least in part from earlier events, including in utero infection.[12] Risk is much higher among very preterm babies and among twins and other multiple fetuses. The search for causes of cerebral palsy goes back many decades—the U.S. Collaborative Perinatal Project (a cohort study of 50,000 pregnant women) was launched in the late 1950s specifically to shed light on cerebral palsy. There have been great strides in understanding its pathology, but its underlying causes remain unknown.

What Are the Biological Links between Birth Length and Infant Mortality?

Body length is a strong predictor of infant mortality independent of birth weight, with short length—and especially long length—associated with increased risk even when controlling for birth weight and gestational age.[13] However, birth length has been much less studied than birth weight. One reason is that data on birth length are less available. Another is that length data are less reliable, especially for ailing newborns who may lack normal muscle tone and thus stretch out more easily for measurement. Birth length also has independent associations with adult health. For example, birth length is more strongly associated with subsequent breast cancer risk than birth weight.[14]

Are There Markers of Female Reproductive Capacity?

Women's fertility declines with age. This happens more rapidly for some women than for others. This fact of aging is becoming more important as women in developed countries increasingly defer their childbearing. In the United States, mean age at first birth has gone from age 21 in 1970 to age 25 in 2005.[15] In Japan and Sweden, the mean age has reached 28. In delaying their childbearing, some women run the risk of bypassing their fertile years altogether. If women had a valid marker of their capacity to conceive—a marker they could monitor over time—they might be able to identify their own decline in fertility and make more informed decisions on when to start their family.

Clinical Practice

Are There Long-Term Consequences of Elective Cesarean Section?

Cesarean section for healthy women and infants is increasingly common. In the United States nearly 30% of babies are delivered by C-section,[15] and in Latin America the proportion is half or more.[16] C-section is undoubtedly a benefit in selected high-risk pregnancies. However, C-sections that are purely elective may deprive the baby (or mother) of hormonal or other exposures during the final stages of labor and delivery that provide unrecognized benefits. For example, fetuses have sterile guts, and the bacteria that first colonize the infant are acquired at delivery. Babies who deliver by C-section have different gut bacteria than those delivered vaginally,[17] which may have implications for later risk of asthma and other illnesses.[18] (Questions might also be raised about the risks and benefits of induction of labor.)

Does Ultrasound Have Long-Term Effects on the Fetus?

Repeated ultrasound examinations of the fetus are now commonplace in many countries, including some developing countries. Familiarity should not be mistaken for safety. (Fluoroscopes, after all, were routinely used by sales clerks in the 1950s to aid in fitting children's shoes.) Although no damaging effects of fetal ultrasound have been identified, there is the suggestion of some central-nervous-system effects, in that boys may be more likely to be left-handed if they are exposed to prenatal ultrasound.[19]

What Are the Long-Term Outcomes for the New Group of Extremely Preterm Babies Now Being Rescued?

The long-term morbidity of infants born at 34 or 35 weeks has been fairly well described.[20] With babies now surviving even at 24 weeks, there are probably additional long-term effects to anticipate and prepare for and to treat early if possible. What might they be?

Are There Long-Term Effects of ART on the Mother or Baby?

In the United States, artificial reproductive techniques (ART) produce at least 20,000 births a year. These interventions occur at a crucial stage of development, exposing the conceptus to unusual levels of hormones and other physiologic stresses. A hard lesson from the experience of DES and thalidomide is that medical therapies can have unintended consequences. What problems might emerge for ART mothers or their infants over their lifetimes?

Are There Long-Term Health Effects for Babies Conceived by ICSI?

Among the ART procedures, intracellular injection of sperm (ICSI) deserves special mention. When carried out as a treatment for male infertility, ICSI allows sperm to fertilize that otherwise may be incapable of fertilization. If the causes of sperm infertility are genetic, these genetic causes will be passed to the sons. Furthermore, those genetic factors may be associated with health problems in addition to infertility. One form of male infertility (congenital absence of the vas deferens) is produced by an allele that also causes cystic fibrosis.[21,22] To the degree that ICSI disrupts the natural imprinting of sperm, this also could have health consequences.[23]

Public Health

Is Fertility Declining over Time?

Concerns have been raised over the possibility that environmental contaminants are eroding humans' capacity to conceive (see Chapter 9).[24] One reason this question remains unanswered is the inherent limitations of epidemiologic methods for studying couple fertility. Careful prospective studies of fecundability would provide valuable information on future developments. Furthermore, new approaches for assessing the latent fertility of men or women (perhaps hormonal or other measures) would be extremely useful—not just for this question but for many others.

What Is the Minimum Possible Infant Mortality?

Forty years ago, as infant mortality in the United States and other developed countries was approaching unprecedented low rates, experts speculated whether infant mortality could ever possibly go as low as 10 per 1,000. Today, rates in the most advantaged countries have fallen below 3 per 1,000 and are still dropping. Although some of this improvement presumably reflects advances in medical care, other strong factors may be at work, as historical patterns suggest.[25]

Is it possible that benefits of prosperity related to nutrition or hygiene (perhaps accumulating biologically over generations[26]) can improve infant survival? If such factors could be identified, they might provide a basis for more targeted public health policies to improve infant mortality in all countries.

How Is Economic Development Related to Infant Mortality?

The correlation between national measures of economic development and infant mortality is remarkably strong (see Fig. 12-7). These data are almost always presented cross-sectionally. Do the factors related to economic factors have their effects immediately, or might there be a lag-time? Air pollution studies have refined the methods for looking at lag times to effect. Such methods could be applied to longitudinal data across nations, with various lag times between changes in annual economic measures and changes in infant mortality. The same general approach could also be applied to economic measures in the birth year of the mother or at various times after her birth. If there are certain lag times or certain ages of the mother at which the correlations with infant mortality are particularly strong, this might provide new clues to the mechanisms of social effects on infant survival.

What Accounts for the High Infant Mortality of Disadvantaged Groups Even within Rich Nations?

One of the most stubborn trends in public health in the United States has been the high mortality among black infants—about double that of whites. While the race difference has decreased in absolute terms as infant mortality has fallen, the relative gap between blacks and whites has widened.[27] Preterm delivery is one element in this black excess risk, but a mortality gap is also seen among term babies. Excess mortality is found among ethnic minorities in many countries, both rich and poor.[28–30] What contributes to this?

Do Prenatal Factors Contribute to the Increase in Testicular Cancer?

Testicular cancer is one of the few cancers that are increasing over time.[31] Given that this disease occurs primarily in young men and is exacerbated by conditions present at birth (such as cryptorchidism), are there prenatal exposures that might be contributing to the increase?

Are There Interventions Specific to Maternal Obesity and Its Effects on Pregnancy?

The rising tide of obesity is well recognized. Although the epidemic seems to have started in the US, it is spreading rapidly to other developed countries and even to developing countries. Maternal obesity has been associated with a spectrum of reproductive problems including neural tube defects,[32] stillbirths,[33] and preeclampsia.[34] Pregnancy not only is affected by obesity but contributes to obesity: weight gained in the first pregnancy is often not fully shed before the next.[35] Thus, women of reproductive age are a particularly appropriate focus for interventions to reduce obesity.

Does Exercise in Pregnancy Affect the Fetus?

In relation to the problem of obesity, moderate exercise during pregnancy is widely recommended by medical professionals.[36] However, the benefits of exercise are difficult to document, and there is some evidence that high-impact exercise may be harmful.[37] Even though much has been published on this topic, the benefits and hazards of physical exercise are not yet fully understood.

Do Prenatal Factors Contribute to the Risk of Autism?

Autism is a difficult outcome to study because it is especially sensitive to changes in diagnostic criteria and thresholds. Although the data are not consistent, there is some evidence that autism may be becoming more prevalent.[38] If rates are truly increasing, this invites hypotheses about the role of exposures that have increased in recent decades, especially exposures found in more well-off segments of the population, among whom autism rates are higher.

Are Prenatal Exposures Contributing to an Increase in Childhood Asthma?

There seems to be little question that allergic asthma has increased in prevalence over the past four decades,[39] although the reasons are unclear. Among the many hypotheses are possible exposures in the prenatal period.[40]

If you have other suggestions for research questions in reproductive epidemiology (and there must be many more), please go to the website accompanying this textbook (www.oup.com/us/fertility). The best nominations will be added to the list, with credit to the nominator. Who knows—your idea may may help stimulate the next great discovery in reproductive epidemiology.

References

1. Wilcox AJ, Baird DD, Weinberg CR. Time of implantation of the conceptus and loss of pregnancy. *N Engl J Med* 1999;340(23):1796–9.
2. Wilcox AJ, Dunson D, Baird DD. The timing of the "fertile window" in the menstrual cycle: day specific estimates from a prospective study. *BMJ* 2000; 321(7271):1259–62.

3. Bigelow JL, Dunson DB, Stanford JB, Ecochard R, Gnoth C, Colombo B. Mucus observations in the fertile window: a better predictor of conception than timing of intercourse. *Hum Reprod* 2004;19(4):889–92.
4. Mai FM. Conception after adoption: an open question. *Psychosom Med* 1971; 33(6):509–14.
5. Martin RH. Meiotic errors in human oogenesis and spermatogenesis. *Reprod Biomed Online* 2008;16(4):523–31.
6. Pacchierotti F, Ranaldi R. Mechanisms and risk of chemically induced aneuploidy in mammalian germ cells. *Curr Pharm Des* 2006;12(12):1489–504.
7. Lie RT, Wilcox AJ, Skjaerven R. Maternal and paternal influences on length of pregnancy. *Obstet Gynecol* 2006;107(4):880–5.
8. Hernandez-Diaz S, Schisterman EF, Hernan MA. The birth weight "paradox" uncovered? *Am J Epidemiol* 2006;164(11):1115–20.
9. Basso O, Wilcox AJ, Weinberg CR. Birth weight and mortality: causality or confounding? *Am J Epidemiol* 2006;164(4):303–11.
10. Kuban KC, Leviton A. Cerebral palsy. *N Engl J Med* 1994;330(3):188–95.
11. Paneth N, Hong T, Korzeniewski S. The descriptive epidemiology of cerebral palsy. *Clin Perinatol* 2006;33(2):251–67.
12. Grether JK, Nelson KB. Maternal infection and cerebral palsy in infants of normal birth weight. *Obstet Gynecol Surv* 1998;53(4):196–8.
13. Melve KK, Gjessing HK, Skjaerven R, Oyen N. Infants' length at birth: an independent effect on perinatal mortality. *Acta Obstet Gynecol Scand* 2000;79(6):459–64.
14. dos Santos Silva I, De Stavola B, McCormack V. Birth size and breast cancer risk: re-analysis of individual participant data from 32 studies. *PLoS Med* 2008; 5(9):e193.
15. Martin JA, Hamilton BE, Sutton PD, et al. Births: final data for 2005. *Natl Vital Stat Rep* 2007;56(6):1–103.
16. Villar J, Valladares E, Wojdyla D, et al. Caesarean delivery rates and pregnancy outcomes: the 2005 WHO global survey on maternal and perinatal health in Latin America. *Lancet* 2006;367(9525):1819–29.
17. Gronlund MM, Lehtonen OP, Eerola E, Kero P. Fecal microflora in healthy infants born by different methods of delivery: permanent changes in intestinal flora after cesarean delivery. *J Pediatr Gastroenterol Nutr* 1999;28(1):19–25.
18. Renz-Polster H, David MR, Buist AS, et al. Caesarean section delivery and the risk of allergic disorders in childhood. *Clin Exp Allergy* 2005;35(11):1466–72.
19. Salvesen KA, Eik-Nes SH. Ultrasound during pregnancy and subsequent childhood non-right handedness: a meta-analysis. *Ultrasound Obstet Gynecol* 1999;13(4):241–6.
20. Moster D, Lie RT, Markestad T. Long-term medical and social consequences of preterm birth. *N Engl J Med* 2008;359(3):262–73.
21. Chillon M, Casals T, Mercier B, et al. Mutations in the cystic fibrosis gene in patients with congenital absence of the vas deferens. *N Engl J Med* 1995;332(22):1475–80.
22. Radpour R, Gourabi H, Dizaj AV, Holzgreve W, Zhong XY. Genetic investigations of CFTR mutations in congenital absence of vas deferens, uterus, and vagina as a cause of infertility. *J Androl* 2008;29(5):506–13.
23. Kurinczuk JJ. Safety issues in assisted reproduction technology. From theory to reality—just what are the data telling us about ICSI offspring health and future fertility, and should we be concerned? *Hum Reprod* 2003;18(5):925–31.

24. Skakkebaek NE, Jorgensen N, Main KM, et al. Is human fecundity declining? *Int J Androl* 2006;29(1):2–11.
25. Wilcox AJ. Infant mortality revisited. *Paediatr Perinat Epidemiol* 1993;7(4):347–8.
26. Pembrey ME, Bygren LO, Kaati G, et al. Sex-specific, male-line transgenerational responses in humans. *Eur J Hum Genet* 2006;14(2):159–66.
27. Singh GK, Yu SM. Infant mortality in the United States: trends, differentials, and projections, 1950 through 2010. *Am J Public Health* 1995;85(7):957–64.
28. Hoa DP, Nga NT, Malqvist M, Persson LA. Persistent neonatal mortality despite improved under-five survival: a retrospective cohort study in northern Vietnam. *Acta Paediatr* 2008;97(2):166–70.
29. Troe EJ, Kunst AE, Bos V, Deerenberg IM, Joung IM, Mackenbach JP. The effect of age at immigration and generational status of the mother on infant mortality in ethnic minority populations in The Netherlands. *Eur J Public Health* 2007;17(2):134–8.
30. Huang W, Yu H, Wang F, Li G. Infant mortality among various nationalities in the middle part of Guizhou, China. *Soc Sci Med* 1997;45(7):1031–40.
31. Bergstrom R, Adami HO, Mohner M, et al. Increase in testicular cancer incidence in six European countries: a birth cohort phenomenon. *J Natl Cancer Inst* 1996;88(11):727–33.
32. Shaw GM, Carmichael SL. Prepregnant obesity and risks of selected birth defects in offspring. *Epidemiology* 2008;19(4):616–20.
33. Little RE, Weinberg CR. Risk factors for antepartum and intrapartum stillbirth. *Am J Epidemiol* 1993;137(11):1177–89.
34. Walsh SW. Obesity: a risk factor for preeclampsia. *Trends Endocrinol Metab* 2007;18(10):365–70.
35. Smith DE, Lewis CE, Caveny JL, Perkins LL, Burke GL, Bild DE. Longitudinal changes in adiposity associated with pregnancy. The CARDIA Study. Coronary Artery Risk Development in Young Adults Study. *JAMA* 1994;271(22):1747–51.
36. *Exercise During Pregnancy*. Washington, DC: American College of Obstetrics and Gynecology, 2009.
37. Madsen M, Jorgensen T, Jensen ML, et al. Leisure time physical exercise during pregnancy and the risk of miscarriage: a study within the Danish National Birth Cohort. *Br J Obstet Gynaecol* 2007;114(11):1419–26.
38. Hertz-Picciotto I, Delwiche LA. The rise in autism and the role of age at diagnosis. *Epidemiology* 2009;20(1):84–90.
39. Platts-Mills TA, Carter MC, Heymann PW. Specific and nonspecific obstructive lung disease in childhood: causes of changes in the prevalence of asthma. *Environ Health Perspect* 2000;108 Suppl 4:725–31.
40. Prescott SL. Maternal allergen exposure as a risk factor for childhood asthma. *Curr Allergy Asthma Rep* 2006;6(1):75–80.

Afterword

This book has had a long gestation.

I was a doctoral student in 1977 when I wrote to one of my advisors suggesting the possibility of a new specialty in epidemiology.

> There is a collection of studies that might be called the epidemiology of reproduction. This includes fertility and infertility, menarche and menopause, contraception, population genetics, fetal loss, infant morbidity and mortality, birth defects.... Currently these subjects are investigated by a motley crowd: epidemiologists, sociologists, demographers, obstetricians, and pediatricians.... No one has identified a common theme in these studies, but I think a sound case could be made for collecting these into a general research area.

I wanted to be a reproductive epidemiologist. Too bad the field did not exist—but, unknown to me, it was being created. The perinatal side of this specialty emerged in the late 1970s, as Zena Stein and Mervyn Susser mobilized a talented group of graduate students at Columbia University to focus on perinatal and neonatal epidemiology. In 1984, Michael Bracken published *Perinatal Epidemiology*, the first textbook devoted to this topic. In 1987, Jean Golding founded the journal *Paediatric and Perinatal Epidemiology*. A new field was born.

Research on the earlier end of the spectrum—fertility and early pregnancy—took longer to develop. I was invited in 1982 to give a talk on the "epidemiology of fertility." I had to tell the meeting organizers that I knew nothing about the topic, to which they replied "No problem—nobody else knows anything about it either." My talk turned into a research plan that kept me occupied for the next 15 years.

There aren't many things more fun than coming into a field as it is unfolding. The problems are fresh, the search is exciting, and the answers are in many ways unexpected. In the process I have had the good fortune of sterling colleagues: Ian Russell, Beth Gladen, Rolv Skjaerven, Rolv Terje Lie, Clare Weinberg, Donna Baird, and Olga Basso, among many others. They have rescued me from the worst of my errors, and they continue to make the journey a joy.

Meanwhile, through these years, this book has been on my mind. I knew it would not be a catalog of facts. Facts are important, but (go ahead, admit it) they can be a bore. Sometimes facts are even unreliable. Our understanding evolves. Much more exciting is the chase—the way epidemiologic thinking can give us glimpses into the marvelous inner workings of biology.

Unlike books, the chase has no end.

Durham, North Carolina

Puzzlers

Selective fertility, natural variability, and shifting denominators are recurring themes in reproductive epidemiology. Now that you have been introduced to these concepts, consider how they might play out in the following problems. Discussion of these problems can be found on www.oup.com/us/fertility.

1. About 1%–2% of pregnancies are ectopic. This is a serious complication when it occurs. If a woman becomes pregnant with an IUD in place, the risk that the pregnancy is ectopic is considerably higher[1]—the package insert for one brand of IUD (Mirena) says up to 50%. Do IUDs increase the risk of ectopic pregnancies? What would be an alternative interpretation? How could you resolve these alternative possibilities?
2. A report from rural China found that perinatal mortality was three times higher for second births than for first births.[2] Usually perinatal mortality declines with second parity (see Fig. 7-7). What conditions in China might lead to this high mortality for second babies?
3. Among couples who seek infertility treatment, suppose that you identify a group in which the male partners are azospermic (without sperm) and another group in which the male partners are severely oligospermic (with very few sperm). If you were to compare the female partners of these two groups of men, would you expect them to have the same fertility? If not, which women would you expect to be more fertile?
4. Suppose you are planning to conduct a prospective study of pregnancy, and you want to include fecundability as one of your study endpoints. You could set your criterion for eligible couples in two ways. One, you could include all couples who are trying to conceive, regardless of how long they have been trying. Alternatively, you could restrict the study to couples who were just starting to try to become pregnant. The advantage of the first is that you would find

many more eligible couples. What would be the disadvantage? If you include couples who have already been trying, what essential additional information would you need?

5. Intercourse has been proposed as a stimulus of labor. Although this hypothesis has some plausibility (there are abundant prostaglandins in semen, and prostaglandins play a role in labor), a randomized clinical trial has failed to show any effect.[3] An epidemiologic study reported a strong association between *lack* of intercourse and preterm delivery.[4] What possible confounders might explain this association?
6. A Swedish study reported that women who took folic acid supplements were more likely to produce dizygotic twins.[5] If the use of folic acid were to increase the chances of twinning, the higher mortality and complications among twins might outweigh the benefits of folic acid for the prevention of neural tube defects. This could argue against fortification of food with folic acid. However, the finding was due to a strong confounding variable overlooked by the authors. The authors controlled for maternal age. Is there another confounding factor that you can think of?
7. Birth defects account for 17% of infant mortality in the United States but only 8% worldwide. Underregistration in developing countries no doubt contributes to this. Is there another contributing factor?

References

1. Mol BW, Ankum WM, Bossuyt PM, Van der Veen F. Contraception and the risk of ectopic pregnancy: a meta-analysis. *Contraception* 1995;52(6):337–41.
2. Wu Z, Viisainen K, Wang Y, Hemminki E. Perinatal mortality in rural China: retrospective cohort study. *BMJ* 2003;327(7427):1319.
3. Tan PC, Yow CM, Omar SZ. Effect of coital activity on onset of labor in women scheduled for labor induction: a randomized controlled trial. *Obstet Gynecol* 2007;110(4):820–6.
4. Sayle AE, Savitz DA, Thorp JM, Jr, Hertz-Picciotto I, Wilcox AJ. Sexual activity during late pregnancy and risk of preterm delivery. *Obstet Gynecol* 2001;97(2):283–9.
5. Ericson A, Kallen B, Aberg A. Use of multivitamins and folic acid in early pregnancy and multiple births in Sweden. *Twin Res* 2001;4(2):63–6.

Glossary

Abortifacient A substance (usually oral) that induces abortion. There is a long history of herbal and other remedies with supposed abortifacient effects; those with any effectiveness usually worked through their extreme toxicity to the mother as well as the fetus. Today, mifepristone is an effective abortifacient that works by competitively blocking the progesterone receptor.

Abruptio placenta (abruption) Detachment or separation of the placenta before delivery. A life-threatening condition for both mother and fetus.

Alpha-fetoprotein (AFP) A protein in fetal blood; small but measurable amounts pass into amnioitic fluid and maternal blood. AFP is one of the proteins measured in maternal blood for pregnancy screening; AFP tends to be increased in the presence of neural tube defects and decreased in the presence of Down syndrome.

Amenorrhea (*see Menstrual cycle*)

Amniocentesis A procedure using a fine needle to sample the fluid around the fetus in order to obtain fetal cells for genetic testing.

Androgen The generic term for hormones that control the development of male sex characteristics. The best-known androgen is testosterone. Androgens are the biochemical precursor of estrogens and are thus also found in women.

Aneuploidy Having too few or too many chromosomes. Aneuploidy is found in about half of clinical miscarriages, about 6% of stillbirths, and much fewer than 1% of live births.[3]

Antepartum During pregnancy, before the onset of labor.

An earlier version of this glossary was published in two parts in the *Journal of Epidemiology and Community Health*.[1,2]

Apgar score Widely used tool for assessment of the newborn, based on infant's heart rate, respiratory effort, muscle tone, reflex irritability, and color. Each sign is scored from zero to 2. Most newborns get a 9 or 10. While "Apgar" may look like an acronym, it was named after its developer, Virginia Apgar.[4]

ART (see *Assisted Reproductive Technologies*)

Assisted reproductive technologies (ART) Clinical and laboratory procedures to aid in fertilization. In vitro fertilization (IVF) was the first and remains the most widely known; other techniques and refinements are intracellular sperm injection (ICSI) and gamete intrafallopian transfer (GIFT).[5,6]

Autosome Any of the ordinary chromosomes (22 in humans), in contrast with the sex chromosomes (X and Y).

Birth interval Time between a mother's deliveries. Interpregnancy interval (the time from delivery to the LMP of the subsequent pregnancy) is often preferred in order to avoid confounding by length of pregnancy.

Blastocyst An early stage of embryonic development in which the cells of the conceptus have formed a hollow ball. Implantation takes place at the blastocyst stage.

Blighted ovum A conceptus with no embryo visible on ultrasound.

Chimerism The condition of carrying cells from two genetically distinct sources.

Chorionic villus sampling A biopsy of the placental tissue for genetic testing. Carried out by needle through the abdomen or small catheter through the cervix.

Clinical pregnancy A pregnancy that lasts long enough to be recognized by the mother or a clinician (sometimes also defined as pregnancies that last 6 weeks or more after last menstrual period). (See *Pregnancy loss.*)

Clinically recognized pregnancy loss Loss of any clinical pregnancy. Can include spontaneous abortions (miscarriages), ectopic pregnancies, and stillbirths.

Conception The fertilization of an ovum by a sperm. The American College of Obstetrics and Gynecology has defined conception as the implantation of the blastocyst,[7] for reasons having chiefly to do with social and political concerns.

Conceptus A generic term for the product of an ovum and sperm, including everything from the preembryonic stages to the fetus at term.

Contraception Any method used by couples to prevent conception. This covers a broad spectrum, from purely behavioral methods (such as the rhythm method), to intercourse-specific methods (such as condom), to woman's systemic use of oral hormones, to postcoital medications.

Corpus luteum A transient hormonally active tissue on the surface of the ovary, formed out of the remnants of the ruptured ovarian follicle. The corpus luteum regulates the second half of the menstrual cycle (the luteal phase) by producing progesterone.

D&C (dilatation and curettage) Surgical procedure to dilate the cervix and scrape the inner surface of the uterus in order to remove products of conception. May be done as an abortion procedure, or after spontaneous abortion to remove retained tissue.

Due date The predicted delivery day, commonly calculated as 40 weeks after the last menstrual period.

Early pregnancy loss (biochemical loss, subclinical loss) Pregnancy ending with vaginal bleeding indistinguishable from menses. Sometimes defined as pregnancy loss within 6 weeks of LMP. Approximately 25% of pregnancies end in early loss.[8]

Ectopic pregnancy Implantation of the conceptus outside the uterus, almost always in the oviduct ("tubal pregnancy").

Embryo Stage of development (from roughly the second through the eighth week of life) during which the major organ systems are established. (The definition of this term is muddled by the fact that infertility specialists use "embryo" to refer to the fertilized egg before implantation but anatomists do not.)

Endometrium The lining of the uterus, which proliferates during each menstrual cycle in preparation for implantation and then is sloughed ("menstrual bleeding") if no pregnancy occurs.

Estrogen Estrogens are a class of steroid hormones that function as the main female sex hormones. These include estrone, estradiol, and estriol.

Fallopian tubes (see *Oviducts*)

Fecundability A couple's probability of conception in one menstrual cycle, assuming regular intercourse and no method of contraception. Mean fecundability is around 25%, with wide variation among couples depending on age, coital frequency, etc.[9]

Fecundability ratio The ratio of fecundability of an exposed group to the fecundability of a comparison group. Unlike most other measures of epidemiologic risk, the fecundability ratio is less than 1.0 when the exposure damages the health endpoint.

Fecundity The capacity to conceive and deliver a baby; fertility.[10]

Fertile window The 6 days of the menstrual cycle ending on the day of ovulation during which intercourse can produce pregnancy.[11]

Fertility The capacity to conceive and deliver a baby. This is the ordinary usage in both colloquial and medical English. Demographers define fertility more narrowly to mean the actual production of a baby. In that sense, fertility is the evidence of fecundity.

Fertilization The combination of the genetic material of an ovum and a sperm to produce a conceptus.

Fetal death An ambiguous term sometimes referring to all deaths of the fetus starting at clinical recognition (including miscarriages but not abortions), and sometimes referring only to stillbirths (starting from the age of viability).

Fetal growth The mostly unobservable development of the fetus prior to birth.

Fetal monitoring Medical interventions to assess well-being and growth of the fetus in utero.

Fetus The stage of development from the end of the embryonic stage (about 8 weeks of life) until delivery.

Follicle-stimulating hormone (FSH) A hormone produced by the pituitary gland that in women promotes the growth of the ovarian follicle in preparation for ovulation.

Follicular phase (menstrual cycle) The first phase of the menstrual cycle, starting with onset of menses and ending on the day before ovulation. Although its mean length is around 17 days, the follicular phase can be highly variable, ranging from 10 to more than 50 days.[12]

FSH (see *Follicle-stimulating hormone*)

Gamete A sperm or ovum.

Genome The total genetic information carried by an individual. Also used more specifically to designate the complete genetic sequence of one set of chromosomes.

Gestational age The duration of pregnancy (and thus an estimate of the age of fetus), measured from the physiologically incorrect but eminently practical LMP. May be adjusted on the basis of ultrasound examination in the first trimester of pregnancy.[13]

Obstetric dates Gestational age expressed in completed weeks rather than ordinal weeks. Thus, a pregnancy at 39 weeks and 5 days is in its fortieth week, but in obstetric week 39.

Gravidity Number of previous pregnancies (distinguished from parity). A **primigravida** is a woman pregnant for the first time. A **multigravida** is a woman who has been pregnant more than once.

hCG (see *Human chorionic gonadotropin*)

Human chorionic gonadotropin (hCG) A hormone secreted by the cells of the blastocyst that later become the placenta. hCG is a mimic of luteinizing hormone and the standard hormonal sign of pregnancy.

Hysterectomy Surgical removal of the uterus. This may include removal of one or both ovaries.

Implantation Attachment of the blastocyst to the uterine lining. In humans implantation typically takes place 6 to 12 days after conception.[14]

In vitro fertilization (IVF) Fertilization by medical procedures outside the body. (Although these babies are colloquially known as "test tube babies", fertilization usually takes place in a flat dish.)

Induced abortion Intentional termination of a pregnancy through either medical or surgical intervention. Abortions are carried out for a wide spectrum of reasons ranging from unwanted pregnancy to malformations of the fetus to the presence of conditions that threaten the life of the mother.

Infant mortality Infant deaths occurring among a defined group of live births during the first year of life. The infant mortality rate is usually defined as the number of infant deaths within a calendar year divided by the number of live births during the same period. Widely used as a measure of national economic development.

Infertility Inability of a woman or a couple to achieve a clinically recognized pregnancy after attempting for more than a year (ACOG)[15] or for more than 2 years (WHO).[16] Fecund couples can be "infertile" if they become pregnant after more than a year of tryijng. **Primary infertility is** the failure of an individual, or couple, to have ever achieved a pregnancy. **Secondary infertility** is the inability of an individual or couple to achieve pregnancy after having had a previous pregnancy. **Subfertility** is an ill-defined condition that indicates less than "normal" fertility.

Interpregnancy interval (see *Birth interval*)

Intracellular sperm injection (ICSI) A variation of in vitro fertilization in which a single sperm is inserted into an ovum. An increasingly common approach for couples with male-factor infertility.[6]

Intrapartum During labor but before the completion of delivery

Intrauterine device Any of several metal or plastic objects that, when inserted into the uterus, prevent pregnancy.

Intrauterine growth retardation (IUGR) A condition in which the fetus fails to reach its expected size during pregnancy. In principle, this can occur to large fetuses as well as small. Frequently (if mistakenly) equated with small-for-gestational-age.

IUD (see *Intrauterine device*)

IUGR (see *Intrauterine growth retardation*)

Lactational amenorrhea (see *Menstrual cycle*)

Last menstrual period (LMP) First day of the most recent menses preceding pregnancy, the standard benchmark to determine gestational age.

LBW (see *Low birth weight*)

LH (see *Luteinizing hormone*)

Live birth An infant born with any sign of life (beating of the heart, pulsation of the umbilical cord, movement of voluntary muscles). Usually restricted to births after 20 or more weeks of gestation.[17]

LMP (see *Last menstrual period*)

Low birth weight (LBW) Birth weight less than 2,500 g. Although LBW is a convenient endpoint for epidemiologic studies, it has come under criticism for being difficult to interpret.[18]

Luteal phase (menstrual cycle) The second major phase of the menstrual cycle, usually starting with the day after ovulation and ending on the day before the onset of next menses. The luteal phase, although more regular than the follicular phase, is not fixed at 2 weeks as is sometimes assumed. Mean length is 13 days with a range of around 11 to 17 days.[12]

Luteinizing hormone (LH) A pituitary hormone that, when stimulated by the rise in ovarian estrogens, undergoes a sharp surge that triggers the rupture of the ovarian follicle and the release of the ovum. LH then promotes the conversion of the ruptured follicle into a corpus luteum.

Maternal mortality Death of a woman from causes related to pregnancy or birth, usually within 42 days of the termination of the pregnancy.[19]

Meiosis A type of cell division unique to the formation of gametes (eggs or sperm), in which the number of chromosomes is reduced to half.

Menarche The sexual maturation of women, marked by the onset of the first menstrual period.

Menopause The cessation of ovarian function. This is usually defined prospectively as the absence of menstruation for at least 12 months. Median age at menopause is around 51, with most women reaching menopause between ages 45 and 55.[20] **Ovarian senescence** refers to age-related depletion of ovarian follicles and the decline of ovarian hormones, culminating in menopause. **Perimenopause** is the time leading up to natural menopause during which ovarian production of estrogen becomes more erratic, and menstrual cycles lengthen and become more variable. **Premature menopause** is natural menopause before the age of 40 (also called premature ovarian failure).[21]

Menstrual cycle Woman's monthly cycle of ovulation and bleeding, comprising the follicular phase, the day of ovulation, and the luteal phase. The onset of menses markes the first day of the menstrual cycle. **Amenorrhea** is a time without menses (at least 3 months, by ACOG definition).[22] **Primary amenorrhea** is the condition of never having had menses among girls who are at least 16 years old.[22] **Lactational amenorrhea** refers to the cessation of menses with regular breast-feeding.[23]

Microchimerism Two genetically distinct populations of cells in one person, derived from different fertilized eggs, where one line of cells is present at very low concentrations. Can occur, for example, when fetal cells pass the placenta and become established in the mother's bone marrow.

Miscarriage (spontaneous abortion) Loss of a clinically recognized pregnancy, usually in the first 20 weeks after LMP. (Later deaths are defined as stillbirths.)

Multigravida (see *Gravidity*)

Multiparity (see *Parity*)

Neonatal mortality Death of a liveborn infant within the first 28 days or (less commonly) the first 7 days of life. The neonatality mortality rate is usually defined as the number of neonatal deaths in a calendar year divided by the number of live births during the same period.

Nulliparity (see *Parity*)

Obstetric dates (see *Gestational age*)

Oocyte The female egg before ovulation.

Oogenesis The process of the formation of the oocyte and ovum.

Ovarian follicle Fluid-filled chambers in the ovary, each encasing an oocyte.

Ovarian senescence (see *Menopause*)

Oviducts Tubes attached to the uterus and opening near the ovaries, through which the ova must travel on their way to the uterus.[24]

Ovulation The release of an oocyte from a mature ovarian follicle.

Ovum The female reproductive gamete, also called the egg. The term is sometimes used more specifically to designate the oocyte after ovulation.

Parity Number of live and stillbirths for a given woman (in contrast with gravidity, which refers to all pregnancies including miscarriages). A **nullipara** is a woman who has never delivered a pregnancy lasting long enough for the fetus to reach the age of viability. A woman pregnant for the first time is nulliparous until she delivers a stillbirth or live birth. A woman who has had three miscarriages is still nulliparous. A **primipara** is a woman who has delivered her first baby, and a **multipara** is a woman who has delivered more than one pregnancy.

Parturition Childbirth.

Pelvic inflammatory disease (PID) Inflammation of the oviducts, usually originating from a sexually transmitted infection. A major cause of ectopic pregnancy and infertility.

Perimenopause (see *Menopause*)

Perinatal The time period immediately prior to, during, and after birth.

Perinatal mortality Stillbirths plus deaths of live births within either the first 7 or the first 28 days after birth.

Pheromone A hormone produced by one person that can change the behavior of another. In humans, pheromones are suspected to play a role in the sexual attractiveness of a woman during her fertile days.

Placenta An organ created by the conceptus and bound to the mother's uterus, providing essential nutrition and oxygenation of the fetus through the umbilical cord.

Placenta previa The condition in which the placenta has grown over the internal cervical opening, presenting a danger of heavy bleeding at labor.

Ponderal index A measure of infant fatness or skinniness, defined as birth weight in grams multiplied by 100 and divided by the cube of crown-heel length in centimeters.[25]

Postneonatal mortality Death to a live birth after 28 days but within the first year. Neonatal plus postneonatal mortality equals infant mortality. Postneonatality rates are usually calculated as the number of postneonatal deaths within a calendar year divided by the number of live births. (Technically, babies who die in the neonatal period should be removed from the denominator, but this nicety is ignored because the adjustment makes so little difference).

Postterm delivery Delivery at 42 or more completed weeks of gestation.[26,27]

Preeclampsia A syndrome of pregnancy defined by hypertension and proteinurea. The progression of preeclampsia to **eclampsia** is a rare but disastrous complication characterized by extreme hypertension, seizures, and sometimes death.

Premature Until 1961, WHO defined "prematurity" as birth weight less than 2,500 g. However, many infants born before 37 weeks weigh more than 2,500 g, and many babies less than 2,500 g are not born early. Because misuse of LBW to mean "premature" has lingered, most perinatal epidemiologists avoid confusion by using "preterm."

Premature menopause (see *Menopause*)

Premature rupture of membranes (PROM) Rupture of the fetal membranes before onset of labor.

Preterm delivery Delivery before 37 completed weeks of gestation.

Preterm premature rupture of membranes (PPROM) Rupture before onset of labor and leading to a preterm delivery.

Primary amenorrhea (see *Menstrual cycle*)

Primary infertility (see *Infertility*)

Primigravida (see *Gravidity*)

Primiparity (see *Parity*)

Puberty Period of rapid growth culminating in sexual maturity. **Thelarche** is the prepubertal onset of breast development. **Menarche** is the event of first menses, marking the onset of a woman's capacity to reproduce.

Puerperal Having to do with the time from delivery of the infant until the uterus has returned to its prepregnant size, usually 3 to 6 weeks.

Secondary infertility (see *Infertility*)

Semen analysis A measure of male fertility based on examination of the seminal fluid. Analysis includes ejaculate volume, sperm concentration, sperm motility, morphology, concentration of white blood cells, and an immunobead or mixed antiglobulin reaction test (WHO[28]).

Sex ratio Ratio of the number of boys to girls, usually restricted to live births. Sex ratio can be expressed as the ratio of boys to girls (e.g., 1.06 boys for every girl) or as the proportion of all births that are boys (e.g., 0.51).

SGA (see *Small for gestational age*)

SIDS (see *Sudden infant death syndrome*)

Small for gestational age (SGA) Typically, the smallest 10% of babies at a given gestational age.

Spermatogenesis The process of the formation of sperm.

Spontaneous abortion Loss of a clinically recognized pregnancy in the first 20 weeks after LMP; miscarriage. "Spontaneous abortion" has been in common medical usage, but there is more recently a preference for "miscarriage," reserving the word "abortion" for induced abortion.[29]

Sterility The complete inability of a person or couple to conceive.

Stillbirth Death of the fetus after it has reached the gestational age of "viability" but with no signs of life after birth. Age of viability was formerly 28 weeks, but this criterion has gradually shifted to earlier ages as medical interventions have improved fetal survival.

Stillbirth rate The number of stillbirths divided by the total number of stillbirths and live births in a given cohort, or in a given year for a population.

Subfertility (see *Infertility*)

Sudden infant death syndrome (SIDS) The unanticipated and unexplained death of an infant between 3 weeks and 9 months of age.[30]

Teratogen An external substance able to disrupt embryonic or fetal development.

Term pregnancy Pregnancy with delivery from 37 to 41 weeks of gestation.

Thelarche (see *Puberty*)

Time to pregnancy Time interval from onset of sexual activity without contraception to the conception of a clinically recognized pregnancy (usually measured in either months or menstrual cycles). Used to estimate fecundability for groups of couples.

Tocolysis Drug treatment to delay delivery in women having preterm labor. Such drugs are available but are limited in their safety and effectiveness.[31]

Trimester One of three roughly-equal time segments of pregnancy, comprising the first 14 weeks, the second 14 weeks and the final 12 weeks of pregnancy.

Tubal pregnancy (see *Ectopic*)

Twins, Dizygous (Fraternal) Two infants in the same pregnancy who arise from two separate ova (which raises the question of "sororal" twins or "trizygous" triplets, neither of which term is used.)

Twins, Monozygous (Identical) Two infants who arise from a single fertilized ovum.

Unplanned (or unintended) pregnancy A combination of mistimed and unwanted pregnancies.[32,33]

Very low birth weight (VLBW) Birth weight less than 1,500 g. Nearly all VLBW babies are preterm.

Weinberg's formula Inference of the rates of monozygotic and dizygotic twins in a population in the absence of individual data, assuming that the number of unlike-sex dizygotic twins equals the number of same-sex dizygotic twins.[34,35]

Zygote A fertilized egg.

References

1. Nguyen RH, Wilcox AJ. Terms in reproductive and perinatal epidemiology: 1. Reproductive terms. *J Epidemiol Community Health* 2005;59(11):916–9.
2. Nguyen RH, Wilcox AJ. Terms in reproductive and perinatal epidemiology: 2. Perinatal terms. *J Epidemiol Community Health* 2005;59(12):1019–21.
3. Kline J, Stein Z, Susser M. *Conception to Birth: Epidemiology of Prenatal Development.* New York: Oxford University Press, 1989.
4. Apgar V. The newborn (Apgar) scoring system. Reflections and advice. *Pediatr Clin North Am* 1966;13(3):645–50.
5. Rowell P, Braude P. Assisted conception. 1-General principles. *BMJ* 2003;327(7418): 799–801.
6. Braude P, Rowell P. Assisted conception. II-In vitro fertilisation and intracytoplastmic sperm injection. *BMJ* 2003;327:852–5.
7. Hughes EC. Gametogenesis and fertilization. In: Hughes EC, Ed. *Obstretric-Gynecologic Terminology.* Philadelphia, PA: FA Davis Company, 1972:299–304.
8. Wilcox A, Weinberg C, O'Connor J, et al. Incidence of early loss of pregnancy. *N Engl J Med* 1988;319:189–94.
9. Weinstein M, Wood J, Ming-Cheng C. Age patterns of fecundability. In: Gray R, ed. *Biomedical and Demographic Determinants of Reproduction.* Oxford: Clarendon Press, 1993;209–27.
10. Wood J. Fecundity and natural fertility in humans. *Oxf Rev Reprod Biol* 1989;11:61–109.
11. Wilcox A, Weinberg C, Baird D. Timing of sexual intercourse in relation to ovulation: effects on the probability of conception, survival of the pregnancy and sex of the baby. *N Engl J Med* 1995;333:1517–21.
12. Baird D, McConnaughey D, Weinberg C, et al. Application of a method for estimating day of ovulation using urinary estrogen and progesterone metabolites. *Epidemiology* 1995;6:547–50.
13. Blondel B, Morin I, Platt R, Kramer M, Usher R, Breart G. Algorithms for combining menstrual and ultrasound estimates of gestational age: consequences for rates of preterm and postterm birth. *Br J Obstet Gynaecol* 2002;109(6):718–20.
14. Wilcox A, Baird D, Weinberg C. Timing of implantation of the conceptus and loss of pregnancy. *N Engl J Med* 1999;340:1796–9.
15. American College of Obstetrics and Gynecology. *Infertility. Precis: An Update in Gynecology and Obstetrics. Reproductive Endocrinology.* 2nd ed. Washington, DC: American College of Obstetrics and Gynecology, 2002.
16. World Health Organization. Reproductive health indicators for global monitoring: *Report of an Interagency Technical Meeting.* Geneva: World Health Organization, 1997.

17. World Health Organization. *ICD-9: International Statistical Classification of Diseases and Health Related Problems.* Geneva: WHO; 1980.
18. Adams M, Andersen A-MN, Andersen P, et al. Sostrup statement on low birthweight. *Int J Epidemiol* 2003;32(5):884–5.
19. World Health Organization. *ICD-10: International Statistical Classification of Diseases and Health Related Problems.* Geneva: WHO; 1992.
20. Luoto R, Kaprio J, Uutela A. Age at natural menopause and sociodemographic status in Finland. *Am J Epidemiol* 1994;139(1):64–76.
21. Luborsky J, Meyer P, Sowers M, Gold E, Santoro N. Premature menopause in a multi-ethnic population study of the menopause transition. *Hum Reprod* 2003;18(1):199–206.
22. American College of Obstetrics and Gynecology. *Disorders of Ovulation and Menstruation. Reproductive Endocrinology: An Update in Obstetrics and Gynecology.* 2nd ed. Washington, DC: American College of Obstetrics and Gynecology, 2002;67–79.
23. von Hertzen H, d'Arcangues C, Van Look P. Methods of the natural regulation of fertility. In: *Annual Technical Report 1995.* Geneva: WHO, 1996;103–20.
24. Khalaf Y. Tubal subfertility. *BMJ* 2003;327:610–13.
25. Chard T, Soc A, Costeloe K. The relationship of ponderal index and other measurements to birthweight in preterm neonates. *J Perinat* 1997;15:111–14.
26. American College of Obstetrics and Gynecology. Diagnosis and management of postterm pregnancy. *ACOG Technical Bulletin no. 130.* Washington, DC: American College of Obstetrics and Gynecology, 1989.
27. Hauth J, Goodman M, Gilstrap LR, Gilstrap J. Post-term pregnancy. *Obstet Gynecol* 1980;56:467.
28. Hirsh A. Male subfertility. *BMJ* 2003;327:669–72.
29. Farquharson RG, Jauniaux E, Exalto N. Updated and revised nomenclature for description of early pregnancy events. *Hum Reprod* 2005;20(11):3008–11.
30. Beckwith J. Defining Sudden Infant Death Syndrome. *Arch Pediatr Adolesc Med* 2003;157(3):286–90.
31. Iams JD, Romero R, Culhane JF, Goldenberg RL. Primary, secondary, and tertiary interventions to reduce the morbidity and mortality of preterm birth. *Lancet* 2008;371(9607):164–75.
32. Abma J, Chandra A, Mosher W, Peterson L, Piccinino L. Fertility, family planning, and women's health: new data from the 1995 National Survey of Family Growth. *Vital Health Stat* 1997;23(19):1–114.
33. Henshaw S. Unintended pregnancies in the United States. *Fam Plann Perspect* 1998;30(1):24–9.
34. Lichtenstein P, Otterblad Olausson P, Bengt Kallen A. Twin births to mothers who are twins: a registry-based study. *BMJ* 1996;312:879–81.
35. Weinberg W. Beitrage zur physiologie und pathologie der mehrlingsgeburten bei menschen. *Pfluegers Arch ges Physiol* 1901;88:346–430.

Appendix

U.S. Birth and Infant and Fetal Death Certificates

Birth Certificate

U.S. STANDARD CERTIFICATE OF LIVE BIRTH

LOCAL FILE NO. BIRTH NUMBER:

CHILD

1. CHILD'S NAME (First, Middle, Last, Suffix)
2. TIME OF BIRTH (24 hr)
3. SEX
4. DATE OF BIRTH (Mo/Day/Yr)
5. FACILITY NAME (If not institution, give street and number)
6. CITY, TOWN, OR LOCATION OF BIRTH
7. COUNTY OF BIRTH

MOTHER

8a. MOTHER'S CURRENT LEGAL NAME (First, Middle, Last, Suffix)
8b. DATE OF BIRTH (Mo/Day/Yr)
8c. MOTHER'S NAME PRIOR TO FIRST MARRIAGE (First, Middle, Last, Suffix)
8d. BIRTHPLACE (State, Territory, or Foreign Country)
9a. RESIDENCE OF MOTHER-STATE
9b. COUNTY
9c. CITY, TOWN, OR LOCATION
9d. STREET AND NUMBER
9e. APT. NO.
9f. ZIP CODE
9g. INSIDE CITY LIMITS? □ Yes □ No

FATHER

10a. FATHER'S CURRENT LEGAL NAME (First, Middle, Last, Suffix)
10b. DATE OF BIRTH (Mo/Day/Yr)
10c. BIRTHPLACE (State, Territory, or Foreign Country)

CERTIFIER

11. CERTIFIER'S NAME: ______________________
TITLE: □ MD □ DO □ HOSPITAL ADMIN. □ CNM/CM □ OTHER MIDWIFE
□ OTHER (Specify)______________________
12. DATE CERTIFIED ____/____/______ MM DD YYYY
13. DATE FILED BY REGISTRAR ____/____/______ MM DD YYYY

INFORMATION FOR ADMINISTRATIVE USE

MOTHER

14. MOTHER'S MAILING ADDRESS: 9 Same as residence, or: State: City, Town, or Location:
Street & Number: Apartment No.: Zip Code:
15. MOTHER MARRIED? (At birth, conception, or any time between) □ Yes □ No
IF NO, HAS PATERNITY ACKNOWLEDGEMENT BEEN SIGNED IN THE HOSPITAL? □ Yes □ No
16. SOCIAL SECURITY NUMBER REQUESTED FOR CHILD? □ Yes □ No
17. FACILITY ID. (NPI)
18. MOTHER'S SOCIAL SECURITY NUMBER:
19. FATHER'S SOCIAL SECURITY NUMBER:

INFORMATION FOR MEDICAL AND HEALTH PURPOSES ONLY

MOTHER

20. MOTHER'S EDUCATION (Check the box that best describes the highest degree or level of school completed at the time of delivery)
- □ 8th grade or less
- □ 9th - 12th grade, no diploma
- □ High school graduate or GED completed
- □ Some college credit but no degree
- □ Associate degree (e.g., AA, AS)
- □ Bachelor's degree (e.g., BA, AB, BS)
- □ Master's degree (e.g., MA, MS, MEng, MEd, MSW, MBA)
- □ Doctorate (e.g., PhD, EdD) or Professional degree (e.g., MD, DDS, DVM, LLB, JD)

21. MOTHER OF HISPANIC ORIGIN? (Check the box that best describes whether the mother is Spanish/Hispanic/Latina. Check the "No" box if mother is not Spanish/Hispanic/Latina)
- □ No, not Spanish/Hispanic/Latina
- □ Yes, Mexican, Mexican American, Chicana
- □ Yes, Puerto Rican
- □ Yes, Cuban
- □ Yes, other Spanish/Hispanic/Latina

(Specify)______________________

22. MOTHER'S RACE (Check one or more races to indicate what the mother considers herself to be)
- □ White
- □ Black or African American
- □ American Indian or Alaska Native (Name of the enrolled or principal tribe)______________
- □ Asian Indian
- □ Chinese
- □ Filipino
- □ Japanese
- □ Korean
- □ Vietnamese
- □ Other Asian (Specify)______________
- □ Native Hawaiian
- □ Guamanian or Chamorro
- □ Samoan
- □ Other Pacific Islander (Specify)______________
- □ Other (Specify)______________

FATHER

23. FATHER'S EDUCATION (Check the box that best describes the highest degree or level of school completed at the time of delivery)
- □ 8th grade or less
- □ 9th - 12th grade, no diploma
- □ High school graduate or GED completed
- □ Some college credit but no degree
- □ Associate degree (e.g., AA, AS)
- □ Bachelor's degree (e.g., BA, AB, BS)
- □ Master's degree (e.g., MA, MS, MEng, MEd, MSW, MBA)
- □ Doctorate (e.g., PhD, EdD) or Professional degree (e.g., MD, DDS, DVM, LLB, JD)

24. FATHER OF HISPANIC ORIGIN? (Check the box that best describes whether the father is Spanish/Hispanic/Latino. Check the "No" box if father is not Spanish/Hispanic/Latino)
- □ No, not Spanish/Hispanic/Latino
- □ Yes, Mexican, Mexican American, Chicano
- □ Yes, Puerto Rican
- □ Yes, Cuban
- □ Yes, other Spanish/Hispanic/Latino

(Specify)______________________

25. FATHER'S RACE (Check one or more races to indicate what the father considers himself to be)
- □ White
- □ Black or African American
- □ American Indian or Alaska Native (Name of the enrolled or principal tribe)______________
- □ Asian Indian
- □ Chinese
- □ Filipino
- □ Japanese
- □ Korean
- □ Vietnamese
- □ Other Asian (Specify)______________
- □ Native Hawaiian
- □ Guamanian or Chamorro
- □ Samoan
- □ Other Pacific Islander (Specify)______________
- □ Other (Specify)______________

Mother's Name ______________

Mother's Medical Record No. ______________

26. PLACE WHERE BIRTH OCCURRED (Check one)
- □ Hospital
- □ Freestanding birthing center
- □ Home Birth: Planned to deliver at home? 9 Yes 9 No
- □ Clinic/Doctor's office
- □ Other (Specify)______________

27. ATTENDANT'S NAME, TITLE, AND NPI
NAME: ______________________ NPI:________
TITLE: □ MD □ DO □ CNM/CM □ OTHER MIDWIFE
□ OTHER (Specify)______________

28. MOTHER TRANSFERRED FOR MATERNAL MEDICAL OR FETAL INDICATIONS FOR DELIVERY? □ Yes □ No
IF YES, ENTER NAME OF FACILITY MOTHER TRANSFERRED FROM:
____

REV. 11/2003

MOTHER

29a. DATE OF FIRST PRENATAL CARE VISIT ___/___/___ MM DD YYYY □ No Prenatal Care

29b. DATE OF LAST PRENATAL CARE VISIT ___/___/___ MM DD YYYY

30. TOTAL NUMBER OF PRENATAL VISITS FOR THIS PREGNANCY ___ (If none, enter A0".)

31. MOTHER'S HEIGHT ___ (feet/inches)

32. MOTHER'S PREPREGNANCY WEIGHT ___ (pounds)

33. MOTHER'S WEIGHT AT DELIVERY ___ (pounds)

34. DID MOTHER GET WIC FOOD FOR HERSELF DURING THIS PREGNANCY? □ Yes □ No

35. NUMBER OF PREVIOUS LIVE BIRTHS (Do not include this child)

35a. Now Living Number ___ □ None

35b. Now Dead Number ___ □ None

36. NUMBER OF OTHER PREGNANCY OUTCOMES (spontaneous or induced losses or ectopic pregnancies)

36a. Other Outcomes Number ___ □ None

37. CIGARETTE SMOKING BEFORE AND DURING PREGNANCY
For each time period, enter either the number of cigarettes or the number of packs of cigarettes smoked. IF NONE, ENTER A0".

Average number of cigarettes or packs of cigarettes smoked per day.

	# of cigarettes		# of packs
Three Months Before Pregnancy	___	OR	___
First Three Months of Pregnancy	___	OR	___
Second Three Months of Pregnancy	___	OR	___
Third Trimester of Pregnancy	___	OR	___

38. PRINCIPAL SOURCE OF PAYMENT FOR THIS DELIVERY
- □ Private Insurance
- □ Medicaid
- □ Self-pay
- □ Other (Specify) ___

35c. DATE OF LAST LIVE BIRTH ___/___ MM YYYY

36b. DATE OF LAST OTHER PREGNANCY OUTCOME ___/___ MM YYYY

39. DATE LAST NORMAL MENSES BEGAN ___/___/___ MM DD YYYY

40. MOTHER'S MEDICAL RECORD NUMBER

MEDICAL AND HEALTH INFORMATION

41. RISK FACTORS IN THIS PREGNANCY (Check all that apply)

Diabetes
- □ Prepregnancy (Diagnosis prior to this pregnancy)
- □ Gestational (Diagnosis in this pregnancy)

Hypertension
- □ Prepregnancy (Chronic)
- □ Gestational (PIH, preeclampsia)
- □ Eclampsia

□ Previous preterm birth

□ Other previous poor pregnancy outcome (Includes perinatal death, small-for-gestational age/intrauterine growth restricted birth)

□ Pregnancy resulted from infertility treatment-If yes, check all that apply:
- □ Fertility-enhancing drugs, Artificial insemination or Intrauterine insemination
- □ Assisted reproductive technology (e.g., in vitro fertilization (IVF), gamete intrafallopian transfer (GIFT))

□ Mother had a previous cesarean delivery
If yes, how many ___

□ None of the above

42. INFECTIONS PRESENT AND/OR TREATED DURING THIS PREGNANCY (Check all that apply)
- □ Gonorrhea
- □ Syphilis
- □ Chlamydia
- □ Hepatitis B
- □ Hepatitis C
- □ None of the above

43. OBSTETRIC PROCEDURES (Check all that apply)
- □ Cervical cerclage
- □ Tocolysis

External cephalic version:
- □ Successful
- □ Failed

□ None of the above

44. ONSET OF LABOR (Check all that apply)
- □ Premature Rupture of the Membranes (prolonged, ∃12 hrs.)
- □ Precipitous Labor (<3 hrs.)
- □ Prolonged Labor (∃ 20 hrs.)
- □ None of the above

45. CHARACTERISTICS OF LABOR AND DELIVERY (Check all that apply)
- □ Induction of labor
- □ Augmentation of labor
- □ Non-vertex presentation
- □ Steroids (glucocorticoids) for fetal lung maturation received by the mother prior to delivery
- □ Antibiotics received by the mother during labor
- □ Clinical chorioamnionitis diagnosed during labor or maternal temperature ≥38°C (100.4°F)
- □ Moderate/heavy meconium staining of the amniotic fluid
- □ Fetal intolerance of labor such that one or more of the following actions was taken: in-utero resuscitative measures, further fetal assessment, or operative delivery
- □ Epidural or spinal anesthesia during labor
- □ None of the above

46. METHOD OF DELIVERY

A. Was delivery with forceps attempted but unsuccessful?
□ Yes □ No

B. Was delivery with vacuum extraction attempted but unsuccessful?
□ Yes □ No

C. Fetal presentation at birth
- □ Cephalic
- □ Breech
- □ Other

D. Final route and method of delivery (Check one)
- □ Vaginal/Spontaneous
- □ Vaginal/Forceps
- □ Vaginal/Vacuum
- □ Cesarean

If cesarean, was a trial of labor attempted?
- □ Yes
- □ No

47. MATERNAL MORBIDITY (Check all that apply) (Complications associated with labor and delivery)
- □ Maternal transfusion
- □ Third or fourth degree perineal laceration
- □ Ruptured uterus
- □ Unplanned hysterectomy
- □ Admission to intensive care unit
- □ Unplanned operating room procedure following delivery
- □ None of the above

NEWBORN

NEWBORN INFORMATION

48. NEWBORN MEDICAL RECORD NUMBER

49. BIRTHWEIGHT (grams preferred, specify unit)
___ 9 grams 9 lb/oz

50. OBSTETRIC ESTIMATE OF GESTATION:
___ (completed weeks)

51. APGAR SCORE:
Score at 5 minutes: ___
If 5 minute score is less than 6,
Score at 10 minutes: ___

52. PLURALITY - Single, Twin, Triplet, etc.
(Specify) ___

53. IF NOT SINGLE BIRTH - Born First, Second, Third, etc. (Specify) ___

54. ABNORMAL CONDITIONS OF THE NEWBORN (Check all that apply)
- □ Assisted ventilation required immediately following delivery
- □ Assisted ventilation required for more than six hours
- □ NICU admission
- □ Newborn given surfactant replacement therapy
- □ Antibiotics received by the newborn for suspected neonatal sepsis
- □ Seizure or serious neurologic dysfunction
- □ Significant birth injury (skeletal fracture(s), peripheral nerve injury, and/or soft tissue/solid organ hemorrhage which requires intervention)
- 9 None of the above

55. CONGENITAL ANOMALIES OF THE NEWBORN (Check all that apply)
- □ Anencephaly
- □ Meningomyelocele/Spina bifida
- □ Cyanotic congenital heart disease
- □ Congenital diaphragmatic hernia
- □ Omphalocele
- □ Gastroschisis
- □ Limb reduction defect (excluding congenital amputation and dwarfing syndromes)
- □ Cleft Lip with or without Cleft Palate
- □ Cleft Palate alone
- □ Down Syndrome
  - □ Karyotype confirmed
  - □ Karyotype pending
- □ Suspected chromosomal disorder
  - □ Karyotype confirmed
  - □ Karyotype pending
- □ Hypospadias
- □ None of the anomalies listed above

56. WAS INFANT TRANSFERRED WITHIN 24 HOURS OF DELIVERY? 9 Yes 9 No
IF YES, NAME OF FACILITY INFANT TRANSFERRED TO: ___

57. IS INFANT LIVING AT TIME OF REPORT? □ Yes □ No □ Infant transferred, status unknown

58. IS THE INFANT BEING BREASTFED AT DISCHARGE? □ Yes □ No

Mother's Name ___

Mother's Medical Record No. ___

Death Certificate (Infant and other)

U.S. STANDARD CERTIFICATE OF DEATH

LOCAL FILE NO. STATE FILE NO.

NAME OF DECEDENT ___
For use by physician or institution

To Be Completed/ Verified By: FUNERAL DIRECTOR:

1. DECEDENT'S LEGAL NAME (Include AKA's if any) (First, Middle, Last)
2. SEX
3. SOCIAL SECURITY NUMBER

4a. AGE-Last Birthday (Years)
4b. UNDER 1 YEAR — Months | Days
4c. UNDER 1 DAY — Hours | Minutes
5. DATE OF BIRTH (Mo/Day/Yr)
6. BIRTHPLACE (City and State or Foreign Country)

7a. RESIDENCE-STATE
7b. COUNTY
7c. CITY OR TOWN

7d. STREET AND NUMBER
7e. APT. NO.
7f. ZIP CODE
7g. INSIDE CITY LIMITS? □ Yes □ No

8. EVER IN US ARMED FORCES? □ Yes □ No
9. MARITAL STATUS AT TIME OF DEATH □ Married □ Married, but separated □ Widowed □ Divorced □ Never Married □ Unknown
10. SURVIVING SPOUSE'S NAME (If wife, give name prior to first marriage)

11. FATHER'S NAME (First, Middle, Last)
12. MOTHER'S NAME PRIOR TO FIRST MARRIAGE (First, Middle, Last)

13a. INFORMANT'S NAME
13b. RELATIONSHIP TO DECEDENT
13c. MAILING ADDRESS (Street and Number, City, State, Zip Code)

14. PLACE OF DEATH (Check only one: see instructions)
IF DEATH OCCURRED IN A HOSPITAL: □ Inpatient □ Emergency Room/Outpatient □ Dead on Arrival
IF DEATH OCCURRED SOMEWHERE OTHER THAN A HOSPITAL: □ Hospice facility □ Nursing home/Long term care facility □ Decedent's home □ Other (Specify):

15. FACILITY NAME (If not institution, give street & number)
16. CITY OR TOWN , STATE, AND ZIP CODE
17. COUNTY OF DEATH

18. METHOD OF DISPOSITION: □ Burial □ Cremation □ Donation □ Entombment □ Removal from State □ Other (Specify):___
19. PLACE OF DISPOSITION (Name of cemetery, crematory, other place)

20. LOCATION-CITY, TOWN, AND STATE
21. NAME AND COMPLETE ADDRESS OF FUNERAL FACILITY

22. SIGNATURE OF FUNERAL SERVICE LICENSEE OR OTHER AGENT
23. LICENSE NUMBER (Of Licensee)

To Be Completed By: MEDICAL CERTIFIER

ITEMS 24-28 MUST BE COMPLETED BY PERSON WHO PRONOUNCES OR CERTIFIES DEATH
24. DATE PRONOUNCED DEAD (Mo/Day/Yr)
25. TIME PRONOUNCED DEAD

26. SIGNATURE OF PERSON PRONOUNCING DEATH (Only when applicable)
27. LICENSE NUMBER
28. DATE SIGNED (Mo/Day/Yr)

29. ACTUAL OR PRESUMED DATE OF DEATH (Mo/Day/Yr) (Spell Month)
30. ACTUAL OR PRESUMED TIME OF DEATH
31. WAS MEDICAL EXAMINER OR CORONER CONTACTED? □ Yes □ No

CAUSE OF DEATH (See instructions and examples)

32. **PART I.** Enter the chain of events--diseases, injuries, or complications--that directly caused the death. DO NOT enter terminal events such as cardiac arrest, respiratory arrest, or ventricular fibrillation without showing the etiology. DO NOT ABBREVIATE. Enter only one cause on a line. Add additional lines if necessary.

Approximate interval: Onset to death

IMMEDIATE CAUSE (Final disease or condition ---------> resulting in death) a.___ ___
Due to (or as a consequence of):

Sequentially list conditions, if any, leading to the cause listed on line a. Enter the **UNDERLYING CAUSE** (disease or injury that initiated the events resulting in death) **LAST**
b.___ ___
Due to (or as a consequence of):
c.___ ___
Due to (or as a consequence of):
d.___ ___

PART II. Enter other significant conditions contributing to death but not resulting in the underlying cause given in PART I

33. WAS AN AUTOPSY PERFORMED? □ Yes □ No
34. WERE AUTOPSY FINDINGS AVAILABLE TO COMPLETE THE CAUSE OF DEATH? □ Yes □ No

35. DID TOBACCO USE CONTRIBUTE TO DEATH? □ Yes □ Probably □ No □ Unknown
36. IF FEMALE: □ Not pregnant within past year □ Pregnant at time of death □ Not pregnant, but pregnant within 42 days of death □ Not pregnant, but pregnant 43 days to 1 year before death □ Unknown if pregnant within the past year
37. MANNER OF DEATH □ Natural □ Homicide □ Accident □ Pending Investigation □ Suicide □ Could not be determined

38. DATE OF INJURY (Mo/Day/Yr) (Spell Month)
39. TIME OF INJURY
40. PLACE OF INJURY (e.g., Decedent's home; construction site; restaurant; wooded area)
41. INJURY AT WORK? □ Yes □ No

42. LOCATION OF INJURY: State: City or Town:
Street & Number: Apartment No.: Zip Code:

43. DESCRIBE HOW INJURY OCCURRED:
44. IF TRANSPORTATION INJURY, SPECIFY: □ Driver/Operator □ Passenger □ Pedestrian □ Other (Specify)

45. CERTIFIER (Check only one):
□ Certifying physician-To the best of my knowledge, death occurred due to the cause(s) and manner stated.
□ Pronouncing & Certifying physician-To the best of my knowledge, death occurred at the time, date, and place, and due to the cause(s) and manner stated.
□ Medical Examiner/Coroner-On the basis of examination, and/or investigation, in my opinion, death occurred at the time, date, and place, and due to the cause(s) and manner stated.

Signature of certifier:___

46. NAME, ADDRESS, AND ZIP CODE OF PERSON COMPLETING CAUSE OF DEATH (Item 32)

47. TITLE OF CERTIFIER
48. LICENSE NUMBER
49. DATE CERTIFIED (Mo/Day/Yr)
50. **FOR REGISTRAR ONLY**- DATE FILED (Mo/Day/Yr)

To Be Completed By: FUNERAL DIRECTOR

51. DECEDENT'S EDUCATION-Check the box that best describes the highest degree or level of school completed at the time of death.
□ 8th grade or less
□ 9th - 12th grade; no diploma
□ High school graduate or GED completed
□ Some college credit, but no degree
□ Associate degree (e.g., AA, AS)
□ Bachelor's degree (e.g., BA, AB, BS)
□ Master's degree (e.g., MA, MS, MEng, MEd, MSW, MBA)
□ Doctorate (e.g., PhD, EdD) or Professional degree (e.g., MD, DDS, DVM, LLB, JD)

52. DECEDENT OF HISPANIC ORIGIN? Check the box that best describes whether the decedent is Spanish/Hispanic/Latino. Check the "No" box if decedent is not Spanish/Hispanic/Latino.
□ No, not Spanish/Hispanic/Latino
□ Yes, Mexican, Mexican American, Chicano
□ Yes, Puerto Rican
□ Yes, Cuban
□ Yes, other Spanish/Hispanic/Latino (Specify) ___

53. DECEDENT'S RACE (Check one or more races to indicate what the decedent considered himself or herself to be)
□ White
□ Black or African American
□ American Indian or Alaska Native (Name of the enrolled or principal tribe) ___
□ Asian Indian
□ Chinese
□ Filipino
□ Japanese
□ Korean
□ Vietnamese
□ Other Asian (Specify)___
□ Native Hawaiian
□ Guamanian or Chamorro
□ Samoan
□ Other Pacific Islander (Specify)___
□ Other (Specify)___

54. DECEDENT'S USUAL OCCUPATION (Indicate type of work done during most of working life. DO NOT USE RETIRED).

55. KIND OF BUSINESS/INDUSTRY

REV. 11/2003

Fetal Death Certificate

LOCAL FILE NO.

US STANDARD REPORT OF FETAL DEATH

STATE FILE NUMBER:

MOTHER

1. NAME OF FETUS (optional-at the discretion of the parents)
2. TIME OF DELIVERY (24hr)
3. SEX (M/F/Unk)
4. DATE OF DELIV ERY (Mo/Day/Yr)

5a. CITY, TOWN, OR LOCATION OF DELIVERY

5b. ZIP CODE OF DELIVERY

6. COUNTY OF DELIVERY

7. PLACE WHERE DELIVERY OCCURRED (Check one)
- □ Hospital
- □ Freestanding birthing center
- □ Home Delivery: Planned to deliver at home? □ Yes □ No
- □ Clinic/Doctor's office
- □ Other (Specify)___________

8. FACILITY NAME (If not institution, give street and number)

9. FACILITY ID. (NPI)

10a. MOTHER'S CURRENT LEGAL NAME (First, Middle, Last, Suffix)

10b. DATE OF BIRTH (Mo/Day/Yr)

10c. MOTHER'S NAME PRIOR TO FIRST MARRIAGE (First, Middle, Last, Suffix)

10d. BIRTHPLACE (State, Territory, or Foreign Country)

11a. RESIDENCE OF MOTHER-STATE

11b. COUNTY

11c. CITY, TOWN, OR LOCATION

11d. STREET AND NUMBER

11e. APT. NO.

11f. ZIP CODE

11g. INSIDE CITY LIMITS? □ Yes □ No

FATHER

12a. FATHER'S CURRENT LEGAL NAME (First, Middle, Last, Suffix)

12b. DATE OF BIRTH (Mo/Day/Yr)

12c. BIRTHPLACE (State, Territory, or Foreign Country)

DISPOSITION

13. METHOD OF DISPOSITION:
□ Burial □ Cremation □ Hospital Disposition □ Donation □ Removal from State □ Other (Specify)___________

ATTENDANT AND REGISTRATION INFORMATION

14. ATTENDANT'S NAME, TITLE, AND NPI
NAME: ___________
NPI:___________
TITLE: □ MD □ DO □ CNM/CM □ OTHER MIDWIFE
□ OTHER (Specify)___________

15. NAME AND TITLE OF PERSON COMPLETING REPORT
Name ___________
Title ___________

16. DATE REPORT COMPLETED
___/___/_____
MM DD YYYY

17. DATE RECEIVED BY REGISTRAR
___/___/_____
MM DD YYYY

18. CAUSE/CONDITIONS CONTRIBUTING TO FETAL DEATH

CAUSE OF FETAL DEATH

18a. INITIATING CAUSE/CONDITION

(AMONG THE CHOICES BELOW, PLEASE SELECT THE ONE WHICH MOST LIKELY BEGAN THE SEQUENCE OF EVENTS RESULTING IN THE DEATH OF THE FETUS)

Maternal Conditions/Diseases (Specify) ___________

Complications of Placenta, Cord, or Membranes
- □ Rupture of membranes prior to onset of labor
- □ Abruptio placenta
- □ Placental insufficiency
- □ Prolapsed cord
- □ Chorioamnionitis
- □ Other Specify)___________

Other Obstetrical or Pregnancy Complications (Specify) ___________

Fetal Anomaly (Specify) ___________

Fetal Injury (Specify) ___________

Fetal Infection (Specify) ___________

Other Fetal Conditions/Disorders (Specify) ___________

□ Unknown

18b. OTHER SIGNIFICANT CAUSES OR CONDITIONS

(SELECT OR SPECIFY ALL OTHER CONDITIONS CONTRIBUTING TO DEATH IN ITEM 18b)

Maternal Conditions/Diseases (Specify) ___________

Complications of Placenta, Cord, or Membranes
- □ Rupture of membranes prior to onset of labor
- □ Abruptio placenta
- □ Placental insufficiency
- □ Prolapsed cord
- □ Chorioamnionitis
- □ Other Specify)___________

Other Obstetrical or Pregnancy Complications (Specify) ___________

Fetal Anomaly (Specify) ___________

Fetal Injury (Specify) ___________

Fetal Infection (Specify) ___________

Other Fetal Conditions/Disorders (Specify) ___________

□ Unknown

Mother's Name ___________

Mother's Medical Record No. ___________

18c. WEIGHT OF FETUS (grams preferred, specify unit)
____
□ grams □ lb/oz

18d. OBSTETRIC ESTIMATE OF GESTATION AT DELIVERY
___________ (completed weeks)

18e. ESTIMATED TIME OF FETAL DEATH
- □ Dead at time of first assessment, no labor ongoing
- □ Dead at time of first assessment, labor ongoing
- □ Died during labor, after first assessment
- □ Unknown time of fetal death

18f. WAS AN AUTOPSY PERFORMED?
□ Yes □ No □ Planned

18g. WAS A HISTOLOGICAL PLACENTAL EXAMINATION PERFORMED?
□ Yes □ No □ Planned

18h. WERE AUTOPSY OR HISTOLOGICAL PLACENTAL EXAMINATION RESULTS USED IN DETERMINING THE CAUSE OF FETAL DEATH? □ Yes □ No

REV. 11/2003

MOTHER

19. MOTHER'S EDUCATION (Check the box that best describes the highest degree or level of school completed at the time of delivery)

- □ 8th grade or less
- □ 9th - 12th grade, no diploma
- □ High school graduate or GED completed
- □ Some college credit but no degree
- □ Associate degree (e.g., AA, AS)
- □ Bachelor's degree (e.g., BA, AB, BS)
- □ Master's degree (e.g., MA, MS, MEng, MEd, MSW, MBA)
- □ Doctorate (e.g., PhD, EdD) or Professional degree (e.g., MD, DDS, DVM, LLB, JD)

20. MOTHER OF HISPANIC ORIGIN? (Check the box that best describes whether the mother is Spanish/Hispanic/Latina. Check the "No" box if mother is not Spanish/Hispanic/Latina)

- □ No, not Spanish/Hispanic/Latina
- □ Yes, Mexican, Mexican American, Chicana
- □ Yes, Puerto Rican
- □ Yes, Cuban
- □ Yes, other Spanish/Hispanic/Latina

(Specify)________________

21. MOTHER'S RACE (Check one or more races to indicate what the mother considers herself to be)

- □ White
- □ Black or African American
- □ American Indian or Alaska Native (Name of the enrolled or principal tribe)________
- □ Asian Indian
- □ Chinese
- □ Filipino
- □ Japanese
- □ Korean
- □ Vietnamese
- □ Other Asian (Specify)________
- □ Native Hawaiian
- □ Guamanian or Chamorro
- □ Samoan
- □ Other Pacific Islander (Specify)________
- □ Other (Specify)________

22. MOTHER MARRIED? (At delivery, conception, or anytime between) □ Yes □ No

23a. DATE OF FIRST PRENATAL CARE VISIT ___/___/____ MM DD YYYY □ No Prenatal Care

23b. DATE OF LAST PRENATAL CARE VISIT ___/___/____ MM DD YYYY

24. TOTAL NUMBER OF PRENATAL VISITS FOR THIS PREGNANCY _____ (If none, enter "0".)

25. MOTHER'S HEIGHT _____ (feet/inches)

26. MOTHER'S PREPREGNANCY WEIGHT _____ (pounds)

27. MOTHER'S WEIGHT AT DELIVERY _____ (pounds)

28. DID MOTHER GET WIC FOOD FOR HERSELF DURING THIS PREGNANCY? □ Yes □ No

29. NUMBER OF PREVIOUS LIVE BIRTHS

29a. Now Living — Number ____ □ None

29b. Now Dead — Number ____ □ None

29c. DATE OF LAST LIVE BIRTH ___/____ MM YYYY

30. NUMBER OF OTHER PREGNANCY OUTCOMES (spontaneous or induced losses or ectopic pregnancies)

30a. Other Outcomes — Number (Do not include this fetus) ____ □ None

30b. DATE OF LAST OTHER PREGNANCY OUTCOME ___/____ MM YYYY

31. CIGARETTE SMOKING BEFORE AND DURING PREGNANCY
For each time period, enter either the number of cigarettes or the number of packs of cigarettes smoked. IF NONE, ENTER "0".

Average number of cigarettes or packs of cigarettes smoked per day.

	# of cigarettes		# of packs
Three Months Before Pregnancy	____	OR	____
First Three Months of Pregnancy	____	OR	____
Second Three Months of Pregnancy	____	OR	____
Third Trimester of Pregnancy	____	OR	____

32. DATE LAST NORMAL MENSES BEGAN ___/___/____ MM DD YYYY

33. PLURALITY - Single, Twin, Triplet, etc. (Specify)______

34. IF NOT SINGLE BIRTH-Born First, Second, Third, etc. (Specify)______

35. MOTHER TRANSFERRED FOR MATERNAL MEDICAL OR FETAL INDICATIONS FOR DELIVERY? □ Yes □ No
IF YES, ENTER NAME OF FACILITY MOTHER TRANSFERRED FROM: __________

MEDICAL AND HEALTH INFORMATION

36. RISK FACTORS IN THIS PREGNANCY (Check all that apply):

Diabetes
- □ Prepregnancy (Diagnosis prior to this pregnancy)
- □ Gestational (Diagnosis in this pregnancy)

Hypertension
- □ Prepregnancy (Chronic)
- □ Gestational (PIH, preeclampsia)
- □ Eclampsia

- □ Previous preterm birth
- □ Other previous poor pregnancy outcome (Includes perinatal death, small-for-gestational age/intrauterine growth restricted birth)
- □ Pregnancy resulted from infertility treatment-If yes, check all that apply:
  - □ Fertility-enhancing drugs, Artificial insemination or Intrauterine insemination
  - □ Assisted reproductive technology (e.g., in vitro fertilization (IVF), gamete intrafallopian transfer (GIFT))
- □ Mother had a previous cesarean delivery
  If yes, how many ______
- □ None of the above

37. INFECTIONS PRESENT AND/OR TREATED DURING THIS PREGNANCY (Check all that apply)

- □ Gonorrhea
- □ Syphilis
- □ Chlamydia
- □ Listeria
- □ Group B Streptococcus
- □ Cytomegalovirus
- □ Parvovirus
- □ Toxoplasmosis
- □ None of the above
- □ Other (Specify)________

38. METHOD OF DELIVERY

A. Was delivery with forceps attempted but unsuccessful?
□ Yes □ No

B. Was delivery with vacuum extraction attempted but unsuccessful?
□ Yes □ No

C. Fetal presentation at delivery
- □ Cephalic
- □ Breech
- □ Other

D. Final route and method of delivery (Check one)
- □ Vaginal/Spontaneous
- □ Vaginal/Forceps
- □ Vaginal/Vacuum
- □ Cesarean
  If cesarean, was a trial of labor attempted?
  - □ Yes
  - □ No

E. Hysterotomy/Hysterectomy
□ Yes □ No

39. MATERNAL MORBIDITY (Check all that apply) (Complications associated with labor and delivery)

- □ Maternal transfusion
- □ Third or fourth degree perineal laceration
- □ Ruptured uterus
- □ Unplanned hysterectomy
- □ Admission to intensive care unit
- □ Unplanned operating room procedure following delivery
- □ None of the above

40. CONGENITAL ANOMALIES OF THE FETUS (Check all that apply)

- □ Anencephaly
- □ Meningomyelocele/Spina bifida
- □ Cyanotic congenital heart disease
- □ Congenital diaphragmatic hernia
- □ Omphalocele
- □ Gastroschisis
- □ Limb reduction defect (excluding congenital amputation and dwarfing syndromes)
- □ Cleft Lip with or without Cleft Palate
- □ Cleft Palate alone
- □ Down Syndrome
  - □ Karyotype confirmed
  - □ Karyotype pending
- □ Suspected chromosomal disorder
  - □ Karyotype confirmed
  - □ Karyotype pending
- □ Hypospadias
- □ None of the anomalies listed above

REV. 11/2003

NOTE: This recommended standard fetal death report is the result of an extensive evaluation process.
Information on the process and resulting recommendations as well as plans for future activities is available on the Internet at: http://www.cdc.gov/nchs/vital_certs_rev.htm.

Index

Note: Page numbers in *italics* refer to figures, and those in **bold** refer to tables.